A Handbook for Dairy Entrepreneurs

About the Authors

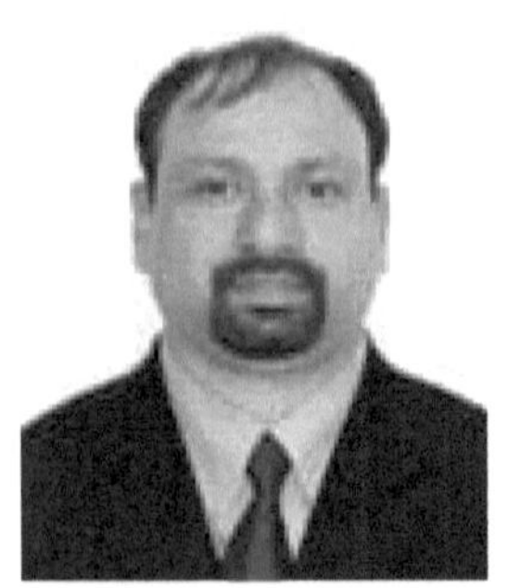

Dr. Pranav Kumar is presently working as Assistant Professor in the Division of Veterinary & A.H. Extension at Faculty of Veterinary Sciences, R.S.Pura, SKUAST-Jammu. He has over twelve years of work experience. He has been engaged in undergraduate & post graduate teaching of Veterinary and Animal Husbandry Extension Education students for the last 8 years. He has graduated from College of Veterinary Sciences, Hyderabad in 2001 and completed Master Degree in Veterinary Extension from IVRI, Izzatnagar in 2005. He has published 22 research papers in NAAS rated journals, 3 review papers, 2 books, 14 book chapters, 20 popular articles and few technical articles. He has authored a book "Handbook for Poultry Entrepreneurs" published by Biotech Books, New Delhi and co – authored a Textbook on "Livestock Entrepreneurship Management" published by NIPA, New Delhi. Recently, he has successfully completed "Organic Leadership Course (OLC) Programme, organised by IFOAM Organics International, Germany and received 'Certificate of Achievement' under the mentorship of Konrad Hauptfleisch, Head of Capacity Development, IFOAM Organics International, Germany.

He has also served as Co-Organizing Secretary of one International Conference and core member committee of one National conference. He was associated with two externally funded research projects as Co-PI funded by National Innovation Foundation (DST) & J&K State Rural Livelihoods Mission (JKSLRM) and presently associated with two on- going projects namely 'Establishment of Women Technology Park in Jammu (funded by DST) and Socio-economic upliftment of rural weaker section (SC/ST) by scientific interventions and amelioration of production diseases in dairy animals (funded by DBT) . He is also a reviewer of different NAAS rated Journals. Dr. Kumar has good exposure of field conditions particularly dairy operations at grassroots level. He has helped in capacity building by forming SHGs of like minded dairy entrepreneurs and linking them to cooperatives under New Generation Cooperatives (NGC) initiative of Mother Dairy. His research work has centered around identification and documentation of indigenous technical knowledge related to low cost treatment of animal ailments, organic dairy farming, SWOT and constraint analysis of dairy cooperatives and entrepreneurial behaviour of rural dairy farmers. He is also involved in research works related to livestock entrepreneurship, ICT enabled web module for Scientific Dairy and broiler farming.

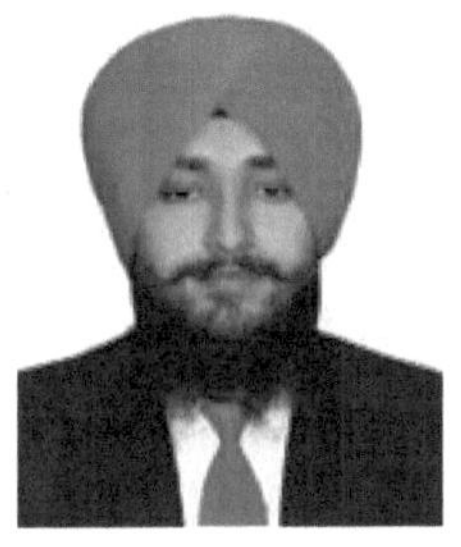

Dr. Amandeep Singh graduated in Veterinary Sciences and Animal Husbandry from Faculty of Veterinary Sciences & Animal Husbandry, Sher-E-Kashmir University of Agricultural Sciences and Technology of Jammu, R.S. Pura, Jammu, Jammu & Kashmir, India. Being from a farming background, he understands the fundamental needs of the farming community and the role of livestock in agrarian society, hence started a web portal www.vetextension.com to cater needs of the rural people involved in livestock rearing by providing information about the same in their hands and pockets all the time through their mobile phones and computers. To his credit he has 02 research papers, 03 review papers, 17 popular articles, 04 case studies and numerous other extension publications. He pitched his idea in "Ideathon-2017" organized by the Department of Biotechnology (DBT), Ministry of Science and Technology, Government of India, in collaboration with Nobel Media AB, Sweden under the Nobel Prize Series-India Programme and got selected for the same. He has also participated in 03 conferences, 03 workshops, 02 national trainings and numerous seminars in the country. He has also participated in 02 international competitions related to sustainable livestock farming. He qualified National Eligibility Test (NET) conducted by University Grants Commission (UGC) with Junior Research Fellowship (JRF).Currently he is pursuing Masters of Veterinary Science in Veterinary Extension Education from Indian Veterinary Research Institute, Bareilly, Uttar Pradesh, India.

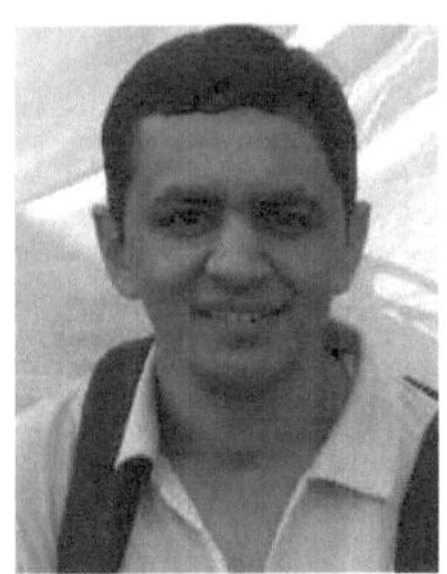

Dr Devesh Thakur is currently working as Assistant Professor in the Department of Veterinary & AH Extension Education, Palampur and Himachal Pradesh. He completed his MVsc & PhD from Indian Veterinary Research Institute Bareilly. He has more than ten years of experience in teaching, research and Extension. He has published more than thirty research publications, forty popular articles & two books. He has worked in the area of entrepreneurship, marketing and business management in agriculture & animal husbandry. His research work includes ICT and social media use in agriculture, livestock based livelihoods, gender issues in animal husbandry, indigenous veterinary practices, socio-psychological factors influencing agriculture & animal husbandry, livestock marketing & market led extension. He has been engaged in formulation and implementation of numerous training programmes to farmers, extension workers, butchers, primary animal husbandry workers, agriculture officers & veterinarians.

A Handbook for Dairy Entrepreneurs

Pranav Kumar
Amandeep Singh
Devesh Thakur

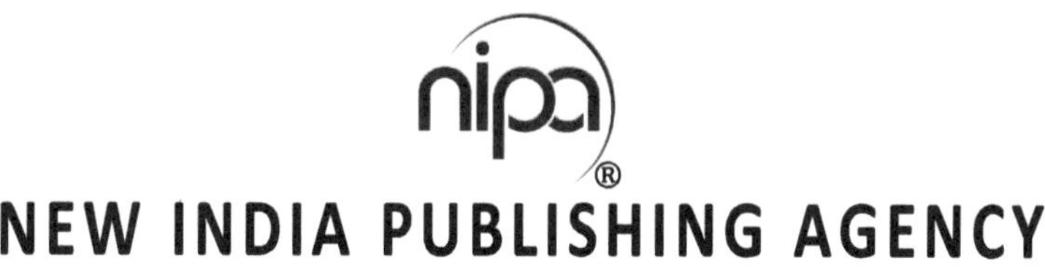

New Delhi – 110 034

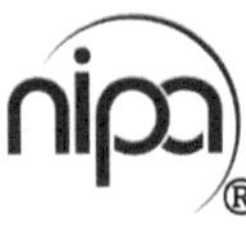

NEW INDIA PUBLISHING AGENCY
101, Vikas Surya Plaza, CU Block, LSC Market
Pitam Pura, New Delhi 110 034, India
Phone: + 91 (11) 27 34 17 17 Fax: + 91 (11) 27 34 16 16
Email: info@nipabooks.com
Web: www.nipabooks.com

Feedback at feedbacks@nipabooks.com

ISBN: 978-93-87973-49-7

Composed and Designed by NIPA

Preface

Development of entrepreneurship is crucial in harnessing vast untapped human resource of a country like India. Given the natural endowment of resources the fact remains that development or under development of any nation is largely the reflection of the abundance or scarcity of entrepreneurship. Entrepreneurship development is an approach of developing human resources. It is concerned with the growth and development of people towards high level of competency, creativity and fulfillment. This approach helps people to grow in terms of self-control, responsibility and other abilities; and then tries to create a climate, in which all the clientele may contribute to the limits of their improved abilities. It is assumed that expanded capabilities and opportunities for people will lead directly to improvement in operating effectiveness.

India is developing very fast and so does the sectors which are related to maximum growth rate. Dairy sector being one of the highest growing sectors provides extensive opportunities to the budding entrepreneurs and also to those farmers who want to take up the business of dairy farming. Milk and milk products are important sources of high quality proteins, fats, minerals and vitamins to balance the human diet. The entrepreneurs are key persons of any country for promoting economic growth and technological change. The appearance of their activities, i.e. the development of entrepreneurship is directly related to the socio-economic development of the society. Entrepreneurship among dairy farmers may be developed through systematic awareness programmes and training interventions. Awareness about latest technologies, opportunities, resource support system and about market potential has to be systematically spread among the rural masses, especially among the farming community. An environment of awareness and need has to be created. This awareness and motivation has to be developed not only among the farmers, but also among the field level extension workers.

This publication "Handbook for Dairy Entrepreneurs" has been written to provide fundamental information to all those farmers who want to take up dairy farming as an entrepreneurial venture for source of their livelihood and income generation. This book covers the basic knowledge about how to start an entrepreneurial dairy farming covering almost all the basic aspects related to the field. It had been taken care that all the information to be scientific and cosmopolitan and a farmer belonging to any region can successfully plan of taking up the business. The information is also provided for small scale dairy farming keeping in view of the landless and poor farmers. This book covers all the elements of dairy production with the goal of helping the dairy owners to keep their animals as healthy as possible. It covers areas including breeds and breeding management, housing and feeding management, basics of dairy animal diseases, disease prevention and control measures etc. This book will serve as a complete encyclopaedia of dairy husbandry practices and will help to guide practicing dairy farmers as well as starter (youth entrepreneur) in starting the dairy entrepreneurial venture from the scratch.

Entrepreneurship is neither a science nor an art. It is a practice. Knowledge in entrepreneurship is the means to an end. It is not a "flash of genius" but purposeful task that can be organized in to systematic work. Entrepreneurship is the buzz word in recent times and also a way for employment generation and hence scaling up the production. Several empirical studies have shown that the entrepreneurs as the human capital have made a large contribution to economic development than non-human capital. Increase in population, which is considered a liability can also contribute positively towards overall national development, only if entrepreneurial qualities are inculcated among the masses. This book provides the insights into the basics of the dairy entrepreneurship and entails the reader to have a brief and significant understanding of the concept of entrepreneurship in general and dairy entrepreneurship in particular. The basics of writing detailed project report (DPR) for financing institutes are also covered.

This book provides the first hand knowledge to the entrepreneurs to start the dairy farming by using the resources present locally. The topics in the book are so designed that even by looking at the pictorial representations one can get the idea of how to start the dairy farming. The book also popularizes the use of non-conventional items present at rural households and their significant use in dairy animal rearing. This book is a collation of information from various sources, and their contributions are gratefully acknowledged, providing an excellent pool of sound information. Most of the topics are aimed specifically at commercial dairy farming, but reference to small dairy farm is also included. Hopefully information provided in this book will be informative enough to encourage healthy dairy farming practices and provide enough mental stimulation to encourage the quest for even more information. This book has been specially written to cater the needs of all those farmers who want to contribute to the ever-increasing field of dairy farming.

The mission of the author will be successful if the youth in rural and semi urban India takes up the subject and practice successful entrepreneurial dairy farming and earn their living. The primary motive of the author is to create awareness among the masses about the benefits of entrepreneurial dairy farming and to take up as a business to alleviate poverty by generation of a sustainable source of income and hence employment.

Authors

Contents

Section B: Dairy Husbandry Information & Practices for Dairy Entrepreneurs

Section A: Dairy Entrepreneurship Approaches

1

Introduction

Twenty first century is the century of entrepreneurship and every individual can be an agent for innovation and change. Entrepreneurship is regarded as one of the most crucial factors in the economic development of every region of the country. It widens the horizons of economic development even in the socially and industrially backward regions. Dynamic entrepreneurs are considered to be the agent of change in a society. Entrepreneurs play a very important role in generating new employment and setting up new business. The problem of poverty, inequality and regional imbalances can be tackled with the development of entrepreneurship. However, in all economic development activities more and more focus is being centered on entrepreneurship of the people. Entrepreneur has been now recognized as a concept, not only for starting industries but also in the development of dairy enterprise. In India, it is believed that tremendous latent entrepreneurial talent exists which, if properly harnessed, could help in solving many of the serious problems facing the country.

Human resources are one of the most strategic and critical determinants of growth. In spite of abundant physical resources, a country cannot make rapid economic and social advancement unless it has enterprising people with necessary knowledge, skills and attitudes. So, it is the supply of people with entrepreneurial thirst that makes nation to march ahead in the process of development. Given the natural endowment of resources the fact that development or under-development of any nation is largely the reflection of the abundance or scarcity of entrepreneurship. Development of entrepreneurship is crucial in harnessing vast untapped human resources of a country like India and this also hold true in the field of dairy where available potential is still to be realized. Several research findings do suggest that entrepreneurship is the dominant variable in the growth process of any society, community or a nation as a whole. Entrepreneurship development among rural people is increasingly being recognized as a means to overall development of the rural community. The problem posing to our rural masses is not so much in terms of creation of productivity and wealth as that of developing the capacities and ensuring utilization of human potential in creating wealth. Motivating the rural folk towards entrepreneurship in the area of agriculture and dairying would go a long way in mitigating their problems of unemployment and poverty.

a. Global Milk Profile

World milk production is forecast to grow by 1.4 per cent to 831 million tonnes in 2017, with output set to expand in Asia and the Americas, stagnate in Europe and Africa, and decline in Oceania. During the first part of 2017 (January to May), prices remained generally stable overall, as recovery of milk deliveries in the EU and continued growth in output in the United States lessened supply concerns. Global trade in dairy products is projected to register a second year of modest growth in 2017, rising by 1 percent to 71.8 million tonnes of milk equivalent. Continued recovery in imports by China, following the substantial drop sustained in 2015, is forecast to be the main engine for growth. Purchases by the Russian Federation, Mexico, Australia, the Philippines, Thailand, Yemen and the Republic of Korea, among others, are also projected to increase. Conversely, a fall in imports is anticipated for Brazil, Saudi Arabia, Malaysia, Viet Nam and Nigeria, while shipments to Indonesia, the United Arab Emirates, the United States and Japan are expected to remain virtually unchanged. Within the overall international market for dairy products, trade flows in skim milk powder (SMP), cheese and butter are anticipated to expand, while those of whole milk powder (WMP) could wane. The EU, the United States, Argentina and Canada are the main exporting countries expected to see increased sales, while New Zealand, Australia and Switzerland are forecast to experience a retrenchment in shipments. Sustained milk output in the EU and a rise in production in the United States are anticipated to be the most dynamic factors affecting the international market in 2017. In Oceania, reduced milk supplies are forecast to constrain its exports, while in Belarus, the level of shipments is expected to remain unchanged, due to limited growth in import demand by the Russian Federation combined with greater competition from other sources of supply.

b. Why to promote Entrepreneurship in Dairying?

It will not be less than correct to mention that entrepreneurship has become the buzzword of the day. Entrepreneurship has now become most important phenomenon for rapid progress in dairy. Today when there is growing concern for greater attention to our rural economy, the dairy sector offers big opportunity to transform our economy by bringing prosperity to the rural sector. The supporting income from animal husbandry and dairying is farmer's cash insurance against any distress caused by the crop failures. The dairy sector provides immense opportunities for eradicating poverty.

There is an urgent need to make dairy development an area of core competence in the national programme of poverty reduction and rural prosperity.

The fact that dairying could play a more constructive role in promoting rural welfare and reducing poverty by generating employment at farm level is increasingly being recognized.

Despite this upside fact about dairying, this sector in India has not picked up on commercial line. But, since Tenth Five Plan onwards Govt. of India, truly focused on animal husbandry and dairying to receive a high priority in the effort for generating income and employment, increasing animal protein availability in the food basket and for generating exportable surplus.

A sustainable and financially viable dairy farming, which will generate income and self employment through entrepreneurship, is need of the day. Market oriented milk production will be key livestock activities to generate income on a steady daily basis for resource poor households. In this context entrepreneur is one of the most important inputs for development of dairying, which may prove phenomenal for economic development of a country or of regions within the country.

c. Factors in Dairy Entrepreneurship

Although, entrepreneurship is a function of several factors, out of those, three sets of factors could be identified, which mainly influence entrepreneurship. These are: i) The individual or Entrepreneur; ii) socio-cultural factors; and iii) support system.

The Individual

The individual constitutes the most important element in entrepreneurship. The entrepreneur as an individual takes the decision to start or not to start dairy as an enterprise. And it is who strives to make it success. Again, three main factors, which influence the individual behaviour are his/her motivational factors, factors concerning various skills that entrepreneur possess, and the factors relating to his knowledge of several relevant aspects that are likely to contribute to success of the entrepreneurial roles. The motivational factors i.e. inner urge of the individual to do something new in a particular field has been found very important. To be successful an entrepreneur needs several kinds of skills; project development skill, enterprise management skill and enterprise building skill. At the same time, an entrepreneur needs to have knowledge about several areas of activity relevant to his domain in dairy enterprise. Knowledge about economic-political environment, financial institution, availability of inputs, technology, development agencies etc. Such knowledge helps him plan his strategy and use skills effectively.

Socio-Cultural Factors

Family background, norms and values of the immediate social circle contribute substantially to entrepreneurship development in dairying. The values and attitude an individual has, are a function of the socio-cultural millieu. Behaviors which reflect inclinations towards initiative and risk taking, dependence or independence, working with one's own hands on tasks requiring manual handling etc. are a result of the socialization process in the family, the school and society. Behaviour rewarded through appreciation, encouragement, and other extrinsic as well as intrinsic devices gets reinforced and related values and norms develop.

Support System

Possibility of the success of dairypreneur generally gets enhanced by efficient and effective operation of the support systems. The list of support systems include family, relatives, commercial bank, cooperative bank, cooperative society, input agencies, animal husbandry and dairy development department, research institute, KVK, veterinary hospital, stockman centre, friends, private money lender, local milk market and local dairy unit.

In the process of entrepreneurship, it is equally important to know that what level of support these support agencies actually extend to the entrepreneurs. Because level of supports extended by them are tangible help received by entrepreneurs. As evident from Figure 1, the cooperatives were extending most tangible support to the entrepreneurs by extending help of multifarious nature. Next comes, input agencies, which support the farmers in running dairy enterprise by supplying important inputs in time. It was quite discouraging to note that government development departments were ranked last on the basis of level of support received and perceived by the entrepreneurs. The general belief of inefficient working of government departments holds true here with great dissatisfaction of entrepreneurs with the kind of support extended by these organizations. Government organization must improve their performance to match their extended level of support with expected degree of importance by the entrepreneurs.

d. Dairying in India

India has outpaced the global milk production with an annual growth rate of 5.53% compared with the 2.09% achieved globally. Milk production, which was around 17-22 million tonnes in the 1960s, has increased to 163.7 million tonnes in 2016-17. Particularly, it has increased by 19% during 2016-17 in comparison to 137.7 million tonnes during 2013-14 recording a growth of 6.26 %, whereas FAO reported 3.1% increase in world milk production from 765 million tonnes in 2013 to 789 million tonnes in 2014 . Similarly, per capita availability of milk has increased from 307 grams in 2013-14 to 351 grams in the year 2016-17. Similarly, the income of dairy farmers increased by 23.77% in 2014-17 compared to 2011-14,

World Milk Day is observed throughout the world on June 1, with an aim to raise awareness about milk and its importance as a global food. Meanwhile, India has witnessed remarkable growth in its production and consumption of milk and dairy products in recent years and this trend is almost certain to continue. India's milk production continues to grow, to the point where it now tops the milk output of all the European Union countries combined. India has been the world's top milk-producing country since 1998, but in the year 2014, for the first time, it beat the entire EU. On a country basis, after India, the US produces the most milk, and China comes in third. This represents a sustained growth in availability of milk and milk products for the growing population in India. Dairying has become an important source of income for millions of rural households engaged in agriculture. This increased consumption of dairy products is also playing a vital role in improving child nutrition and boosting the livelihoods of smallholder farmers across the region, as they are the source of production for the vast amount of milk and dairy products. The success of the dairy industry has resulted from the integrated co-operative system of milk collection, transportation, processing and distribution, conversion of the same to milk powder and products, to minimise seasonal impact on suppliers and buyers, retail distribution of milk and milk products, sharing of profits with the farmer, which are ploughed back to enhance productivity and needs to be emulated by other farm produce/producers. The most crucial reason for India to be the highest producer of milk is that India has had a successful decades-long programme to source milk from small farmers through cooperatives. One of the prime examples is AMUL. It's worth noting that the majority of Indian milk comes from buffaloes, not cows (the US is still the number one cow-milk-producing country in the world). According to the joint OECD-UN FAO Agricultural Outlook for 2014, most of India's milk is consumed fresh (as opposed to powdered or canned).

The per capita availability of milk in the country which was 130 gram per day during 1950-51 has increased to 355 gram per day in 2016-17 as against the world average of 293.7 grams per day during 2013. This represents sustained growth in the availability of milk and milk products for our growing population. Dairying has become an important secondary source of income for millions of rural families and has assumed the most important role in providing employment and income generating opportunities particularly for marginal and women farmers. Most of the milk is produced by animals reared by small, marginal farmers and landless labourers. About 15.46 million farmers have been brought under the ambit of 165835 village level dairy corporative societies up to March

2015. Government of India is making efforts for strengthening the dairy sector through various Central sector Schemes like "National Programme for Bovine Breeding and Dairy Development", National Dairy Plan (Phase-I) and "Dairy Entrepreneurship Development Scheme".

Dairy activities have traditionally been integral to India's rural economy. The country is the world's largest producer of dairy products and also their largest consumer. Almost its entire produce is consumed in the domestic market and the country is neither an importer nor an exporter, except in a marginal sense. Despite being the world's largest producer, the dairy sector is by and large in the primitive stage of development and modernization. Though India may boast of a 200 million cattle population, the average output of an Indian cow is only one seventh of its American counterpart. Indian breeds of cows are considered inferior in terms of productivity. Moreover, the sector is plagued with various other impediments like shortage of fodder, its poor quality, dismal transportation facilities and a poorly developed cold chain infrastructure. As a result, the supply side lacks in elasticity that is expected of it. On the demand side, the situation is buoyant. With the sustained growth of the Indian economy and a consequent rise in the purchasing power during the last two decades, more and more people today are able to afford milk and various other dairy products. This trend is expected to continue with the sector experiencing a robust growth in demand in the short and medium run. If the impediments in the way of growth and development are left unaddressed, India is likely to face a serious supply – demand mismatch and it may gradually turn into a substantial importer of milk and milk products.

e. Advantages of Dairying

1. Important human food: Milk is palatable, easy to digest and highly nutritious.
2. Milk, a nearly perfect food: It contains fat, milk sugar, proteins, minerals and liberal source of many vitamins but it is deficient in vitamin C and iron.
3. Milk as a protective and balanced food: Milk and its products are the only source of animal protein in vegetarian diet. Hence, Nutritional Advisory Committee of ICMR recommended 285 gm. of milk/ day/per capita to balance the diet for supply of essential amino acids.
4. Sources of draft power for various agricultural operations. Some of the excellent draft breeds supply good quality bullocks—the source of draft power which brings savings in energy resources like petroleum products and coal.

5. **Suited to agricultural operations**: Due to small sized holdings of farmers all agricultural operations can best be completed by bullocks.
6. **Provides organic manure:** Which is the best means of maintaining soil fertility and organic farming.
7. Opportunity of making use of barren/unfertile land for housing of animals.
8. Dairying under Indian conditions fits well with agriculture as mixed farming and provides protective and balanced farming.
9. **National income:** Dairying contributes little more than 7 per cent to the national income.
10. Offers opportunity of earning foreign exchange worth Rs. 5,213.8 crores by export of poultry, hides, bones, hair, etc.
11. Offers opportunity of proper utilization of by-products and industrial wastes as cheaper source of feeds for animals.
    - Utilization of agriculture waste by-products like wheat bhusa, paddy straw, rice polish, wheat bran, cakes, chunis, etc.
    - Utilization of milk by-products like whey, butter milk for feeding to calves and other growing stock.
    - Utilization of animal by-products like bone meal, fish meal, meat meal; blood meal, etc.

- Utilization of industrial by-products like molasses, grain, go down sweepings etc.

12. Dairying offers opportunity of getting income round the year.

Indian dairying is emerging as a sunrise industry. It is crucial for rural economy and livelihood. India represents one of the world's largest and fastest growing markets for milk and milk products due to the increased disposable incomes among the 250 million strong middle class.

e. Profile of the Indian dairy industry

- India is the world's largest producer and consumer of dairy. The dairy industry in India was worth INR 5,000 billion in 2016.
- India is also globally the largest milk producing country since 1998.
- In India, the co-operatives and private dairies have access to only 20% of the milk produced.

- Approximately, 34% of the milk is sold in the unorganized market while 46% is consumed locally. This is in comparison to most of the developed nations where almost 90% of the surplus milk is passes through the organized sector.
- India ranks first in Total Livestock Population, Milk Production, Cattle Population, Buffalo Population and Total Bovine Population

Commodity	Total Production (per year)	Per Capita Availability	ICMR Recommendations
	(2016-17)	(2016-17)	
Milk	165.4 MT	355 grams/day	280 grams/day

Important figures	
Percentage of total world milk produced in India	18.5 per cent
Highest milk producing state	Uttar Pradesh
State with highest per capita availability of milk	Punjab (1075 g)
Highest Cross-bred or exotic cows	Tamil Nadu
Highest number of livestock	Uttar Pradesh
Highest cattle population	Madhya Pradesh
Highest buffalo population	Uttar Pradesh
Highest Share of milk in Total Milk Production of India:	Uttar Pradesh (16.8%)
Growth Rates of milk production in India	5.3 per cent
Highest growth rate in milk production	Andhra Pradesh (12.6%)
Value output of Milk and Milk Products out of the total output from livestock rearing	65.05 per cent
Total livestock population	512.05 million
Milch animals	118.59 million
Total bovine population:	299.99 million
Total cattle population	190.90 million
Total indigenous cattle	151.17 million
Total buffalo population	108.70 million
Percentage Distribution of Cattle population	37. 28 per cent
Percentage Distribution of Buffalo population	21.23 per cent
Percentage of the World Livestock Present in India: Total Livestock	11.54 per cent
Percentage of the World Livestock Present in India: Buffalo	56.7 per cent
Percentage of the World Livestock Present in India : Cattle	12.5 per cent

Demographic Dependence on Livestock

- Livestock sector employs 8 per cent of total Indian Workforce
- Percentage of population dependent on agriculture for livelihood: 49.8 per cent

- Percentage of livestock owned by marginal, small and semi-medium farmers: 87.7 per cent
- Percentage of area used for all types of livestock farming: 1.69 per cent

The world dairy is zooming on India for its rapidly growing markets and ever increasing share in the GDP contributing > 25 % of total value of output from agriculture and allied sector. The changing international dairy trade pattern following GATT and the emergence of the World Trade Organization (WTO) offers to the Indian diary industry an opportunity to take its bow as an exporter. India's enthusiasm to integrate with the world economy is reflected in the technological upgradation, professional excellence and a cost effective approach. It is already recognized as a sourcing center for exports of products and services to countries in Asia – the powerhouse of fastest growth in the world. Its central geographical location in the region gives it an extra competitive edge.

Two main reasons for the world focus on India are: one, the low cost economy; and two, the liberalization process initiated since 1991. Other important factors include low inflation rate, inexpensive labour, the presence of the world's third largest pool of technical manpower, the world's largest democracy and an independent judiciary, well established and free from government interference and ease in communication due to wide spread use of English among the educated and the professional class.

g. Dairying for inclusive growth

The following characterizes India's dairy farming and its relevance to inclusive growth

- Small and marginal farmers own 33 percent of land and about 60 percent of female cattle and buffaloes.
- Some 75 percent of rural households own, on average, two to four animals.
- Dairying is a part of the farming system, not a separate enterprise. Feed is mostly residual from crops, whereas cow dung is important for manure.
- Dairying provides a source of regular income, whereas income from agriculture is seasonal. This regular source of income has a huge impact on minimizing risks to income. There is some indication that areas where dairy is well developed have less incidence of farmer suicide.
- About a third of rural incomes are dependent upon dairying.
- Livestock is a security asset to be sold in times of crisis.

Dairy has a lot of potential to improve rural incomes, nutrition and women empowerment, and hence is a very critical area for investment. A well-developed industry will enable millions of farmers to capitalize on the emerging opportunities and make a significant impact on rural incomes. On the flip side, weak efforts towards dairy development also can have a significant but negative impact on the dairy industry. The growth rate has been sluggish over the past few years. With an increase in demand on one hand and sluggish supply on the other, there is a likely shortfall in demand in the coming years.

Emerging situation

Dairy is currently the top-ranking commodity in India, with the value of output in 2004 at 1.179 billion rupees (US$39 million), which is almost equal to the combined output value of rice and wheat. Despite the importance of the dairy sector in overall GDP, it receives less government budgeting than the agriculture sector. Further, there has been no concentrated investment in the development of value-added or innovative products, nor any serious effort to support and modernize the informal sector.

In light of the increasing demand driven by the growing population, higher incomes and more health consciousness, the slowdown in dairy industry growth is severely worrisome. Based on estimates by the National Dairy Development Board (NDDB), the demand for milk is likely to reach 180 million tonnes by 2022. To supply the market, an average incremental increase of 5 million tonnes per annum over the *next* 15 years is required – a doubling of the average incremental rate achieved over the *past* 15 years. In the absence of sufficient increased production, India will need to rely on the world market for imports. And because of the huge volume required, it will affect global milk prices. Thus, focusing on areas for local dairy development is critical.

h. SWOT analysis of dairy farming business

Strengths

The Indian dairying with its vastness contributes rather uniquely to the nation's health and wealth. Factors that give strength include:

- The vast livestock population of the country could prove to be a vital asset for the country and unlike many other natural resources which will deplete over the years, a sustainable livestock production system will continue to propel Indian economy.
- Dairying is crucial in providing employment and supplementary income to the bulk of rural families. The main beneficiaries are woman who contribute over 70 per cent of labour in cattle rearing.

- Dairying as a small enterprise is mostly common with landless labourers, marginal and small farmers, the progress in this sector result in more balanced development of the rural economy, particularly in reduction of poverty ratio.
- This is the sector where poor contribute to growth directly instead of getting benefit from growth generated elsewhere.
- Dairy farming helps directly in increasing crop production by making available draught power, manure and cash income on day- today basis.
- As the milk productivity of our animals is low, there is a vast scope for improvement of the milk production and consequently increased marketable surplus of milk for processing.
- **Availability of raw material:** Abundant. Presently, more than 80 per cent of milk produced is flowing into the unorganized sector, which requires proper channelization.
- Purchasing power of the consumers is on the upswing with growing economy & continually increasing population of middle class.
- Milk consumption in India is regular part of the dietary programme irrespective of the region and hence demand is likely to rise continuously.
- Indian dairy farming thrives largely on crop residues and agricultural byproducts keeping the input costs low. Labour cost is also fairly low making the industry fairly cost competitive.
- Industry continues to grow and the margins are still fairly reasonable. Indian dairy farmers do not receive any subsidy and when the world dairy market opens up post-WTO negotiations, our products could compete on the price front
- Large number of dairy plants both in public and cooperative sectors besides several others in the private sector is coming up.
- **Technical manpower:** Vast pool of professionally- trained and qualified technical manpower built over last 40 years is available at all levels to support R&D as well as industry operations.
- Crop residues and by-products fed to the cattle form the basis of "grain-saving" dairying, appropriate to the mixed farming system.
- The buffalo is India's milking machine, accounting for more than half of the country's milk production. It is notable for its efficiency as a converter of coarse feeds into rich milk. It is preferred by the dairy processors not only for its higher total solids but also for its higher fat content.

- Whitening property of buffalo milk makes it more suitable for manufacture of some dairy products and its acceptance as fluid milk is high.
- Cooperative dairying has increased milk production.
- Dairying provides regular and additional income which helps in improving the quality and standard of life in rural areas.
- Involvement of large number of small and marginal farmers in dairying
- An effective marketing channel helps to meet the demands of the urban consumer
- Increased involvement of private and multinational companies such as Reliance, Dabur, ITC, JP group, Sahara India and many more in milk production, procurement, processing and marketing other than enhanced presence of established brands such as Amul, Nestle, Mother Dairy and other dairy cooperatives & private dairies at both national level and globally.
- **Margins:** Quite reasonable, even on packed liquid milk.
- **Flexibility of product mix:** Tremendous. With balancing equipment, one can keep on adding to product line.

Weaknesses

The dairy sector is not without its share of constraints. Some weaknesses include:

- **Perishability:** Milk being the perishable item, setting up of Bulk Milk Coolers (BMCs) at village level, milk chilling plants at major places, pasteurization facilities has overcome this weakness partially. UHT gives milk long life. Surely, many new processes will follow to improve milk quality and extend its shelf life.
- **Lack of control over milk yield:** Theoretically, there is little control over milk yield. However, increased awareness of developments like embryo transplant, artificial insemination and properly managed animal husbandry practices, coupled with higher income to rural milk producers should automatically lead to improvement in milk yields.
- **Competition:** With so many newcomers entering this industry, competition is becoming tougher day by day. But then competition has to be faced as a ground reality. The market is large enough for many to carve out their niche.
- Quality dairy animals (heifers) are in short supply. Though cross breeding programmes have significantly improved animal productivity, milk production system in many parts of the country is still largely dominated

by low yielding animals. Artificial insemination service for breeding better cattle has limited coverage, barely reaching an estimated 10 per cent of bovines

- Poor condition of roads and erratic power supply remain a major challenge for procurement and supply of good quality raw milk. Furthermore, raw milk collection systems in certain parts of the country remain fairly underdeveloped.
- **Logistics of procurement:** Woes of bad roads and inadequate transportation facility make milk procurement problematic. But with the overall economic improvement in India, these problems would also get solved.
- Maintenance of cold chain is still a major handicap. For organized marketing of milk, the milk produced is required to be transported to nearby processing plant which incurs cold storage and transportation costs which are quite high.
- The immediate problem of Indian dairy industry is not just short fall in milk availability but poor infrastructure for transporting, processing and distributing rurally produced milk to major consumer centers in urban areas posing problems to procurement and distribution.
- **Problematic distribution:** Yes, all is not well with distribution. But then if ice creams can be sold virtually at every nook and corner, why can't we sell other dairy products too? Moreover, it is only a matter of time before we see the emergence of a cold chain linking the producer to the refrigerator at the consumer's home!
- Majority of milk producers is unaware about scientific dairy farming, clean milk production and value chain. Farmer's access to training in modern cattle management is limited.
- The rural women, an invisible partner need access to training in modern cattle management to maximize returns.
- Despite the vast potential and huge resource base available, entrepreneurial ability is lacking among milk producers.
- Seasonal fluctuations in milk production pattern, regional imbalance of milk supply and species-wise variation (buffalo, cow, goat etc.) in milk quality received by milk plants continue to pose serious handicaps.
- Absence of comprehensive and reliable milk production data, impact assessment studies are almost non-existent, investments in dairy research is also not commensurate with returns and potential.

- Large share of milk (70–85%) of marketable surplus goes through informal channel where quality is a big concern. Sometimes quality is an issue in the formal channel as well.
- Green fodder and quality feed availability to cattle throughout the year is not adequate.
- Animal health care activities are not adequate. The animal health cover is getting increasingly neglected. In many states, over 70-80 per cent of the veterinary budget is used for the staff salaries and jeeps with little left to buy medicines and other supplies.
- Limited marketing support handicaps rural milk producers seriously.
- Poor infrastructure in many areas for transporting rurally-produced milk to major processing centers. Dairy producers in remote areas are neglected.
- Limited investment or delay in the availability of funds in setting up or expansion of milk procurement.
- Farmers do not share in the benefits and profits of high demand because of poor governance of cooperatives
- Milk production is scattered over a large number of farmers producing miniscule quantities
- Milk distribution is limited to urban and peri-urban areas
- Low milk prices because of lower prices declared by cooperatives, which results in low prices of milk paid by all players
- Adhoc export policies and a ban on exports
- Quality of milk and milk products are a barrier to entry to the export market, especially the EU and the USA
- Lack of policy focus on strengthening indigenous breeds
- Non-existent of livestock extension facilities and delivery system at ground level.
- Farmers' milk prices are not based on fat and SNF measurement, which affects their profitability.
- Because of low access to credit and risk-taking ability, farmers cannot increase their herd size.

Opportunities

"Failure is never final, and success never ending". Dr Kurien bears out this statement perfectly. He entered the industry when there were only threats. He met failure head-on, and now he clearly is an example of 'never ending successes! If dairy entrepreneurs are looking for opportunities in India, the following areas must be tapped:

- **Value addition:** There is a phenomenal scope for innovations in product development, packaging and presentation. Given below are potential areas of value addition:
    - Steps should be taken to introduce value-added products like *shrikhand*, ice creams, *paneer, khoa*, flavored milk, dairy sweets, etc. This will lead to a greater presence and flexibility in the market place along with opportunities in the field of brand building.
    - Addition of cultured products like yoghurt and cheese lend further strength - both in terms of utilization of resources and presence in the market place.
    - A lateral view opens up opportunities in milk proteins through casein, caseinates and other dietary proteins, further opening up export opportunities.
    - Yet another aspect can be the addition of infant foods, geriatric foods and nutritionals.
- **Export potential:** Efforts to exploit export potential are already on. Amul is exporting to USA, UK, European countries, Bangladesh, Sri Lanka, Nigeria, and the Middle East. Following the new WTO agreements, opportunities will increase tremendously for the export of agri-products in general and dairy products in particular.
    - The mass production of indigenous milk based sweets in modern dairy plants can tap its growing demand by value addition. With more than 150 million NRI overseas the scope for their export is promising.
    - Expanding market will see creation of enormous job and self employment opportunities.
    - Economy is growing at the rate of nearly 8% of GDP. Consequently, the investment opportunities are also increasing continually.
    - Entry of large corporations in retailing such as Reliance, Dabur, ITC, JP group, Sahara India and many more which can lead to more investment

- Demand for dairy products is income elastic. Continued rise in middle class population will see shift in the consumption pattern in favour of value added products besides the growth in demand for liquid milk.
- Cost of milk production in India is low. So more opportunities for export of quality milk products at competitive price in international market.
- Greatly improved export potential for indigenous as well as western milk products.
- Opening of the world market offers opportunities for utilization of byproducts of the dairy industry for manufacturing value added products for import substitution.
- India has been described by one FAO expert as a "slumbering giant" of the international dairy trade.
- Increased farmer income by exploiting the ever increasing high demand for milk and milk products.
- Increased consumer sophistication and awareness of quality reception of quality packaged products (though slowly).
- Immense scope to enhance governance of dairy farmer organizations and thus enable dairy farmers to demand higher prices.
- Overall positive growth environment, which is triggering the Government to enhance infrastructure.
- Scope exists for higher milk yield through better use of crop residues and other feeds, upgrading cattle through planned cross breeding and improving availability of animal health care facilities.
- Better returns from clean and organic milk production because of increased awareness in consumers about quality and health consciousness.

Threats

Dairying is also facing threats from many quarters. These include:

- A large cattle population (mostly unproductive and low milk yielder) grazes on uncultivated lands, forest areas and common property resources. This imposes a heavy social cost, leading to degradation and denudation of land and loss of natural resources base.
- Indiscriminate crossbreeding for raising milk productivity could lead to disappearance of valuable indigenous breeds.

- Organized dairy industry handles only 15% of the milk produced. Cost effective technologies, mechanization, and quality control measures are seldom exercised in unorganized sector and remain key issues to be addressed.
- Large portion of the population does not care about quality issues in milk as there is a gross lack of awareness among farmers about the quality parameters, including microbiological and chemical contaminants as well as residual antibiotics.
- Middlemen still control a very large proportion of the milk procurement. Serious efforts need to be taken to eliminate them from the supply chain.
- Export of quality feed ingredients viz., cakes, molasses etc. is making the domestic producers rely on low energy fodders.
- Entry of multinationals could result in a large portion of milk being diverted towards value added products which, though it augers well for the producers, is likely to affect the availability of liquid milk supply for mass consumption especially for the poor urban class as well as because of high price sensitivity for dairy products, poor and lower middle class people are not able to pay for quality products marketed by multinationals at a very exorbitant price.
- A parallel economy is thriving on adulterated liquid milk including synthetic milk in certain pockets which needs to nip in the bud.
- Significant increase in maize and other concentrate feed prices can increase the milk production cost.
- Large informal markets that extend credit are constraining farmers. The high cost of credit is another adverse factor that reduces the viability of the dairy projects.
- Low productivity and scattered production leading to high cost of transportation.
- Emphasis on milk fat and not on SNF content maintaining relatively lower prices of milk.
- Competition between organized and un-organized sectors resulting in unhealthy business practices / lowering values (quality/service/ethics).
- Inadequate Regulatory staffs / food inspectors to monitor quality of imported / indigenous products.

- Possibility of importing substandard or low-priced milk products that can destabilize dairy sector because of corrupt regulatory staff.
- Natural calamities like floods, drought, diseases that can affect feed to cattle/cattle population.
- Seasonal fluctuations in milk production.
- **Milk vendors, the un-organized sector:** Today milk vendors *(Dudhia)* are occupying the pride of place in the industry. Organized dissemination of information about the harm that they are doing to producers and consumers should see a steady decline in their importance.

The study of SWOT analysis shows that the 'strengths' and 'opportunities' far outweigh 'weaknesses' and 'threats'. Strengths and opportunities are fundamental and weaknesses and threats are transitory. Any investment idea can do well only when you have three essential ingredients: entrepreneurship (the ability to take risks), innovative approach (in product lines and marketing) and values (of quality/ethics).

The Indian dairy industry, following its delicensing, has been attracting a large number of entrepreneurs. Their success in dairying depends on factors such as an efficient yet economical procurement network, hygienic and cost-effective processing facilities and innovativeness in the market place. All that needs to be done is: to innovate, convert products into commercially exploitable ideas. All the time keep reminding yourself: Benjamin Franklin discovered electricity, but it was the man who invented the meter that really made the money!

Thus, SWOT analysis, indicate if the strengths and opportunities are understood the weaknesses and threats can be managed to make Dairy Farm Sector into a profit oriented business.

- ***Strengths*** and ***Weaknesses*** refer to issues under the direct control of the farm or agribusiness. ***Strength*** is something the business is good at; a ***Weakness*** is something the business is not good at. For example, the managers of a dairy may boasts of having excellent dairy breeds of animals at their farm (***Strength***), but erratic power supply (hindrances to milking oprations) and poor road to transport the milk to city consumers (***Weakness***) to fetch premium price of their
- ***Opportunities*** and ***Threats*** refer to issues the business has no direct control over. A new milk plant opening in the area would be an example of an ***Opportunity*** for a dairy, because it may give the managers "opportunity" to exercise more negotiating power. ***Threats*** are external influences that may adversely affect the dairy. If a country which normally imports dairy

products is in a recession, it may not be able to buy as many dairy products from the usual exporting country. This "threat" may hurt the farm if it results in a decreased milk price or decrease in demand.

i. Important 4 P's for Dairy Entrepreneurs

In addition to the SWOT analysis, the successful Dairy Entrepreneur must have a proper understanding of the four 'P': Procurement, Production, Processing and Promotion.

Procurement: It covers collection of milk from rural producers or contractors including setting up of chilling centers, provision of laboratory equipment and supplies, milking machines, cattle welfare, including feed and fodder and last but not the least the transportation.

Production: It includes activities of producing various types of liquid milks like the conventional whole, toned and standardized as well as innovative like milk with extra nutrition for school children, pregnant mothers, the aged and the infirm: low fat milk for the calorie conscious. The key is to sale milk also as a **fun product** and not merely as something, which is good for health.

Processing: Processing of products such as butter and cheese spread, pre-sliced butter and cheese, dairy whiteners, milk beverages (Plain and Carbonated), butter oil as a cooking medium, whip-and-serve milk shake powders, wet and dry kulfi and ice cream mix, high protein whey drinks for sports man, milk sweets, Shrikhand, dried condensed milk, dried khoa and many more can be added the list.

Promotion: It covers activities like brand promotion, setting up of dairy parlours, buying milk in bulk and repacking to sell, distribution, devising attractive packaging and other such activities, which will result in building an image either nationally or even regionally and enhance the marketing of the products.

Agriculture and animal husbandry in Indian context is considered as a family tradition and majority of the farmers continue to practice what their forefathers did or their neighbours do. Rearing farm animals besides agriculture is routine activity of farming community in India and a large number of farmers depend on animal husbandry for their livelihood. The word 'entrepreneur' is derived from the French verb 'enterprendre' which means, "To undertake". In the present era, it is increasingly being realized that entrepreneurship contributes to development of a country in several ways, viz. assembling and harnessing the various inputs, bearing the risks, innovating and imitating the techniques of production to reduce the cost and increase quality and quantity, expanding the horizons of the market and coordinating and managing the manufacturing unit at various levels. The development of entrepreneurship is directly related to the socio-economic development of the society. Dairy as an enterprise is increasingly being recognized could play a more constructive role in promoting rural welfare and reducing poverty by generating employment at farm level. A sustainable and financially viable dairy farming, which will generate income and self employment through entrepreneurship, is the need of the day

j. STEEP analysis of Dairy Entrepreneurship

STEEP analysis: It refers to as a tool used to get an insight into past, current and future of the external environment developments which impact an organization/enterprise. It consists of five drivers namely:

- **Sociological drivers:** This includes factors like consumer behavior demographics, religion, lifestyles, values and advertising;
- **Technological drivers:** It focuses highly on technological advancements. It includes factors like innovation, communication technology, packaging technology, cold chain technology etc.
- **Economical drivers:** it is strongly associated with consumers buying position. It includes interest rates, financing facilities, cooperatives, market demand etc.
- **Environmental drivers:** it includes environmental factors that affect the dairy sector.
- **Political drivers:** It includes various govt. policies that affect the dairy sector

STEEP analysis of dairy entrepreneurship: The opportunities can be captured through timely understanding of the drivers of dairy entrepreneurship from present to future. The drivers will provide momentum and direction to growth of the dairy entrepreneurship. The driving factors have potential to turnaround the weaknesses and threats of the dairying into opportunity and strength of organic dairy entrepreneurship.

Sociological Drivers

1 Favourable demographic factors for milk consumption

2 Changing consumption pattern due to rise in more middle class income group and urbanisation

3 More awareness about health consciousness in people around the globe

4 Goal of sustainable nutritional and food security

5 Enhanced training, exposure and improvement in social conditions due to improved communication and interaction among academia, govt. farmers and industries.

6 Increased consumers autonomy /choice in selection of food items.

7 Enhanced consumer confidence/ ability in purchase of both indigenous and imported milk and milk products.

8 Source of employment generation for unemployed youth in both rural and urban areas as dairy farming provides more remunerative business opportunities.

9 No social taboo towards dairy farming.

10 Dairy farming being an age old practice.

Technological Drivers

1 Provision of cold chain technology (bulk milk coolers) for milk storage at village level provides time utility of dairy business enterprise.

2 Increased dependence on electronic dairy equipments like automatic milk collection unit (AMCU), electronic milk tester , electronic weighing balance etc removes malpractice and adulteration of milk which gives boost to young entrepreneur to enter into dairy business.

3 Automation of indigenous milk and milk products manufacturing like curd, ghee, butter etc.

4 Technological up gradation of Indigenous milk product making.

5 Awareness creation for throughout the year green fodder cultivation and green fodder conservation through Hay and Silage making – an important aspect of dairy farming.

6 Technological advancement in feed technology for different categories of dairy animals.

7 Increased documentation and validation of indigenous technical knowledge (ITKs) for treatment of various ailments of livestock. Therefore, relying less on antibiotics, steroids and hormones.

8 Improved packaging technology for milk and milk products like tetra pack.

9 Dairy productivity enhancement techniques like application of balanced ration, organic green and dry fodder, indigenous technical knowledge (ITKs) for treatment of various ailments of livestock.

10 Availability of refrigerated vans for milk transport.

11 Appropriate technology access and transfer of milk related data and information through internet and mobiles.

Economical drivers

1 Foreign Direct Investment (FDI) in dairy industry and collaboration with more developed countries in terms of dairy farming.

2 More trained & skilled human resources for dairy operations.

3 Increased involvement of private and multinational companies such as Reliance, Dabur, ITC, JP group, Sahara India and many more in milk production, procurement, processing and marketing other than enhanced presence of established brands such as Amul, Nestle, Mother Dairy and other dairy cooperatives at both national level and globally will lead to more involvement of these MNC's to enter into more lucrative milk production.

4 Large and untapped rural and urban market in country for milk and milk products.

5 Improved credit/finance – facilities / availability and accessibility for dairy entrepreneurship through Govt. Schemes like *Dairy Entrepreneurship Development Scheme* (DEDS).

6 Improvement in marketing and retail chain- both at rural and urban areas

7 Low cost skilled human resource for dairy operations.

8 More demand of milk from urban areas for producing dairy products.

9 Commercialization of indigenous dairy products.

10 WTO's Sanitary & Phyto-Sanitary (SPS) measures and demand by private agencies for clean milk at premium price leading to improvement in clean milk production habit of milk producers.

11 Assured income generation through dairying for women dairy farmers as well as small and marginal farmers.

Environmental drivers

1 Importance given to milk and milk products due to increased health consciousness.

2 Improved technologies for dairy waste management.

3 Increased conversion of dairy waste into commercial products.

4 Emission norms and obligations set up by environment protection agencies

5 Vermi-compositing as a means for manufacturing manure.

6 Biogas plants for pollution free cooking gas as well as for lightening purpose.

7 Medicinal use of urine and cow dung of indigenous cattle.

Political drivers

1. Availability of easy bank loans for various dairy operations.
2. Livestock insurance schemes for dairy animals.
3. Supportive and encouraging Govt. policies for dairy farming and dairy related operations.
4. World fame 3-tier Dairy Cooperative model- AMUL.
5. Establishment of various training institutes for organic dairy entrepreneurs.

2

Key Concepts in Dairy Entrepreneurship

a. Dairy entrepreneurship

A dairy entrepreneur is a person who undertakes dairy based activities such as rearing of milch animals, production of milk, processing of milk, manufacture of milk products and marketing of milk and milk products and also involved in buying and selling of other inputs of dairy business. He finds ways and means to create and develop a profitable dairy business. Dairy entrepreneurs see their farming as a business and as a means of earning profits. So they are willing to take calculated risks to make profits and to grow their businesses. They are also motivated to improve dairy production through mechanization and application of technologies in the field of dairy and allied enterprises.

b. Technical skills required by a Dairy entrepreneur

Technical competencies are needed particularly in five areas:

1. Managing inputs
2. Managing production
3. Managing marketing
4. Financial Management
5. Labor Management

1. Managing inputs

The dairy-entrepreneur is good at identifying, sourcing and acquiring inputs for the farm. To manage inputs successfully, the farmer needs to know what inputs are required for each enterprise, where to get them and how to use them. He always looks for better quality inputs, lower input prices and more efficient alternatives. The dairy-entrepreneur is ready to experiment and learn.

2. Managing production

The entrepreneurial farmer knows the most profitable and sustainable way to produce. Every dairy entrepreneur should have all the production skills needed to produce good volume of milk like scientific knowledge about breeding, feeding, housing and health care management of their dairy animals. He should keep correct records for all the production activities. The entrepreneurial farmer is aware of time – doing things now rather than later. The entrepreneurial farmer is also ready to experiment with alternative production systems. Managing production involves animal production skills as well as ability to make most of the modern technologies which can help farmers to improve their production processes.

3. Managing marketing

In order to make profits, produce has to be marketed and sold. Farmer-entrepreneurs know where the most profitable market is for each product. They are good at negotiating contracts. Keep records of transactions. They look for more profitable markets. Adapt quickly to market changes and market opportunities Large scale dairy businesses require marketing management skills, market and customer orientation, identifying market opportunities, sales management, customer management; assessing customer needs through dialogue and feedback.

Besides these skills two more important skills of financial and labour management are also important such as

4. Financial management

This involves accountancy and financial skills. Financial Management is important because profit can be determined only if income and costs are accurately recorded.

5. Labour Management

This is important especially, as the farm business grows, it will have more employees. This is important for production management, as well as for risk management. Hiring the wrong laborer can quickly change profits into losses This involves determination of job requirements of different types of work, determine cost of labor, recruitment, selection, orientation and training, working with employees, motivating employees and evaluating employees.

c. Managerial/Management skills required by a Dairy entrepreneur

The successful dairy-entrepreneur uses farm resources effectively and efficiently. Two farms, with the same physical resources, markets, labour availability and capital base can generate very different levels of profits and income. Managerial functions are diagnosis, planning, organizing, leading, controlling and evaluating. The dairy entrepreneur performs these functions in each of the key areas of the farm business such as managing inputs, production and marketing.

1. **Diagnosis:** Entrepreneurial farmers have the analytical skills to understand the farm business and its enterprises very well. They are able to identify the constraints and opportunities that affect profitability. This involves understanding of the input, production and marketing requirements of each enterprise. They regularly analyze the farm business to identify problems and opportunities as well as form solutions and perform actions to minimize or remove the problems and grab the opportunities with both hands.
2. **Planning:** Planning involves identifying and selecting actions to take to achieve a goal. Thus it involves having knowledge about the goals and objectives and identifies, evaluate and choose alternatives to achieve those goals. It also involves outlining the steps and resources needed to implement alternatives
3. **Organizing:** Know what and when resources and materials are needed and where to get them. It includes obtaining the inputs and materials necessary to put the plan into effect.
4. **Directing** This involves motivating, enabling and drawing out the talent of people to achieve the goals of the farm business. Motivation is done through good communication; building of trust and confidence, creating a climate that encourages good performance and developing the capabilities, skills and competencies of staff.
5. **Evaluating:** Evaluation is assessing the outcomes of the farm business and the impact of decisions. It involves making comparisons of the farm business performance over time and with other farms. The results are used to identify strengths and weaknesses and plan for the future. Successful farmer-entrepreneurs are careful and objective evaluators.

d. Dairy entrepreneurs can effectively contribute to the society in the areas mentioned below:

- Creates jobs for the large section of unemployed educated youth.
- Creates market opportunities for the indigenous products through product diversification and innovative marketing.
- Utilizes the non-conventional resources like solar energy, rain water, agricultural by products and other locally available resources.
- Entrepreneurs introduce new technologies and new products through entrepreneurial spirit.
- Reducing poverty, nutritional hunger through dairy development (Increase income and equity).

- Export orientation of the dairy products (food safety and quality). Export of animals, milk products.
- Surveillance and monitoring of emerging livestock disease due to decline in genetic diversity.
- Developing breeding policy/conservation of elite indigenous germplasm.
- Integrating small holder dairy production in value chain.
- Adapting dairy production to climate change (methane mitigation, housing scheme).
- Sustainability of commercial dairy production.

e. Scope of Dairy Entrepreneurship Development

1. Ration Balancing Advisory Services

Ration given to animals usually comprises one or two locally available concentrate feed ingredient(s), seasonal grasses and crop residues. This leads to imbalanced feeding which adversely affects the health and productivity of animals in various ways and also reduces the net daily income to milk producer from dairying. At times, overfeeding of animals can also raise the cost of milk production. Therefore, milk producers need to understand the implications of imbalanced feeding and recognize the importance of giving balanced ration to their animals. Keeping this in view, NDDB has developed software for ration balancing, which will guide the milk producer about scientific animal feeding.

Implementation of RBP optimizes milk production of milk animals at the least cost by proper utilization to available feed ingredients, so as to provide them adequate amounts of proteins, minerals, vitamins as well as energy. This requires creation of a delivery system that provides advices to the producers and also arranges sale of feed and feed supplements that helps in sustaining the activity.

2. Field Artificial Insemination Services

High levels of productivity in dairy cattle can be achieved by bringing larger proportion of breedable female bovines under artificial insemination (A.I.) services. This opens a wide opportunity for entrepreneurs who can become Mobile A.I. Technicians (MAITs). MAITs can provide quality A.I. services at the farmer's doorstep.

Other Opportunities

- Operating one's own dairy farm, involving milk production activities.
- Working as dairy farm managers.
- As dairy herdman.
- As milkers.
- As testers.
- As Stockman.
- As Manager in a Cooperative set up.
- Manufacture of cattle feeds and other value added products.
- Veterinary services for animal health and breeding.
- Import-Export (Machinery/Ingredients/Products).
- Use of automation and information technology.
- As fieldsmen for dairy organisations.
- As fieldsmen for pure breed associations.
- As technical staff for research organisations.
- Teachers.
- Dairy extension worker—imparting vocational training.
- Writers for technical journals/magazines.
- Opportunities for leadership, dairy development.

3

Entrepreneurship Project on Dairy Farming

The total milk production in the country for the year 2013-14 has been estimated at 126 million metric tonnes and the demand is expected to be 180 million tonnes by 2020. To achieve this demand annual growth rate in milk production has to be increased from the present 2.5 % to 5%. Thus, there is a tremendous scope/ potential for increasing the milk production through profitable dairy farming.

a. Requirements of project report for setting up dairy units

Project report can be prepared by a beneficiary after consulting local technical persons of State Animal Husbandry Department, DRDA, Dairy Co-operative Society / Union / Federation / commercial dairy farmers. .

Items of Finance

1. The items of finance would include capital asset items such as purchase of milch animals, construction of sheds, purchase of equipments etc.
2. The feeding cost during the initial period of one/two months is capitalised and given as term loan.
3. Cost towards land development, fencing, digging of well, commissioning of diesel engine/pumpset, electricity connections, essential servants' quarters, godown, transport vehicle, milk processing facilities etc. can be considered for loan.
4. Cost of land is not considered for loan.

Proposed Dairy Project

5. The proposed dairy project should include information on land, dairy markets, availability of water, feeds, fodder, veterinary aid, breeding facilities, marketing aspects, training facilities, experience of the farmer and the type of assistance available from State Government, dairy society/ union/federation.

6. The scheme should also include information on the number and types of animals to be purchased, their breed, production performance, cost and other relevant input and output costs with their description. Based on this, the total cost of the project, margin money to be provided by the beneficiary, requirement of bank loan, estimated annual expenditure, income, profit and loss statement, repayment period, etc. can be worked out and shown in the Project report.
7. If possible, the beneficiaries should also visit progressive dairy farms and government / military / agricultural university dairy farms in the vicinity and discuss the profitability of dairy farming. A good practical training and experience in dairy farming will be highly desirable. The dairy co-operative societies, if existing in the villages would provide all supporting facilities particularly for marketing of fluid milk. Nearness of dairy farm to such a society, veterinary aid centre, artificial insemination centre should be ensured. There is a good demand for milk, if the dairy farm is located near urban centre

b. Technical Feasibility of proposed dairy project

This includes information on availability of good quality animals in nearby dairy market, availability of good grazing grounds and lands, availability of green/dry fodder, availability of concentrate feed, medicines etc. Further availability of veterinary aid, animal breeding (AI) centre, milk collection and marketing centre are also important.

c. Economic Viability of the project

Under this, information about the unit cost of animals, various input and output costs are provided.

Input costs involve cost of (feed and fodder, veterinary aid, breeding of animals, insurance, labour and other overheads) whereas output costs involve (sale price of milk, manure, gunny bags, male/female calves, other miscellaneous items etc). Further income expenditure statement, annual gross surplus, cash flow analysis is prepared to ensure economic viability of the project.

After ensuring technical feasibility and economic viability, the project is sanctioned by the bank. The loan is disbursed in kind in 2 to 3 stages against creation of specific assets such as construction of sheds, purchase of equipments and machinery, purchase of animals and recurring cost on purchase of feeds/ fodders for the initial period of one/two months. The end use of the funds is verified and constant follow-up is done by the bank.

The dairy project so formulated is submitted to the nearest branch of the bank. The bank's officer can assist in preparation of the project or filling in the prescribed application form. The bank examines the proposed dairy project for its technical feasibility and economic viability. Borrower need to deposit margin money from 5 to 25% along with security. Repayment period depends upon the gross surplus in the project. The loan will be repaid in suitable monthly/quarterly installments usually within a period of five to seven years Other documents such as loan application form, security aspects, margin money requirements etc. are also examined. A field visit to the proposed project area is undertaken for conducting a techno-economic feasibility study for appraisal of the project. The animals and capital assets may be insured annually or on long term master policy, whichever is applicable.

4

Format for Project Report Preparation of A Dairy Farm

1. General

In this the nature of objectives of the enterprise i.e. setting up a dairy farm, details of proposed investments, specification of the project area, name of the financing bank branch, status of beneficiary: (Individual/Partnership/Company/ Corporation/Co-operative Society / Others) details of borrowers profile in terms of capability, experience, financial soundness, technical / other special qualifications are mentioned.

2. Technical Aspects

a) **Location, Land and Land Development:** This involves the site details of the proposed project. The total land area and its cost. Also, particulars of land development such as fencing, boundary wall, gates are mentioned in it. Thus, site map is also mentioned in this subheading.

b) **Civil Structures:** Several structures like sheds, milking room, store room, quarters for dairy farm manager / labourers are also to be constructed. So, their measurements as well as approximate costs need to be mentioned.

c) **Equipment/Plant and Machinery:** Several equipments are also needed such as chaff cutter, silo pit, milking machine, feed grinder and mixer, milking pails/milk cans, biogas plant, bulk coolers, manufacturing equipments of dairy products and a vehicle such as truck/van. The price quotations for the above equipments should be given.

d) **Housing:** This would cover the housing design loose/conventional barn, head to head or tail to tail, the proposed area for different categories of animals such as adults, heifers (1-3 years), calves (less than 1 year) etc.

e) **Animals:** This subheading should cover the type of animal species and breeds to be maintained in the farm. Further the source of purchase as well as the individual animal cost should also be provided

f) **Production parameters:** The information about production parameters like order of lactation, milk yield, lactation days, dry days, conception rate, mortality percentage in young and adult stock is given in this subheading

g) **Herd projection :** based on all assumptions

h) **Feeding:** This would include information on the source of feed and fodder such as dry fodder, green fodder, concentrates, type of crop rotations followed e.g. Rabi and Kharif. Also requirement and costs including fodder cultivation costs is also given.

Quantity required (kg./day)

	Cost(Rs. / Kg)	Lactating animal	Dry animal	Young Stock
Green Fodder				
Dry Fodder				
Concentrates				

Details about breeding facility (AI, Natural Service), Veterinary aid, electric supply, water, and marketing facility also need to be mentioned.

3. Financial Aspects

i) Project Cost

Sr. No.	Item	Physical Unit and Specification	Cost (Rs.)
	Capital Costs		

	Total Capital Costs(A)		
	Recurring Costs		

	Total Recurring Costs (B)		
	Total Project Cost (A+B)		

ii) Down payment/margin/subsidy (Indicate source & extent of subsidy):

iii) Financial viability (comments on the cash flow projection on a farm model/ unit and enclose the same.)

Particulars

a) Internal Rate of Return (IRR)

b) Benefit Cost Ratio (BCR)

c) Net Present Worth (NPW)

a. Techniques for Economic Analysis: Break-Even Analysis

Break-even analysis determines the level at which the gains and losses are equal. This level of values and quantities is known as the break-even point. Generally, break-even analysis is done by manipulating the most uncertain key factor.

E.g. Determination of timing for culling of dairy cows

The dairy farmer is interested to know at what age the maintenance cost of the cow will be equal to the value of milk from the cow. Break-even point indicates the time at which a farmer should sell the cow. At break-even point, benefits = costs, above break-even point, benefits > costs and below break-even point benefits < costs.

Break-even price: It is the price at which the farm's given level of output, if sold would equable the farmer to at least recover costs.

Break-even output: It is level of production that would enable the farmer to recover costs if the products were sold at the given or prevailing price.

Importance of Break-even analysis

- It is used as a measure of risk
- It yields the minimum or maximum value of the critical factor at which a new technology is expected to become or stop being beneficial to the farmer

Advantages

1. Instead of calculating a fixed value, the result of a budget analysis can be assured in terms of probabilities.
2. If the break-even value is very high or very low, conclusions can be made about the profitability of the change with a high degree of confidence.

BEP: The **break-even point** in economics is the point at which cost or expenses and income are equal – there is no net loss or gain, one has "broken even"

The point at which a firm or other economic entity breaks even is equal to its fixed costs divided by its contribution to profit per unit of output, which can be shown by the following formula:-

$$\textbf{Break-even point} = \frac{\text{Fixed costs}}{\text{Contribution per unit output}}$$

The break-even point is also the point on a chart indicating the time when something has broken even, and is a general term for not having gained or lost something in a process.

The contribution per unit can be worked out using

Contribution = Price per unit - Variables costs per unit

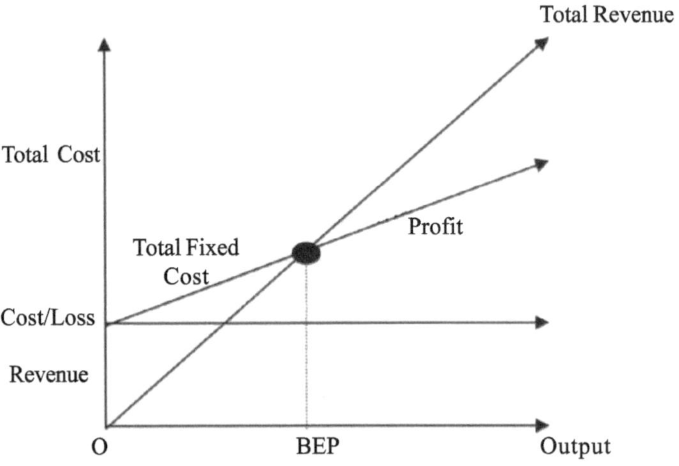

Graphical representation

In any business, there is a point where total costs become equal to total revenues and that point is called as Break Even point and the corresponding output is known as Break Even output (BEO). This means that at this point, the business is making neither profit nor loss. Break-even point is the minimum point of average total cost. A farmer must produce at least this amount of product or out put to cover the total cost of production. Whatever is produced above this point will be the profit for the farmer. The point where the farmer recoups his investment is the Break even point. The investment is in the form of fixed cost and variable cost which constitutes the total cost. When the total cost is equal to total revenue it is Break even point.

$$\textbf{Break Even Quantity} = \frac{\text{Total Fixed Cost}}{\text{(Selling price/unit of output)} - \text{(Variable cost/unit of output)}}$$

$$\text{Break Even Price} = \frac{\text{Total Fixed Cost}}{1 - \left\{\dfrac{\text{Variable cost/unit of output}}{\text{Selling price/unit of output}}\right\}}$$

Margin of safety

The margin of safety of a farmer is the difference between its normal capacity and break even output. Margin of safety indicates the shock absorbing capacity of the farmer in terms of risk and uncertainty. In other words it reflects the financial strength of the enterprise.

Margin of safety = Normal capacity – Break even output

Margin of safety in monetary terms = Revenue of the total output - Revenues from Break even output

Percentage of margin of safety

In physical terms = {Break even output/Normal capacity} × 100

In monetary terms = (Revenues from break even output/Revenues of the total output } × 100

Further, the break even analysis is also useful to know the output to be produced to make fixed amount of profits in the business.

Q_t = TFC + Profit/P-V

b. Project Feasibility Report

(Investment Analysis/ Capital Budgeting/Project Appraisal)

Generally in agricultural or livestock development projects, the investments are made during different time periods and the associated benefits are also spread overtime. These investments and returns are not comparable as such without adjusting for their time value. Thus the time value of money has to be necessarily taken into reckoning in the investment analysis of agricultural projects.

The project appraisal techniques are broadly classified under two heads namely:

1. Undiscounted Measures
2. Discounted Measures

1. Undiscounted Measures

They are the simple methods of ranking the projects. The three important undiscounted measures are

a. Payback period

b. Proceeds per rupee of outlay

c. Average annual proceeds of rupee outlay

a. Payback Period

Pay back period is a simple technique of ranking projects based on the actual period of time in which one can get back total investment.

$$P = \frac{I}{E}$$

Where, P is the payback period

I is the total investment made in the project and

E is the net cash revenues / net revenues per annum.

b. Proceeds per rupee of outlay

This is measured by dividing the total proceeds by the total investment. The projects are ranked by the highest magnitude of the parameter.

$$\text{Proceeds per rupee of outlay} = \frac{\text{Total Proceeds}}{\text{Total investment}}$$

c. Average annual proceeds of rupee outlay

This is another method of evaluating the projects. The average annual proceeds of rupee outlay is calculated by the following formula

$$\text{Average annual proceeds of rupee} = \frac{\text{Total proceeds / life span of project}}{\text{Total investment}}$$

The projects are estimated by the magnitude of the Average annual proceeds of rupee.

The major drawback of the undiscounted measures is that for the same data of the project, we will get different rankings. Thus undiscounted measures are inconsistent and incompatible in ranking.

2. Discounted Measures

Here the cash flows, which are accrued in the project, are discounted with an appropriate discount rate. Generally the existing interest rate is taken as discount rate for this purpose. The discount rate cash flows are the best estimates to measure the worth of the projects. The three important discount rate measures are

a. Net Present Worth (NPW)

b. Benefit Cost Ratio (BCR)

c. Internal rate of Returns (IRR)

a. Net Present Worth

The Net Present Worth also called as Net Present Value (NPV) is the present value/worth of the cash flow stream in the project. The cash flow in the project is the difference between cash inflow and cash outflow. The investments made in the projects are generally called costs or cash outflows. The receipts that accrued during different time periods are called as cash inflows or gross returns. The cash flows discounted with an appropriate discount rate will give the net present worth of the project.

NPW can be calculated by using the formula:

$$NPW = \sum_{t=1}^{n} B_t / (1+r)^t - \sum_{t=1}^{n} C_t / (1+r)^t$$

Bt is cash flows in t^{th} year, C_t is cash outflows in t^{th} year, t is 1 to 10 years that is life span of the project and r is the rate of interest.

The choice criterion using NPW is that the project with positive NPW is accepted for implementation and the project with negative NPW is rejected. If the NPW is zero, the entrepreneur is left in indifference. If he is to choose among different projects, the project with highest NPW has to be chosen.

b. Benefit Cost Ratio (BCR)

BCR is worked out by dividing the present value of cash inflows by the present value of cash outflows. If the BCR of a project is more than one, then that project is accepted and if BCR is less than one the project is rejected. Among the different projects, the project with highest BCR is to be selected. The BCR is calculated by

$$BCR = \sum_{t=1}^{n} \frac{B_t/(1+r)^t}{C_t/(1+r)^t}$$

c. Internal Rate of Returns (IRR)

It is the rate of return per rupee invested in a project over its life span. For example, if the IRR is 30 per cent in a livestock project, it means that this project gives an average annual return of Rs. 30 per Rs. 100 invested in the project over its life span. It is the rate of return at which the present value of total cash flows in a project is equal to zero. In other words, it is the discount rate, at which the NPW of the project is zero.

IRR could be calculated at by using the formula:

$$IRR = \sum_{t=1}^{n} B_t / (1+r)^t - \sum_{t=1}^{n} C_t / (1+r)^t = 0$$

For a project to be viable it should have a

- BCR of one or greater than one at the opportunity cost of capital
- NPW of zero or greater than zero at the opportunity cost of capital and
- IRR should be greater than the opportunity cost of capital

The NPW is inversely related to the discount rate. Higher the NPW lower the discount rate and lower the NPW higher the discount rate and vice versa.

5

Dairy Entrepreneurship Training and Development Programmes

Introduction

Demand of dairy products is on the rise in India. India's demand forecast for milk and milk products is more than the current supply of these products. To meet this demand entrepreneurship initiatives are need of the hour. Further, younger generations of India are more interested in commercial dairy farming rather than subsistence based farming. Therefore, scientific as well as commercial dairy entrepreneurial training to farmers about advanced technology used in breeding, feeding, housing and healthcare is essential.

a. Barriers for Entrepreneurship in dairy

An average dairy entrepreneur faces several barriers to start a new enterprise. Some of them are as under

1. ***Lack of financial support:*** A major stumbling block for many dairy farmers to expand production or diversify into new high value enterprises is lack of access to finance. Farmers who are starting new enterprises often face difficulty raising investment capital.

2. ***Lack of training facilities:*** To have a healthy dairy farming sector, training facilities and support must be easily available to the upcoming dairy entrepreneurs. Effective institutions need to be developed to provide education and training at the right time, in the right place, and with the right balance of technical knowledge and practical skills.

3. ***Lack of support services and trained extension staff:*** Dairy farmers advancing through the different stages of entrepreneurship will need information, advice and support. Extension services are needed to advice and support farmers in identifying, preparing, designing and implementing efficient dairy farm businesses. Advice and support to dairy farmers must cover areas beyond the traditional production-led services. The support needs of farmers are much wider covering all aspects of running a profitable, market oriented dairy farm business.

4. ***Marketing constraints:*** When running a dairy farm business, production must always be linked to a market. Access to markets is often constrained by a number of factors. These include poor communications, infrastructure and marketing facilities, lack of reliable and timely market information, limited purchasing power and even negative attitudes of buyers.
5. ***Social barriers:*** There are also social barriers to entrepreneurship that farmers faces. The concept of entrepreneurship is not common to every culture or society. The fear of failure can be a barrier. Creativity and innovation are not always valued traits. Some countries have social systems that create dependence and hopelessness. Women in business are often not supported or are even discouraged. In some cultures community enterprises may be more acceptable than individual businesses.

b. Entrepreneurship Skills

Capacity building of entrepreneurs involves a combination of efforts including education, training, information dissemination and extension. Entrepreneurial training in animal husbandry can aim to improve following skills of a prospective dairy entrepreneur:

A. Professional skills

a. Animal production skills (more important if the entrepreneur does not have any previous experience)

b. Technical skills: ability to know and handle new technology applicable to his enterprise (e.g. Milking machine, AMCU (Automatic Milk Collection Unit), Green fodder cultivation through hydroponic system, use of RFID tag, newer dairy equipments, ICT tools, software for dairy herd management etc)

B. Management skills

a. Financial management and administration skills

b. Human resource management skills

c. Customer management skills: Market and customer orientation

d. General planning skills

e. Recognising business opportunities

f. Awareness of threats

g. Innovation skills

h. Risk management skills

C. Strategic skills

a. Skills in receiving and making use of feedback

b. Reflection skills

c. Monitoring and evaluation skills

d. Strategic management (Planning, decision making) skills

e. Goal setting skills

D. Cooperation / networking skills

a. Skills in cooperating with other farmers and companies

b. Networking skills

c. Team Working

6

Prevailing Support System for Dairy Entrepreneurship

1. Technical support
2. Financial support

1. Technical support

A. Institutes for Professional skills in dairy based enterprises:

Several institutions offer training programmes in dairy based enterprises:

I. Society for Innovation & Entrepreneurship in Dairying (SINED)

Society for Innovation & Entrepreneurship in Dairying (SINED) is registered under society regulation act 1860, hosted by National Dairy Research Institute, Karnal for promotion of entrepreneurship in dairying. The major activity of the society is to administer a Technology Business Incubator which provides support for technology based entrepreneurship in Dairying.

Objectives

- To promote National development through creation and development of technology driven new enterprises and generation of highly skilled employment.
- To create awareness on self employment and entrepreneurship in unemployed graduates and graduating students.
- To assists the potential entrepreneurs to identify and evaluate the technology and know-how.
- To conduct research and develop educational material on topics related to innovations and their evolution into viable enterprises
- To disseminate research findings and related information on the management of innovation, incubation and entrepreneurship.

- To deploy new tools of technology transfer for speedy commercialization of R&D outputs.
- To help the entrepreneur to conduct their feasibility study, project appraisal, market research and economic study.
- To help the existing units and entrepreneurs by training their employees to improve their technical, financial, marketing and management skills.

Technology Business Incubator

TBI is an entity generated to create successful, viable and free standing business within a certain time frame. The TBI has the broad objective of promoting knowledge-based and innovation-driven dairy enterprises in the country. It facilitates an atmosphere congenial for their survival and growth. It provides all the necessary support and facilities required for a budding entrepreneur like infrastructure support, technology/prototype development support, research assistance, help in getting funding, business consulting assistance, marketing assistance and any other consultation required to set up an enterprise

Globally, the concept of Technology Incubation has proven to reduce the failure rate of new start up companies. In doing so, they create employment and assist local and regional economic development. TBI is designed to support and nurture industries in the area of Dairy and Food Processing, Feed Technology, Dairy Farming, Fish farming, Apiculture & Honey Processing, Biofertilizers, Biopesticides & Panchgavya products based on dung and urine. TBI is located in National Dairy Research Institute (NDRI), a source of technology and knowledge. Locating TBI in country's premier Dairy Research Institute reduces the time lag between technology development and its commercialization.

Vision

To provide a holistic enabling environment to potential entrepreneurs and graduating students so as to translate knowledge and innovation into creation of successful entrepreneurs.

Mission

To create an ecosystem that will foster the entrepreneurial spirit among youth through consultancy, research, training, promotion and incubation in high-tech technologies or ideas thereby promoting innovation and knowledge-based entrepreneurship in dairying leading to the self employment, creation of wealth and social values.

Incubation Programme

Technology Business Incubator (TBI) at National Dairy Research Institute Campus, Karnal provides incubation support to innovative projects. The TBI provides budding entrepreneurs all necessary infrastructure support, technology/ prototype development support, research assistance, marketing assistance and do whatever is necessary to make up a success.

The TBI is designed to support and nurture industries in the following areas

- Commercial Dairy Processing
- Commercial Dairy Farming
- Commercial Food Processing
- Commercial Feed Technology

Incubation Process

SINED-TBI is designed to provide a launch pad to budding entrepreneurs who wish to launch themselves into the world of technology based business careers. The incubator is designed to provide entrepreneurs all the support to make technology based business ventures successful. An entrepreneur makes fewer mistakes when he operates in highly innovative and supportive environment of TBI.

Membership Criteria

A panel of eminent technocrats consisting of experienced and qualified professionals from dairy industry, leading bankers, seasoned venture capitalists and academicians of repute will process the applications of potential entrepreneurs for membership in TBI. The panel will select the ventures for incubation after carefully evaluating the business idea, capability for business viability & growth prospects, market availability, potential value of the technology, innovative content and promoter team. The expert committee will assess this through personal interview, review of past activities, background check, references etc

Who are covered?

Any innovative Indian- a student, dairy/food technologist, engineer, scientist, retired scientist, unemployed youth/housewife, etc., can be member of the TBI. The individual must have an innovative idea/project, which has the potential of commercial utility and/or societal absorption. The TBI is conducting counseling sessions every Saturday for the young innovators.

How to Join

One can join the TBI if you have a viable project idea having high technology content covered under thrust areas which requires incubation facilities. The Application form to become a member of TBI and Format to submit business plan can be obtained from TBI office or downloaded from the site. (www.**ndri**.res.in/**ndri**/De**sign**/**TBI**.html) (http://www.ndritbi.com/)

Pre-Incubation Programme

Entrepreneurship Awareness Camps

SINED-TBI conducts Entrepreneurship Awareness Camps for the benefit of students every year. Experienced entrepreneurs, industry experts, officials from various agencies like banks, district industry centre and venture funding companies interact with our students and provide them with valuable inputs. Such programs are held to identify potential candidates for incubation.

Entrepreneurship Development Programmes (EDP)

Educating and training people for developing entrepreneurial capabilities through positive training interventions is the core strategy of SINED-TBI. It acts as facilitator and resource institution to motivate, guide and help prospective and existing entrepreneurs in their entrepreneurial endeavors/efforts through positive training interventions. Entrepreneurship Development Programmes (EDPs) are well formulated and suitably structured programmes conducted with the aim of new enterprise creation.

Programme provides details on institutional linkages and assistance, business opportunities, achievement motivation, technical orientation, factory visits, market survey, project report preparation, marketing management aspects, financial aspects, Factory Acts and Labour Laws, etc.

Entrepreneurship Development Programme (EDP) conducted by SINED-TBI at NDRI, Karnal

i) Entrepreneurship Development Programme on Commercial dairy Farming

ii) Entrepreneurship Development Programme on Clean Milk Production

iii) Entrepreneurship Development Programme on Milk and Milk Products Processing

Technology Entrepreneurship Training

Any student of NDRI, who considers himself as a true high-potential entrepreneur, want to access rapidly to leadership positions without wasting personal and professional assets, want to launch his own venture or begin a new professional career as a corporate entrepreneur, have an idea or product in mind, or look for an Idea or an opportunity, here is a unique opportunity to shape his dreams! He will spend 4 hours per week over a period of 2 years working very hard to acquire the skills and behavior that can enable him to make his project happen by the time he finishes his studies. This unique learning experience can transform both personal and professional lives of a student.

The programme is centered upon

Competencies specific to entrepreneurial actions: communication, negotiation, Opportunity Identification, Marketing Accounting, Finance, Environmental Scanning- documents and procedures (business plan and techniques for project evaluation), project management etc.

My Idea Programme

SINED-TBI organizes "My Idea Programme" to promote a sustainable culture of innovation and entrepreneurship among student community. In this programme, idea contests are organized and selected students are recognized with certificates and cash prizes.

Incubation of start-up ventures

SINED-TBI assists potential and qualifying ventures / incubatees by supporting them in ***Different Stages of Business Development.*** The role of SINED-TBI will depend on the individual cases, their strengths, weaknesses and extent of support required by the tenet incubatees. SINED-TBI can only assist the venture promoters through various stages of development, but can never replace entrepreneurship demanded from the promoters for business. Hence, the entrepreneurship of the promoters plays a very important role in success of these ventures. To encourage entrepreneurship, SINED-TBI will train the potential entrepreneurs and guide them through the process of business venturing through interactive workshops and constant nurturing. Broadly all the business activities can be summed up in following four stages:

- Ideation / Innovation stage
- Incubation Stage
- Implementation Stage
- Take off stage

Services at Different Stages

SINED-TBI will offer services to venture start-ups during the following stages of development:

A. Ideation / Innovation stage

- Concept development / Opportunity spotting
- Market assessment / Competition analysis
- First level Business Planning / Business Modeling
- Founding Team formation
- Intellectual property safe guarding
- Seed Funding

B. Incubation Stage

- Counseling
- Mentoring
- Advisory board
- Proof of Concept/ Prototyping
- Financing
- Test marketing
- Full scale business planning

C. Implementation Stage

- Pitching for Venture Funding
- Scaling up operations
- Large scale commercialization
- Mature Team Formation

D. Take off stage

- Going National
- Initial Public Offering
- Exit provisioning for Venture Capitalists
- Full scale business Graduation

Preparation of Business Plan

TBI will extend all assistance helping the entrepreneurs build their business plans using the panel of mentors and consultants.

Mentoring

SINED-TBI has a panel of mentors and consultants who assist the entrepreneurs admitted to TBI. Following are the areas where SINED-TBI has mentors and consultants available to assist the entrepreneurs:

- Mentors
- Angel investors
- Venture capitalists
- Finance consultants
- Accounting & audit services
- Academic activities
- Technical consultants
- Quality consultants
- Management consultants
- Marketing assistance
- Legal assistance
- HR consultants
- Training consultants
- Media Consultants

Financing

A nominal license fee is charged each month based on the module occupied. Additional costs include charges you incur for usage of special equipment, telephone, internet, postage, etc. Charges are collected using a monthly billing cycle. Incubatees will be provided with the opportunity to get financial assistance from the Department of Science & Technology (DST), Department of Scientific & Industrial Research (DSIR), Technology Information Forecasting and Assessment Council (TIFAC), Ministry of Food Processing Industries & other related services as and when needed.

Introduction to Banks / Venture Capitalists

SINED-TBI has entered into partnership with various venture capitalists. All these institutions will be empanelled by TBI to support the entrepreneurs. The TBI is helping the incubatees in finding seed capital and working capital assistance from venture capitalists.

i. **State Agricultural Universities**: SAU's through its directorate of extension education and KVK (Krishi Vigyan Kendras) organize several training programmes to farmers, dairy owners, rural youth for skill development in agriculture including dairy farming.

ii. **State animal husbandry department** also have mandate for capacity building programmes for dairy owners.

iv. **Indira Gandhi National Open University** (IGNOU): Indira Gandhi National Open University IGNOU offers several diploma programmes on training in dairy entrepreneurship for farmers and rural youth. Some of these programmes are

   i. Diploma in Dairy Technology

   ii. Training skills in Dairy entrepreneurship

   iii. Awareness Programme on Dairy Farming for Rural Farmers (APDF)

v. **National Social Entrepreneurship Forum (NSEF)** is a non-profit organization supporting youth-driven social innovations & entrepreneurship in India. (http://nsef-india.org). National Social Entrepreneurship Forum was founded by Yashveer Singh and Srikumar in 2009 at Bangalore. Since its inception, NSEF has undertaken social entrepreneurial activities in several academic institutes and cities across India and has worked in collaboration with various organizations such as Villgro, Samhita Social Ventures, NASSCOM Social Innovation Honours, Ashoka Innovators for the Public, and Sankalp Forum to enable youth-driven social innovations and young social entrepreneurs. NSEF has trained thousands of students through its programs across India.

Programs

- NSEF Idea Conferences - A platform to educate students about social innovations and to provide them with a launch pad for their social entrepreneurial ideas.
- NSEF Authors of Change Program - A solutions delivery program for key challenges that social organizations are facing, by connecting them to student talent from across the country through internships.

- NSEF Fellowship - A support program for students who start social ventures after completing college, to connect them with the resources and network they would need to grow their ventures.

vi. **Skill India** is an initiative of the Government of India. It was launched by Prime Minister Narendra Modi on 16 July 2015 with an aim to train over 40 crore people in India in different skills by 2022. The initiatives include National Skill Development Mission, National Policy for Skill Development and Entrepreneurship 2015, Pradhan Mantri Kaushal Vikas Yojana (PMKVY) scheme and the Skill Loan scheme.

B. Institutes for Management and Strategic Skills

Several institutes help to build management and strategic skills required by a budding entrepreneur. Some of them are

National Level Training Institutes

- National Institute of Micro, Small and Medium Industry Extension Training(NIMSMIET), Hyderabad
- National Institute for Entrepreneurship and Small Business Development (NIESBUD), at NOIDA, which conducts national and international level training programmes in different fields and disciplines.
- Indian Institute of Entrepreneurship (IIE), Guwahati. The main objective of the institute is to act as a catalyst for entrepreneurship development with its focus on the North East.

Other Associated Agencies

- National Small Industries Corporation (NSIC) for technology and marketing support
- Small Industries Development Bank of India (SIDBI) an apex bank set up to provide direct/indirect financial assistance under different schemes to meet credit needs of the small-scale sector and to coordinate the functions of other institutions in similar activities.
- Khadi and Village Industries Commission (KVIC) assist the development and promotion and disbursal of rural and traditional industries in rural and town areas.

State Level Institutional Support

- State Government executes different promotional and developmental projects/schemes and provides a number of supporting incentives for development and promotion of MSME sector in their respective States.

- These are executed through State Directorate of Industries, who has District Industries Centers (DICs) under them to implement Central/State Level schemes.
- The State Industrial Development & Financial Institutions and State Financial Corporations also look after the needs of the MSME sector.

Let us discuss few of them in detail

1. National Small Industries Corporation Limited (NSIC) 1955 provides for technology and marketing support to entrepreneurs.

i. NSIC directly markets the Micro, Small & Medium Enterprises (MSME) product in the national and international market.

ii. It manages single point registration scheme for manufacturers for government purchases. Enterprises registered under this scheme obtain the benefit of free tender documents and exemption from earnest money deposit and performance guarantee.

2. National Institute for Entrepreneurship and Small Business Development (NIESBUD), NOIDA (nisebud.nic.in)

It is an apex organization established by Ministry of Industries, Govt. of India. This body organizes national as well as international training programmes in Entrepreneurship Development in different fields such as computer courses, beauty, Bakery Product, fashion designing as well as dairy entrepreneurship courses.

3. Entrepreneurship Development Institute of India, Ahmedabad

The Entrepreneurship Development Institute of India (EDI), an autonomous and not-for-profit institute, set up in 1983, is sponsored by the IDBI Bank Ltd., IFCI Ltd., ICICI Bank Ltd. and State Bank of India (SBI).

It offers a two-year, full-time, residential programme Post Graduate Diploma in Management - Business Entrepreneurship (PGDM-BE) that has been designed for entrepreneurs and entrepreneurial managers.

4. National Institute of Micro, Small and Medium Enterprises (NIMSME), Hyderabad

It focuses on entrepreneur skills for Food Processing, agro and Food Enterprises, Promotion of Micro Enterprises, Empowerment of Women through Enterprises.

5. National Institute of Rural Development, Hyderabad

It offers entrepreneurship programmes on middle and senior level managers and officers in following areas.

a. Microfinance for poverty alleviation

b. Participatory rural development

c. Management of rural drinking water and sanitation projects

d. Natural resources management for sustainable rural livelihood

e. Geo informatics applications in rural development

f. Strategies for sustainable agriculture and rural development

g. Planning for poverty reduction and sustainable development

h. Information Technology for rural development

6. Micro, Small and Medium Enterprises – Development Organisation (MSME-DO)

[earlier known as Small industries Development Organisation (SIDO)

- SIDO was established in 1954 on the basis of the recommendations of the Ford Foundation. Over the years, it has seen its role evolve into an agency for advocacy, hand holding and facilitation for the small industries sector.
- It has over 60 offices and 21 autonomous bodies under its management. These autonomous bodies include Tool Rooms, Training Institutions and Project-cum-Process Development Centres. SIDO provides a wide spectrum of services to the small industries sector.
- These include facilities for testing, training for entrepreneurship development, preparation of project and product profiles, technical and managerial consultancy, assistance for exports, pollution and energy audits, etc.

7. National Institute For Small Industry Extension Training (NISIET)

- The NISIET, since its inception in 1960 by the Government of India, has taken gigantic strides to become the premier institution for the promotion, development and modernization of the SME (Small and Medium Scale Enterprises) sector.
- An autonomous arm of the Ministry of Small Scale Industries (SSI), the Institute strives to achieve its avowed objectives through a gamut of

operations ranging from training, consultancy, research and education, to extension and information services.

8. MANAGE (National Institute of Agriculture Extension Management) Hyderabad

Manage through its Agri-clinics and Agri-business centres (ACABC) scheme – 2010 offers two month training programme for Graduates in veterinary and animal sciences and allied subjects from SAUs/ Central Agricultural Universities/ Universities recognized by ICAR/ UGC Nodal Training Institutes (NTIs) and motivating them for setting up of Agri-Clinics and Agri-Business Centres.

Entrepreneurship training and support to veterinarians

The veterinarians willing to start self employment ventures in veterinary, dairy, fisheries, poultry, allied enterprises can begin their venture through support under Agri-clinics and Agri-business centres (ACABC) scheme 2010).Under this scheme credit support as well as basic two months training is given to prospective veterinarian entrepreneur.

Credit support

Credit support upto 20 lakh for an individual and up to 100 lakh for a group project is provided. Further, In case of loans up to 5 lakh, no margin money is required as per present norms. Back ended Composite Subsidy" upto 44% of project cost for women, SC/ST & all categories of candidates from NE and Hill states and 36% of project cost for all other candidates have been given. Thus, bank do not charge interest on the subsidy component of the loan.

Training

The selected potential entrepreneurs also have to undergo two month training programme in veterinary and animal sciences and allied subjects from SAUs/ Central Agricultural Universities/ Universities recognized by ICAR/ UGC Nodal Training Institutes (NTIs) and motivating them for setting up of Agri-Clinics and Agri-Business Centres. The notable feature of scheme is that there is no age bar for enrolling in training programme. Many young veterinary graduates, retired veterinarians have benefitted from the scheme and have started successful dairy and agri based enterprises.

Entrepreneurship training and support to farmers

Government support is needed for entrepreneurship training and development programmes. Realizing this, Government of India has started dairy entrepreneurship development programmes which have been described as under:

1. Dairy entrepreneurship development scheme
2. "Salvaging and Rearing of Male Buffalo Calves

b) Financial support

1. Bank support for Dairy Entrepreneurship in India

Setting up dairy enterprise be it a small dairy unit, goat unit, milk and meat processing plant, selling parlor requires capital. Lack of access to credit to expand the herd is a critical problem for farmers. There is little access to formal credit through the cooperatives or banks. Informal credit is available from private traders and agents of private companies, but the interest rate is very high. Keeping this situation in mind and to provide financial support from banks few major dairy entrepreneurship schemes have been developed and implemented by banks with the support of state animal husbandry departments across different parts of the country. National Bank on agriculture and Rural Development (NABARD) is the lead bank for financial support of such schemes.

2. Dairy entrepreneurship development scheme

Dairy Entrepreneurship Development Scheme (DEDS) was started in September, 2010 with the objective for promotion of private investment in dairy sector in order to increase the milk production in the country and helping in poverty reduction through self employment opportunities. This scheme is being implemented through NABARD which provides financial assistance to commercially bankable projects with loan from Commercial, Cooperative, Urban and Rural banks with a back ended capital subsidy of 25% of the project cost to the beneficiaries of general category and 33.33% of the project cost to SC & ST beneficiaries. The scheme has approved for continuation with certain modifications and the budget provision of Rs 1,400 crore during 12th five year plan. Since inception, against the total release of Rs 871.29 crore, NABARD has disbursed Rs 823.14 crore as back ended capital subsidy to the beneficiaries for setting up of 2,24,402 dairy units upto 31st December, 2014.

Under these scheme farmers, individual entrepreneurs, NGOs, companies, groups of unorganized and organized sector including self help groups, dairy cooperative societies, milk unions and milk federations are eligible for financial assistance from banks to set up following type of dairy based enterprise:

---

1. Establishment of small dairy units with crossbred cows/ indigenous descript milch cows like Sahiwal, Red Sindhi, Gir, Rathi etc / graded buffaloes upto 10 animals.

Bank supports cheap credit upto Rs 6.00 lakh (earlier Rs 5 lakh) for 10 animal units.

2. Rearing of heifer calves – cross bred, indigenous descript milch breeds of cattle and of graded buffaloes – upto 20 calves. Bank supports cheap credit upto Rs 5.30 lakh (earlier Rs 4.80 lakh) for 20 calf units
3. Vermicompost with milch animal unit (to be considered with milch animals and not separately), bank supports cheap credit up to Rs 22,000/- (earlier Rs 20,000/-)
4. Purchase of milking machines /milkotesters/bulk milk cooling units (upto 5000 lit capacity, earlier 2000 lit capacity), bank supports cheap credit upto Rs 22 lakh
5. Purchase of dairy processing equipment for manufacture of indigenous milk products, bank supports cheap credit upto Rs 13.20 lakhs.
6. Establishment of dairy product transportation facilities and cold chain, bank supports cheap credit upto Rs 26.50 lakh (earlier Rs 24 lakh)
7. Cold storage facilities for milk and milk products, bank supports cheap credit upto Rs 33 lakh (earlier Rs 30 lakh)
8. Establishment of private veterinary clinic, bank supports cheap credit upto Rs 2.60 lakh (earlier Rs 2.40 lakh) for mobile clinic and Rs 2 lakh (earlier Rs 1.80 lakh) for stationary clinic
9. Dairy marketing outlet / Dairy parlour, bank supports cheap credit upto Rs 1 lakh (earlier Rs 56,000/-)

Funding pattern

1. Entrepreneur contribution (margin) - 10 % of the outlay (minimum)
2. Back ended capital subsidy of 25 %(33.33 % for SC/ST beneficiaries of the project cost.

Banking Requirements for the Scheme:

Procedure for Sanction of project and availing subsidy through banks

Step 1: Beneficiary should apply to the bank for sanction of the project

Step 2: The bank shall approve the project of the eligible as per their norms and sanction the total outlay excluding the margin, as the bank loan.

Step 3: The loan amount is disbursed in suitable installments depending on the progress of the unit.

Dairy Entrepreneurship Development Scheme (DEDS)

S. No	Component	Unit Cost	Pattern of Assistance
i.	Establishment of **small dairy units** with crossbred cows/ indigenous descript milch cows like Sahiwal, Red Sindhi, Gir, Rathi etc / graded buffaloes upto 10 animals, (for SHGs, Cooperatives societies, Producer Companies unit size will be 2-10 animals per member)	Rs. 6.00 lakh for 10 animal unit-minimum unit size is 2 animals with a n upper limit of 10 animals	25% of the project cost (33.33% for SC/ST farmers), as back ended capital subsidy. Subsidy shall be restricted on prorata basis to a maximum of 10 animals subject to a ceiling of Rs. 15,000 per animal, (Rs 20,000 for SC/ST farmers) or actual whichever is lower.Beneficiaries may purchase animals of higher costs, however, the subsidy will be restricted to the above ceilings
ii.	Rearing of **heifer calves** – cross bred, indigenous descript milch breeds of cattle and graded buffaloes – upto 20 calves	Rs. 5.30 lakh for 20 calf unit with an upper limit of 20 calves	25 % of the project cost (33.33 % for SC/ST farmers) as back ended capital subsidy. Subsidy shall be restricted on prorata basis to a maximum of 20 calf unit subject to a ceiling of Rs 6,600/- per calf (Rs 8, 800 for SC/ST farmers) or actual, whichever is lower.
iii.	**Vermicompost** with milch animal unit (to be considered with milch animals/ small dairy farm and not separately)	Rs. 22,000	25% of the project cost (33.33 % for SC /ST farmers) as back ended capital subsidy subject to a ceiling of Rs. 5,500/- (Rs7300/- for SC/ST farmers) or actual whichever is lower.
iv.	Purchase of **milking machines / milkotesters / bulk milk cooling units** (upto 5000 lit capacity)	Rs. 20 lakh	25% of the project cost (33.33 SC/ST farmers) as back ended capital subsidy subject to a ceiling of Rs 5.0 lakh (Rs.6.67 lakh for SC / ST farmers) or actual whichever is lower.
v.	Purchase of **dairy processing equipment** for manufacture milk products.	Rs.13.20 lakh	25% of the project cost (33.33 % for SC/ST farmers) as back ended capital subsidy subject to a ceiling of Rs. 3.30 lakh (Rs. 4.40 lakh for SC/ST farmers) or actual whichever is lower.

Contd.

S. No	Component	Unit Cost	Pattern of Assistance
VI.	Establishment of **dairy product transportation facilities** and cold chain	Rs. 26.50 lakh	25% of the project cost (33.33 % for SC/ST farmers) as back ended capital subsidy subject to a ceiling Rs. 6.625 lakh (Rs. 8.830 lakh for SC/ST farmers) or actual whichever is lower.
VII.	**Cold storage facilities** for milk and milk products	Rs 33 lakh	25% of the project cost (33.33% for SC/ST farmers) as back ended capital subsidy subject to a ceiling of Rs. 8.25 lakh (Rs. 11.0 lakh for SC/ST farmers) or actual whichever is lower.
VII	Establishment of **private veterinary clinic**	Rs. 2.60 lakh for mobile clinic and Rs 2.0 lakh for stationary clinic	25% of the project cost (33.33% for SC /ST farmers) as back ended capital subsidy subject to a ceiling of Rs. 65,000/- and Rs. 50.000/- (Rs. 86,600/- and Rs. 66.600/ - for SC/ST farmers) respectively for mobile and stationary clinics or actual whichever is lower.
IX.	Dairy marketing outlet / **Dairy parlour**	Rs.1.0 lakh/-	25% of the project cost (33.33 % for SC /ST farmers) or actual whichever is lower.

Step 4: The bank shall apply to the concerned Regional Office of NABARD for sanction and release of subsidy in the specified format, after the disbursement of first installment of loan.

Time limit for Completion of the project

It is maximum of 9 months from the date of disbursement of the first installment of loan which may be extended by a further period of 3 months, if reasons for delay are considered justified by the concerned financial institution

3. State level Entrepreneurship Development Institute

i) JKEDI (Jammu and Kashmir Entrepreneurship Development Institute) in J&K

JKEDI was established by Government of J&K to impart entrepreneurial training to the general public in March 1997. It started its regular activities in February 2004 and has positioned itself as a state of the art learning centre. One can connect with JKEDI through internet also. JKEDI run training courses for dairy development for the farmers who have a keen interest in this industry. Likewise other entrepreneurship development schemes are undertaken by different EDIs in different states.

Some tips for starting a dairy farm

First look at various aspects before you leap into the dairy farming trade business

Do's

- Ensure the availability of land at properly raised place and away from residential area (at least 300 m) / water bodies (at least 250 m)
- Build sheds with mud. This will keep them warm.
- Purchase cross bred cows. Choose from Jersey and Holstein Friesian breed because only they thrive in the moderate climate of the Kashmir Valley.
- Cross bred Jersey cow is more preferable because of low green feed requirements and high fat content in milk.
- Select healthy, high yielding cows with the help of veterinary/animal husbandry officer of state government, experts etc.
- Purchase freshly calved cows/in late pregnancy. Age should be 3-4 years or should be in 2nd or 3rd lactation.
- Get the building permission from the local body

Don’ts

- Don’t construct concrete sheds because low temperature will threaten the survival of animal.
- Don’t hire or purchase land without proper legal documentation.
- Don’t construct sheds on marshy or swampy land.
- Don’t purchase cows without expert help.
- Don’t get tempted to purchase pure breed with high milk yield

7

Preparing Projects for Bank Appraisal and Banking Requirements for the Dairy Entrepreneurship Projects

Any farmer/Entrepreneur who wishes to avail bank loan for starting or expanding his dairy enterprise should apply for loan to the nearest branch of a commercial bank, regional rural bank or co-operative bank in their area in the prescribed application form which is available in the branches of financing banks.

Preparing Projects for Bank Appraisal

1. The entrepreneur can prepare the project or Scheme report after consulting local technical persons of State Animal Husbandry Department, DRDA, Dairy Co-operative Society / Union / Federation / commercial dairy farmers.

2. The project report should have mention about practical training and experience in dairy farming. So in order to meet this requirement the inexperienced entrepreneurs can visit progressive dairy farms and government / military / agricultural university dairy farms in the vicinity to have first hand information about the enterprise. Nowadays several online portals (www.aaqaa.com.) also provide useful guidance and information on setting up dairy based enterprise.

3. The report should mention about distance of enterprise to nearest selling facility, support services such as veterinary aid centre, artificial insemination centre/feed unit etc.

4. The scheme should include information on land, dairy markets, availability of water, feeds, fodder, veterinary aid, breeding facilities, marketing aspects, training facilities, experience of the farmer and the type of assistance available from State Government, dairy society/union/federation.

5. The scheme should also include information on the number and types of animals to be purchased, their breed, production performance, cost and other relevant input and output costs with their description.

Banking Requirements for the Project

While approving a dairy entrepreneurship projects bank has to look upon the techno economic feasibility of the enterprises under different conditions. The technical analysis examines the possible technical aspects of a proposed dairy project. This involves potential of region for dairy production, water availability which includes both natural (rainfall, and its distribution) and supplied (the possibilities for developing irrigation, with its associated drainage works) form; the type of dairy species and breeds suited to the area; the availability and supply of input related to dairy production; constraints(diseases etc.) prevalent in the area and the kinds of dairy support services (vaccination, veterinary cover). On the basis of these and similar considerations, the technical analysis will determine the potential yields from the dairy, the coefficients of production, and the possibilities for further expansion. The technical analysis will also examine the marketing and storage facilities required for the successful operation of the project, and the processing systems that will be needed.

Scrutiny of Schemes By Banks

The scheme so formulated should be submitted to the nearest branch of a bank. The bank's officers would assist in preparation of the scheme for filling in the prescribed application form. The bank will then examine the scheme for its technical feasibility and economic viability.

8

Technical and Economic Feasibility of Entrepreneurship Project (Dairy Farm)

1. Technical Feasibility of Dairy Unit

This includes following information such as

1. Availability of good quality animals in nearby dairy market,
2. Availability of good grazing grounds and lands,
3. Availability of green/dry fodder,
4. Availability of concentrate feed, medicines etc.
5. Further availability of veterinary aid, dairy breeding (AI) centre, milk collection and marketing centre are also important.
6. Nearness of the selected area to veterinary/breeding/milk collection centre and the financing bank's branch.
7. Capability of the owner and employees such as technical knowledge and skill.

2. Economic Viability of the Project

Under this information about the unit cost of animals, various input and output costs are provided . Input costs involve cost of (feed and fodder, veterinary aid, breeding of animals, insurance, labour and other overheads) whereas output costs involve (sale price of milk, manure, gunny bags, male/female calves, other miscellaneous items etc).Further income expenditure statement, annual gross surplus, cash flow analysis, repayment schedule of loan is prepared to ensure economic viability of the project. Other documents such as loan application forms, security aspects, margin money requirements, etc. are also examined. A field visit to the scheme area is undertaken for conducting a techno-economic feasibility study for appraisal of the scheme. Break Even Point, Investment Analysis (particularly, IRR), Payback period, Marketing process are also considered.

3. Sanction of Bank Loan and its Disbursement

1. After ensuring technical feasibility and economic viability, the scheme is sanctioned by the bank.
2. The items of finance would include capital asset items such as purchase of milch animals, construction of sheds, purchase of equipments etc.
3. The feeding cost during the initial period of one/two months is capitalized and given as term loan.
4. Cost towards land development, fencing, digging of well, commissioning of diesel engine/pumpset, electricity connections, essential servants' quarters, godown, transport vehicle, milk processing facilities etc. can be considered for loan.
5. Cost of land is not considered for loan.
6. The loan is disbursed in kind in 2 to 3 stages against creation of specific assets such as construction of sheds, purchase of equipments and machinery, purchase of animals and recurring cost on purchase of feeds/ fodders for the initial period of one/two months.
7. The end use of the fund is verified and constant follow-up is done by the bank.
8. Margin money depends on the category of the borrowers (marginal/small/ large farmers) and range from 5 to 25%).
9. Repayment period depends upon the gross surplus and cash flow in the scheme. The loan will be repaid in suitable monthly/quarterly installments usually within a period of five to seven years.
10. The animals and capital assets may be insured annually or on long term master policy, where ever it is applicable.
11. After ensuring technical feasibility and economic viability, the scheme is sanctioned by the bank.
12. The loan is disbursed in kind in 2 to 3 stages against creation of specific assets such as construction of sheds, purchase of equipments and machinery, purchase of animals and recurring cost on purchase of feeds/ fodders for the initial period of one/two months.
13. Rate of interest on the loans shall be as per RBI guidelines and declared policy of the bank in this regard. The bank may charge interest on the entire loan amount till the subsidy is received and from the date of receipt of subsidy by the implementing branch, interest has to be charged only on the effective bank loan portion i.e. outlay excluding the margin and subsidy
14. The end use of the fund is verified and constant follow-up is done by the bank.

9

Entrepreneurial Funding

According to a recent study, over 94% of new businesses fail during first year of operation. Lack of funding turns to be one of the common reasons. Money is the bloodline of any business. The long painstaking yet exciting journey from the idea generation to revenue generating business needs a fuel named capital. That's why, at almost every stage of the business, entrepreneurs find themselves asking – *How do I finance my startup?*

Now, when an entrepreneur require funding depends largely on the nature and type of the business. Here is a comprehensive list of funding options for startups that will help the entrepreneur to raise capital for business.

1) Bootstrapping

Self-funding, also known as bootstrapping, is an effective way of startup financing, especially when you are just starting your business. First-time entrepreneurs often have trouble getting funding without first showing some traction and a plan for potential success. You can invest from your own savings or can gct your family and friends to contribute. This will be easy to raise due to less formalities/compliances, plus less costs of raising. In most situations, family and friends are flexible with the interest rate.

Self-funding or bootstrapping should be considered as a first funding option because of its advantages. When you have your own money, you are tied to business. On a later stage, investors consider this as a good point. But this is suitable only if the initial requirement is small. Some businesses need money right from the day-one and for such businesses, bootstrapping may not be a good option.

Bootstrapping is also about stretching resources – both financial and otherwise – as far as they can.

2) Crowdfunding

Crowdfunding is one of the newer ways of funding a startup that has been gaining lot of popularity lately. It's like taking a loan, pre-order, contribution or investments from more than one person at the same time.

This is how crowdfunding works – An entrepreneur will put up a detailed description of his business on a crowdfunding platform. He will mention the goals of his business, plans for making a profit, how much funding he needs and for what reasons, etc. and then consumers can read about the business and give money if they like the idea. Those giving money will make online pledges with the promise of pre-buying the product or giving a donation. Anyone can contribute money toward helping a business that they really believe in.

Why you should consider Crowdfunding as a funding option for your business:

The best thing about crowd funding is that it can also generate interest and hence helps in marketing the product alongside financing. It is also a boon if you are not sue if there will be any demand for the product you are working on. This process can cut out professional investors and brokers by putting funding in the hands of common people. It also might attract venture-capital investment down the line if a company has a particularly successful campaign.

Also keep in mind that crowdfunding is a competitive place to earn funding, so unless your business is absolutely rock solid and can gain the attention of the average consumers through just a description and some images online, you may not find crowdfunding to work for you in the end. Some of the popular crowdfunding sites in India are Indiegogo, Wishberry, Ketto, Fundlined and Catapooolt.

In US, Kickstarter, RocketHub, Dreamfunded, Onevest and GoFundMe are popular crowdfunding platforms.

3) Angel Investment in your startup

Angel investors are individuals with surplus cash and a keen interest to invest in upcoming startups. They also work in groups of networks to collectively screen the proposals before investing. They can also offer mentoring or advice alongside capital.

Angel investors have helped to start up many prominent companies, including Google, Yahoo and Alibaba. This alternative form of investing generally occurs in a company's early stages of growth, with investors expecting upto 30% equity. They prefer to take more risks in investment for higher returns. Angel Investment as a funding option has its shortcomings too. Angel investors invest lesser amounts than venture capitalists.

The popular Angel Investors in India – Indian Angel Network, Mumbai Angels, Hyderabad Angels.

4) Venture Capital

Venture capitals are professionally managed funds who invest in companies that have huge potential. They usually invest in a business against equity and exit when there is an IPO or an acquisition. VCs provide expertise, mentorship and acts as a litmus test of where the organisation is going, evaluating the business from the sustainability and scalability point of view.

A venture capital investment may be appropriate for small businesses that are beyond the startup phase and already generating revenues. Fast-growth companies like Flipkart, Uber, etc with an exit strategy already in place can gain up to tens of millions of dollars that can be used to invest, network and grow their company quickly.

However, there are a few downsides to Venture Capitalists as a funding option. VCs have a short leash when it comes to company loyalty and often look to recover their investment within a three- to five-year time window. If you have a product that is taking longer than that to get to market, then venture-capital investors may not be very interested in you.

They typically look for larger opportunities that are a little bit more stable, companies having a strong team of people and a good traction. You also have to be flexible with your business and sometimes give up a little bit more control, so if you're not interested in too much mentorship or compromise, this might not be your best option.

Some of the well known Venture Capitalists in India are – Nexus Venture Partners, Helion Ventures, Kalaari Capital, Accel Partners, Blume Ventures, Canaan, Sequoia Capital and Bessemer Ventures.

5) Business Incubators & Accelerators

Early stage businesses can consider Incubator and Accelerator programs as a funding option. Found in almost every major city, these programs assist hundreds of startup businesses every year. Though used interchangeably, there are few fundamental differences between the two terms. Incubators are like a parent to a child, who nurture the business providing shelter tools and training and network to a business. Accelerators so more or less the same thing, but an incubator helps/assists/nurtures a business to walk, while accelerator helps to run/take a giant leap.

These programs normally run for 4-8 months and require time commitment from the business owners. You will also be able to make good connections with mentors, investors and other fellow startups using this platform.

In US, companies like Dropbox and Airbnb started with an accelerator – Y Combinator. In India, popular names are Amity Innovation Incubator, Angel Prime, CIIE, IAN Business Incubator, Villgro, Startup Village and TLabs.

Popular business accounting software – Profit Books is also a part of Washington based accelerator Village Capital.

6) Raise Funds By Winning Contests

An increase in the number of contests has tremendously helped to maximize the opportunities for fund raising. It encourages entrepreneurs with business ideas to set up their own businesses. In such competitions, you either have to build a product or prepare a business plan.

Winning these competitions can also get you some media coverage.

You need to make your project stand out in order to improve your success in these contests. You can either present your idea in person or pitch it through a business plan. It should be comprehensive enough to convince anyone that your idea is worth investing in.

Some of the popular startups contests in India are NASSCOM's 10000 startups, Microsoft BizSparks, Conquest, NextBigIdea Contest, and Lets Ignite. Check out the latest startup programs & contests in your area.

7) Raise Money Through Bank Loans

Normally, banks are the first place that entrepreneurs go when thinking about funding.

The bank provides two kinds of financing for businesses. One is working capital loan, and other is funding. Working Capital loan is the loan required to run one complete cycle of revenue generating operations, and the limit is usually decided by hypothecating stocks and debtors. Funding from bank would involve the usual process of sharing the business plan and the valuation details, along with the project report, based on which the loan is sanctioned.

Almost every bank in India offers SME finance through various programs. For instance, leading Indian banks – Bank Of Baroda,HDFC, ICICI and Axis banks have more than 7-8 different options to offer collateral free business loans. Check out the respective bank sites for more details.

In US, sites like Kabbage can help you get working capital loan online in minutes. Unlike traditional lenders, Kabbage approve small business loans by looking at real-life data, not just a credit score.

8) Get Business Loans From Microfinance Providers or NBFCs

What do you do when you can't qualify for a bank loan? There is still an option. Microfinance is basically access of financial services to those who would not have access to conventional banking services. It is increasingly becoming popular for those whose requirements are limited and credit ratings not favoured by bank.

Similarly, NBFCs are Non Banking Financial Corporations are corporations that provide Banking services without meeting legal requirement/definition of a bank.

9) Government Programs that offer Startup Capital

The Government of India has launched 10,000 Crore Startup Fund in Union budget 2014-15 to improve startup ecosystem in India. In order to boost innovative product companies, Government has launched 'Bank Of Ideas and Innovations' program.

Government backed 'Pradhan Mantri Micro Units Development and Refinance Agency Limited (MUDRA)' starts with an initial corpus of Rs. 20,000 crore to extend benefits to around 10 lakhs SMEs. You are supposed to submit your business plan and once approved, the loan gets sanctioned. You get a MUDRA Card, which is like a credit card, which you can use to purchase raw materials, other expenses etc. Shishu, Kishor and Tarun are three categories of loans available under the promising scheme. Learn more about MUDRA.

Also, different states have come up different programs like Kerala State Self Entrepreneur Development Mission (KSSEDM), Maharashtra Centre for Entrepreneurship Development, Rajasthan Startup Fest, etc to encourage small businesses.

SIDBI – Small Industries Development Bank Of India also offer business loans to MSME sector.

In US, there is a small business lending fund and dedicated portal for Government grants available for local businesses.

If you comply with the eligibility criteria, Government grants as a funding option could be one of the best. You just need to make yourself aware of the various Government initiatives.

10) Quick ways to raise Money For Your Business

There are few more ways to raise funds for your business. However, these might not work for everyone. Still, check them out if you need quick funds.

Product Pre-sale: Selling your products before they launch is an often-overlooked and highly effective way to raise the money needed for financing your business. Remember how Apple & Samsung start pre-orders of their products well ahead of the official launch? Its a great way to improve cashflow and prepare yourself for the consumer demand.

Selling Assets: This might sound like a tough step to take but it can help you meet your short term fund requirements. Once you overcome the crisis situation, you can again buy back the assets.

Credit Cards: Business credit cards are among the most readily available ways to finance a startup and can be a quick way to get instant money. If you are a new business and don't have a tons of expenses, you can use a credit card and keep paying the minimum payment. However, keep in mind that the interest rates and costs on the cards can build very quickly, and carrying that debt can be detrimental to a business owner's credit.

10

Preparing Project Report of A Dairy Plant

The Feasibility study of dairy project cover capital investment on land, building, infrastructure, working capital, manufacturing and marketing cost, and financial projections to work out its viability. Once viability is established, a detailed project report should include the following ten steps for project planning and implementation:

First Step: This step involves appointing a consultant to plan the project in relation to the design the dairy plant, proposed market and select an architect and a structural consultant. Prepare tender documents for civil works and plant equipment. Study the demand-supply of target products through a market survey to formulate the suitable product mix in terms of volume and range. e.g. study of various dairy products e.g. Khoa, ghee, Ice cream. The capacity of the plant and the provision of various facilities would be determined by the products demand.

Second Step: After qualifying the product mix work out the process flow diagram showing the material balances. This will also lead to:

a) Assessing the requirement of raw materials, including milk procurement;

b) Formulating specifications for raw materials, required; and,

c) Identifying sources of their supply

Third step: formulate dairy plant specifications. The proposed design should include:

a) Space required (floor area)

b) List of equipments, their specifications and capacities

c) Prepare the plant layout, including process, service and storage

d) Provide for service requirements like refrigeration, boiler, electricity, pressurized (compressed) air, water supply equipment and specification and the effluent treatment facilities.

Fourth Step: prepare for plant construction by attending to the following:

a) Selection of site;

b) Survey the availability of essential services like water, electricity, all-weather road, communication, etc; and

c) Tender for civil works, equipment supply and installation, and the subsequent award of contracts.

Fifth Step: Formulate the marketing plans for design of brand name, logo, packaging and labeling materials. Appointments of core staff, including plant manager, administration and marketing personnel.

Sixth Step: Arrange for sanctions/approvals/clearances by the central/state/ local statutory authorities.

Seventh Step: Coordinate the civil construction work with the suppliers for timely installation of the dairy equipment and machinery.

Eighth Step: Complete the civil construction to the stage when equipment can be installed.

Ninth Step: Select and appoint supervisors and the operating staff. Election, Installation and commissioning of the plant and machinery.

Tenth Step: Place the products in the market through well established market channels.

11

Financial Credit and Financial Management

a. General Principles and practices

b. Analyzing project appraisals and reports

c. Capital Expenditure decisions, reinvestment and payback

d. Assessing project profits.

a. Financing the dairy enterprise

Dairy rearing provides triple benefits of income, employment and nutritional security to the society and is important source of subsidiary income to small/ marginal farmers and agricultural laborers. Finance is a prerequisite and of paramount importance for setting up of a dairy enterprise whether a dairy farming unit for milk production, sheep or goat unit/piggery unit, dairy/poultry processing unit etc. Decisions about credit are often most important judgments that people in the agricultural industry must make. These decisions often determine whether individuals operating in input, production, processing, and services based dairy enterprise would succeed in making profit.

b. Importance of credit in dairy entrepreneurship

Credit helps to overcome shortage of equity capital in dairy enterprise. Restricted credit, changing interest rates, lack of credit information are most common problems faced by a dairy entrepreneur. Credit serves many purpose of an entrepreneur such as

1. Start up and increase production.
2. Improvement in quality of what is being produced
3. Revise operations to make them more profitable.

The money borrowed must generate enough additional income to pay for the cost of the borrowed money (interest) and to ensure that principle is repaid according to specified terms of the loan.

Credit is normally needed in three broad expenses in an enterprise: Fixed expense, operating expenses and start up expenses. Fixed expenses are items which can be used over and over for a long period of time incurring the same price (expense) each year. Examples are land, buildings, machinery, equipment, tools and machinery. Operating expenses are needed to run an enterprise e.g. production entrepreneur would need money to buy feed and fodder, manpower expenses to run his dairy enterprise. In dairy sales enterprise operating expenses would need communication, transportation, fuel, advertising expenses. Start up expenses is before the business begins operation. It may include cost of construction of farm housing, fees to architects and construction work etc.

c. Type of Credit requirement in dairy enterprise

The financial credit needs of farmers according to length of the loan period can be classified into three parts:

(1) **Short Term Credit:** Short term credit is required for a period of six to 12 months. These type of credit is needed for maintenance expenses as well as to purchase items like feed and fodder of dairy, fodder seeds, feed additives, medicines for animals. Short term credit is important for survival of dairy enterprise as it finances everyday operations of the firm which generate the cash flow in the business. Such type of credit is taken from money lenders, relatives, friends and the co-operative societies. To maintain good flow of credit these loans should be repaid upon receipt of money at harvest or auction time.

(2) **Medium Term Credit :** These loans are needed from 1 to 10 years. These types of loans are needed by farmers to purchase cattle, repair and construction of irrigation system, housing of animals, fencing, sophistication in dairy enterprise, purchase of dairy implements such as milking machine /milk tester/bulk milk cooling unit, cold storage facilities for milk and milk products, purchase of dairy processing equipment for manufacturing indigenous milk products. Such type of credit is taken from money lenders and the commercial banks Bank or lender may require collateral when considering a loan application.

(3) **Long term Credit:** Loans that extend over 10 years are long term credit. Long term credit is especially important when starting a dairy enterprise. The entrepreneur has to determine how much land and what type of building are suitable to the scale of operations. In fact startup of dairy venture depends on whether a lender is willing to extend this credit. Loan repayment of long term credit depends on funds left over after deductions of all expenses for the year.Net income are examples of sources of repayment for long term loans.

d. Sources of Farm Credit

The different sources for agriculture can be obtained from formal and informal sources.

i) **Formal sources** include Credit co-operatives, commercial banks, government, Regional Rural Banks.

ii) **Informal sources** include money lender, Friends and relatives, traders and Landlords.

e. Credit analysis and Loan Rationality for an Entrepreneur

Banks while lending loan look into credit analysis and loan rationality which is done by taking into three considerations (R's and C's) of credit. Three 'R's of credit are Returns, Repayment capacity and Risk bearing ability. Three 'C's of credit are character, capacity and capital.

i. **Returns:** Borrowing money i.e. credit should increase net returns and make profit. Each investment from credit should be made after analyzing its ability to repay back the borrowed money (credit) The bank as well as entrepreneur should be well satisfied that the proposed enterprise would generate enough returns to repay the loan and sustain the enterprise .Selection of enterprise; determining most economic optimum production techniques and size of enterprise affect the returns

ii. **Repayment ability:** Priority is given to loans which have earning capacity. e. g. borrowing for dairy cows would take priority over borrowing for automatic feeders to replace hand feeding. The automatic feeder generates no direct income unlike the sale of milk from the dairy cows.

iii. **Risk bearing ability:** Borrowers with strong assets can take on more risk than those with few assets. It also depends upon character of entrepreneur.

Three 'C's of credit are character, capacity and capital.

i. Character implies the borrower's moral qualities, such as honesty, integrity and sense of responsibility which all influence the risk bearing ability and repayment.

ii. Capacity signifies the potential of the borrower to repay the loan, when it is due and depends upon his income.

iii. Capital reflects the net worth of the borrower (assets minus liabilities) which also reflects his repayment and risk bearing ability.

f. Methods of Repayment of Credit

There are three ways of repayment:

a) Credit or loan can be repaid back as straight end or lump sum payment in which loan is paid as lump sum after expiry of the term. Interest is however paid every year.

b) In partial repayment method, a part of the loan together with a part of the interest on the loan is paid up every year.

c) In Amortized even repayment an equal amount is repaid every year. This includes a larger proportion of the principal and a smaller amount of interest in each succeeding installment of payment. This method of payment is suitable when income is likely to flow at a constant rate throughout the period.

12

Financial Analysis in Dairy Enterprise

Financial analysis of a dairy enterprise can be done with following major tools:

1. Balance sheets
2. Cash flow records:
3. Income statements
4. Break Even analysis
5. Budgets

a. Balance Sheets or Net worth Statement

Balance sheet is the list of assets and liabilities owned by a business. It helps to calculate the growth in net worth of the business by calculating the change in assets less the change in liabilities. They represent the financial foundation on which the business is built.

The term 'balance sheet' implies some sort of balance as part of the document. That balance represents the relationship between assets on one side, and liabilities on the other, and the basic accounting principle that assets always equal liabilities plus equity. Since it is simply a list of assets owned and debts owed, at a given time, with monetary values attached, we must understand the concepts of assets and liabilities.

Assets are resources owned by or owed to the business such as dairy, equipment, real estate, and notes receivable. Assets are those parts of the business that are owned or controlled. They include any property/resource owned by a person or business e.g. cash, land, buildings, dairy, farm equipment and dairy-related share. Assets are usually listed on the top or on the left hand side of the balance sheet. They are classified in following ways

Current Assets: Assets that can be quickly monetized or converted to cash. Current assets are those assets which can be converted into cash during one normal operating cycle of the business. In the normal course of business current assets could be converted into cash within one year.

Examples of Current assets include cash on hand, bills receivable, account deposits in banks, marketable securities (shares/bonds), short-term notes receivable, prepaid expenses and inventory – items that are held for sale i.e., crop and dairy produce and those items to be consumed in the process of producing dairy products to be sold i.e., fodder seeds, feed and fuel, lubricants, feed additives etc.

Intermediate assets are those that can impact on the business after one year but within 10 years. This category includes assets used to produce income, such as breeding dairy, retirement accounts and longer-term securities. They also include plant and equipment such as fixed farm machinery (milking machines, vats, forage and other feed-processing machinery), tractors, farm vehicles, motorbikes and also any equipment with a reasonable asset value, such as cultivation and spray equipment. These values are also used to calculate depreciation

Fixed assets/Long term assets: These are those items owned by business firm that have a relatively longer life and takes long time to convert into cash. They include land, buildings, cattle sheds, machinery and equipments, implements and tools, dairy furniture and fixtures. They are normally not for resale. They are recorded in the Balance Sheet at their net cost less accumulated depreciation.

Other assets: These include any intangible assets, such as patents, copyrights, other intellectual property, royalties, exclusive contracts, and notes receivable from officers and employees.

Liabilities

The debts that the business owes to creditors are called liabilities. These are the dues/loans/borrowings of business/credit outstanding etc. Liabilities are generally located in the middle section or on the right side of the balance sheet. Legally creditors of the business would have first claim against any of its assets.

Current Liabilities are those liabilities that will come one normal operating cycle i.e. due within 1 year. Thus current liabilities are to be paid during the year or yet to be paid even though their goods and services have been delivered. These are accounts/bills payable i.e., items purchased on credit, short term loans, notes payable, taxes payable, wages and salaries payable, specific portion of any long term and debt that will come due within a year, accrued interest, taxes, rents and leases.

Long term liabilities: These are liabilities that will come due after more than 1 year in the future. They include bonded indebtedness, mortgages, long term loans, cattle loans, poultry loans, tractor loans, land development loans, dairy machinery loans. Thus, Long-term liabilities are due to be paid in more than one year.

Equity or net worth

Calculation of equity, or the owner's share of the farm assets, is one of the key functions of balance sheets. As equity (which is sometimes called net worth) is the difference between what you own and what you owe, it is the difference between total assets and total liabilities. If the equity is positive, the business is solvent. It is the difference between the total assets and total liabilities in the business. The most liquid current asset is cash in hand and the least liquid current asset is inventory. Eg. Milk can. The most liquid current liability is money at call and the least liquid asset is long term loans.

Equity (and net worth) is expressed in monetary terms while equity can also be expressed as a percentage as follows:

Net worth or Equity = (Assets -Liabilities), in local currency units

$$\text{Equity (\%)} = \frac{\text{Assets} - \text{Liabilities}}{\text{Assets}} \text{X } 100$$

Some creditors use equity on property as a guide to how much liability (or mortgage) debtors can secure against the value of their land.

Assets are calculated the following way

Assets − Liabilities + Net worth

All balance sheets contain the same categories of assets, liabilities and net worth figures.

Assets are arranged in decreasing order of their liquidity. Liabilities are listed in the order of how soon they must be repaid, followed by retained earnings (net worth of owner's equity).

Importance of Balance Sheet

Basic building blocks for financial analysis

1. Balance sheet is an indicators of the business's ability to handle risk
2. The first step in analyzing the debt position of the business.
3. The net result of past decisions
4. Very important ways to track and monitor financial progress

Summarized form of Balance sheet

Balance sheet of farmer (Name ....) as on date:

A.	Assets	Value (Rs.)	B	Liabilities	Value (Rs.)
a)	Current assets		e)	Current liabilities	
b)	Fixed assets		f)	Long term liabilities	
c)	Other assets		g)	Total liabilities	
d)	Total assets= (a+b+c)		h)	Net worth (d-g)	
			i)	Retained earnings	

Total assets = (balancing figure) = (g +h)

Features of Balance sheet

1. Balance sheet is also known as *Net Worth statement.*
2. In a typical Balance sheet, the assets are listed on the left hand side and liabilities are listed on the right hand side.
3. Apart from this, at the bottom of right hand side of balance sheet Net worth or Equity is mentioned.
4. Generally the left hand side values are equal or balances the right hand side values and hence this statement is called as Balance sheet.

b. Income Statement

It is also called profit and loss statement. It states the source of firm's incomes, describes the nature of the expenses, and shows the net profit earned (or net loss incurred) during an accounting period. It is supporting evidence to balance sheet, in the sense, that it explains the change in retained earnings on the balance sheet

The format of a profit & loss statement varies from business to business but such statement generally begins with sales and subtracts the appropriate expenses with profit showing as a remainder.

A farm income statement is broadly divided into two areas income and expenses. Both of these sections are divided into a section of cash entries and noncash adjustments.

Income section: In these sources of income such as sale of dairy products, payments received are entered. In the second part of this section adjustments due to change in market value of inventories like dairy, feed etc. are included

Expenses section: In this cash expenses incurred for operation of business during current year is added. This may include anything purchased, insurance premium, interest paid on loans, rent/lease payments. Purchase of capital assets like land, machinery, dairy losses is not included. In the second part of this section adjustments for reduction in value of feed inventories and depreciations are added.

Once all the income and expenses are accounted for, total farm expenses are subtracted from total farm income and Net cash income is calculated. Often frequently, net farm income which is calculated from subtracting total fixed expenses from net operating income is calculated which is Thus, there are three major sections of the income statement, namely receipts, expenses and adjustments and net income. The adjustments are necessary to convert cash flow to annual earnings by including inventory change, accounts payable and receivable and depreciation. From these income is calculated.

Importance of income statement

The income statement is the only tool of farm business analyses that measures profitability. Budgets, the balance sheet and cash flow projections are essential management tools, but do not indicate if the business is profitable. Income statements are also called profit and loss statement

c. Cash Flow Statement

This is the third financial statement which summarizes all cash receipts or cash flows and cash expenditures or cash inflows in a particular year. It does not indicate profitability but shows the sources and uses of cash .It also helps to assess the time at which funds are required for enterprise. It also indicates the sources from which funds can be raised, the purpose for which the loan is required, the need of sale and purchase of capital assets, the time and quantum of repayment, etc.

Preparation of Cash Flow Statement

In this financial statement, account of cash receipts and cash expenses is maintained. Cash receipts are maintained through cash income, sale of capital assets, new loans received, non farm income and cash balance in the beginning .In, cash outflows records of total cash expense, purchase of capital assets, principals repaid, on farm expenses, cash at the end of year are maintained.

Cash Flow Statement

	Cash Inflows	Cash Outflows
1. Cash income and cash expenses.		
1a)Total Cash Income	E	
1b)Total Cash Expense		v
2. Sale and Purchase of capital assets		
2a)Sales of capital assets	E	
2b)Purchase of capital assets		E
3. New loans received and principal repaid		
3a)New loans received	E	
3b)Principal repaid		E
4. Non Farm income and expenses		
Nonfarm income Nonfarm expenses	E	
5. Cash on hand		
Beginning of the year	E	
End of the year		E

Advantages of cash flow statement

1. To estimate the total credit needs (Short term, Medium term and Long term) of the farmer along with time and quantum;
2. To plan the repayment schedule,
3. In making purchases and sales at the appropriate time thereby helping to minimize the credit dependence, so that the farmers can keep limits to avoid wastages
4. To keep ready input requirements well in advance so that the last minute rush can be avoided
5. To know the farm household's expenditure pattern and enable the farmer to exercise a check on farm costs,
6. the farmer in preparing the farm business plans for the ensuing years,
7. the banker for revising the scale of finance, rescheduling loans, etc., and finally, as a tool of financial control to the farmer.

d. Break Even analysis

Break even analysis is important for undertaking enterprise analysis. Break even point refers to a point when total cash receipts are equal to cash expenses. A break even point indicates the output and price at which there is no profit or loss because the costs are equal to the income. It is important because it shows the minimum output that should be sold for the farm not to operate at a loss. It therefore gives information to be used in production and pricing decisions

a. Break even yield = Total costs divided total production

b. Break even sale price = Total costs/sales price

Break even analysis

Determination of break even point of a firm is an important factor in assessing its profitability e.g. breakeven point of a dairy processing plant would help us to know the profitability of plant and plan accordingly.

Break even point

Break even point is an important yardstick used by bankers and other proponents to decide the viability of a new project/or a new activity in a project. Break even point establishes the level of output/production which evenly breaks the costs and revenues. It is the level of production where a total cost is equals to sales i.e. the point of zero profit and zero loss and the unit starts making profits.

From the banker point of view the project should achieve a break even position within a reasonable time from the start of production. The project which reaches its break even point earlier is considered a viable project. This is because the banker's can expect earlier payment of their advances in those projects and also those projects are likely to adapt themselves to the day to day developing technology.

Calculation of Break even point: BEP can be calculated in terms of physical units and in terms of sales turnover.

i) In terms of physical units

The number of units required to be sold to achieve the breakeven point can be calculated using the following formula:

Break even point: Fixed Costs/Selling price-Variable costs i.e. contribution per unit

Let us take an example suppose a dairy entrepreneur engaged in pasteurized milk selling had Rs 100000 as fixed costs for machinery, building etc. His per unit i.e. per liter variable costs is Rs 20 and selling price is 25 liters.

Maximum capacity is 60,000 liters of pasteurized milk per year

BEP =100000/25-20=20,000 litres of milk (i.e.One third of the capacity)

ii) In terms of sales volume

BEP in terms of sales volume can be calculated using the following formula:

BEP=Selling price per unit (Fixed costs/Selling price per unit-Variable costs per unit)

Or another formula is

BEP=Fixed Expenses X Sales/Total contribution

13

Livestock Insurance

Dairy rearing is central to livelihoods and survival of millions of people of India. It is estimated that approximately 100 million people derive their live hood from dairy rearing as primary or secondary source of income. Dairy related activities help to maintain regular in flow of income for these households. Small farmers in India generate nearly half of their income from dairy and the value of cattle represents a significant part of their wealth, so the death of cattle poses a significant risk and affects farmers' net worth and income.

a. Type of risks to dairy based livelihoods

Large animal's are expensive and thus carry higher risk exposure. Dairy losses due to the disease, accident, theft, natural calamity can cause significant losses to these household. Sometimes owners are forced to sell their animals due to loss due to incurable disease/ disorder/ fodder and water scarcity and they are unable to rebuild their stock. Many times animal losses force them into poverty trap from where they are unable to recover.

Risks faced by dairy owner's dairy dependent livelihoods can be classified into two broad categories

1. Production risk
2. Price risk

1. Production risk: These include

1. Lack of nutrition: It may be due to non availability of imputes (dry and green fodder for animals)
2. Morbidity: (Cattle disease like mastitis, FMD, HS result in reduction or stoppage of milk production, loss of animal value due to permanent loss in productivity, fertility and hide value of animal.
3. Cattle morality: It may be accidental or natural loss of asset is biggest challenge for cattle owner as there is dramatic fall in income.

2. Price Risk

1. Fluctuation in the costs of cattle and its products during disease outbreaks
2. Changes in demand supply equation of dairy production leading to reduced demand / lower price which results in income losses to farmers.

b. Livestock Insurance in dairy risk management

Dairy risk management would involve two components-risk reduction and risk transfer. Risk reduction mechanisms through government owned veterinary services have limited impact due to shortage of manpower, timely nature of veterinary services, remoteness of famer's location, poor delivery of services etc. Therefore, role of risk transfer in the form of dairy insurance becomes importance. Dairy insurance would not only minimize the economic losses due to animal loss but also it may incentivize the dairy owner to rear quality animals in the wake of adequate risk protection mechanism through dairy insurance.

c. Livestock Insurance in India

Introduction

Pioneering effort to create a market for dairy insurance was started by Government of India in 1971 with the help of small farmers Development agency (SFDA).Subsequently several scheme e.g. Integrated Rural Development Programmes (IRDP) were launched at the national level to provide safety nets for all dairy rearing farmers in the country. In these schemes cattle insurance was tied with rural credit delivery programs. Thus, insurance remained scheme driven and mandatory in nature with little awareness among the customers. Also, public players remained the only sources of dairy insurance in India till 2003.However, private players like ICICI Lombard, IFFCO Tokio etc. entered in dairy insurance since 2003.

Livestock Insurance Scheme: A Centrally Sponsored Scheme

Government of India introduced a Centrally Sponsored Scheme (CSS) on Livestock Insurance on a pilot basis during 2005-06 & 2006-07 in 100 selected districts of the Country. The scheme is restricted to high yielding cattle and buffaloes only (1500 litre per lactation). This scheme is reviewed from 100 districts to 300 districts and eventually to all the districts and includes five milch animals from two animals. The scheme is implemented in all the districts of the Country from 21.05.2014. Animals covered under any other insurance scheme would not be considered under this scheme. The involvement of veterinary officer in the scheme is from beginning to end. Under the scheme, the crossbred and high yielding cattle and buffaloes are being insured at maximum of their current market price. The premium of the insurance is subsidized to the tune of 50%. The entire cost of the subsidy is being borne by the Central Government. The benefit of subsidy is being provided to a maximum of five animals per beneficiary for a policy of maximum of three years. The scheme is being implemented in all states except Goa through the State Livestock Development Boards of respective states. The scheme is now subsumed as a component titled Risk Management and Insurance under the sub-mission on livestock development of National Livestock Mission.

The Livestock Insurance Scheme has been formulated with the twin objective of providing protection mechanism to the farmers and cattle rearers against any eventual loss of their animals due to death and to demonstrate the benefit of the insurance of livestock to the people and popularize it with the ultimate goal of attaining qualitative improvement in livestock and their products.

Objectives of Scheme

The Dairy Scheme has been formulated with the twin objective of providing protection mechanism to the farmers and cattle bearers against any eventual loss of their animals due to death and to demonstrate the benefit of the Insurance of dairy to the people and popularize it with the ultimate goal of attaining qualitative improvement in dairy and their products.

Features of the scheme

1. Under the scheme, the crossbred and high yielding cattle and buffaloes are being insured at maximum of their current market price. The premium of the Insurance is subsidized to the tune of 50%. The entire cost of the subsidy is being become by the central Government.
2. The benefit of subsidy is being provided to a maximum of 2 animals per beneficiary for policy of maximum of three years.
3. Animal to be covered under the scheme and selection of beneficiaries:
4. All those female cattle / buffalo yielding at least 1500 Littre of milk per lactation are to be considered high yielding and hence can be insured under the scheme for maximum of their current market value.
5. Animals covered under any other Insurance scheme / plan scheme will not be covered under scheme.
6. Benefit of subsidy is to be restricted to two animals per beneficiary and is to be given for one time Insurance of an animal up to a maximum period of three years.

7. The farmer will have to be encouraged to go for a three year policy which is likely to be more economical and useful for getting the real benefit of on occurrence of natural calamities like flood and drought etc, However , if a dairy owner prefers o have an Insurance policy for less than three years period for valid reasons, benefit for valid reasons, benefit of the subsidy under the scheme would be available to them also , with the restriction that no subsidy would be available of further extension of the policy.
8. The animal insured will have to be properly and uniquely identified at the time of Insurance claim. The ear tagging should, therefore, be fool proof as ear as possible. The traditional method of ear tagging or the recent technology of fixing microchips could be used at the time of taking the policy.
9. The cost of fixing the identification mark will be borne by the Insurance companies and responsibility of its maintenance will be mutually agreed by the beneficiaries and the Insurance Company.
10. The Veterinary practitioners may guide the beneficiaries about the need and importance of the tags fixed for settlement of their claim so that they proper care for maintenance of the tags.
11. It has been decided to pay an honorarium of Rs-/- per animal at the stage of insuring the animal and Rs-100/- per animal at the stage of issuing veterinary certificate in case of any insurance claim

Central assistance

Benefit of subsidy is to be restricted to 5 animals per beneficiary per household for all animals except sheep, goat, pig and rabbit. In case of sheep, goat, pig and rabbit the benefit of subsidy is to be restricted based on “Cattle Unit” and one cattle unit is equal to 10 animals i.e a total of 50 animals. If a beneficiary has less than 5 animals / 1 Cattle Unit, s/he can also avail the benefit of subsidy.

Component	Pattern of assistance
Premium rates **Premium rates for one year policy in** Normal Areas - 3.0% NER / Hill areas / LWE affected areas -3.5%,	**Normal areas** Central share 25%, State share 25% and Beneficiary share 50% for APL, and Central share 40%, State share 30%, and Beneficiary Difficult areas - 4.0 % share 30% for BPL / SC / ST
Premium rates for three year policy in Normal Areas - 7.5%, NER / Hill areas / LWE affected areas - 9.0% Difficult areas - 10.5 %	**NER / Hill areas / LWE affected areas** Central share 35%, State share 25% and Beneficiary sh are 40% for APL, and Central share 50%, State share 30%, and Beneficiary share 20% for BPL / SC / ST **Difficult Areas** Central share 45%, State share 25% and Beneficiary share 30% for APL, and Central share 60%, State share 30%, and Beneficiary share 10% for BPL / SC / ST

#NER: North Eastern Region
#LWE: Left Wing Extremism

Scope of cover/insurance coverage

i. Accident (Inclusive of flood, cyclone, famine) or any other fortuitous circumstances (fortuitous means accidental in origin)

ii. Diseases (Inclusive of Rinder-pest, Black Quarter, Hemorrhagic Septicemia, Foot and Mouth disease subject to vaccination against this disease).

iii. Surgical operations

iv. Strike riot and civil commotion and terrorism.

v. Earthquake.

Animals are identified by way of ear tagging. The policy covers both scheme and non-scheme animals. Scheme animals are those animals, which are sponsored by the Government agencies and are financed by some financial institutions, which may or may not involve any subsidy. Master Policy arrangements are usually done with DRDA, Bank, and Cooperative Societies etc.

Conditions for Livestock insurance

Livestock owners are required to fulfill the following conditions;

1. Provide suitable housing accommodation.
2. Offer good and balance feed to the animal.

3. Animals should be free from ecto and endo-parasites and should be periodically treated for parasites.
4. Animals must be protected against bacterial and viral diseases.

Requirements of livestock insurance

1. Health certificate: It is obligatory on the part of the owner to produce a certificate from a qualified veterinarian to the effect that this animal is healthy and free from any disease. The owner is required to pay a fee for this certificate as prevailing rates by government/ insurance company.
2. Identification of animal: is of great importance. Emphasis has to be given on breed, age, sex, body color, shape of horns, height and identification marks. Tagging must be done by veterinarian. The animal owner should note the number of ear tag of his animal. If the ear tag falls or lost due to tearing of ears while rubbing, the fallen tag should be preserved and must be reported to bank or insurance company in writing.
3. Principle of No tag-No claim: nowadays insurance companies have adopted the principle of no claim i.e; no claim is paid if the specific ear tag is not submitted.
4. Insurance policy: livestock can be through to type of policy – proposal cum policy and master policy agreement. The owner is required to fill the pro-forma called personal cum policy (either by himself or agent of insurance company or veterinarian) with recipient and veterinary certificate. The pro-forma contains information about; owner-his name address and occupation, period of insurance, particulars of animal- species breed sex color age identification height purpose for which used date of last calving, present market value, sum for which to be insured, location of dairy farm.
5. Premium amount.
6. No. of animals lost during past three years and its cause.
7. Special remarks if any.

Procedure of Dairy Insurance in India

1. Normally dairy insurance covers following category of animals whether indigenous, exotic or cross-bred.
   a. Milch Cows and Buffaloes
   b. Calves / Heifers

c. Stud Bulls

d. Bullocks (Castrated Bulls) and Castrated Male Buffaloes.

2. Animals within a specified age group are accepted under the Standard Insurance Scheme.
3. Sum Insured under the policy will be the Market Value of the animal.
4. Indemnity under the policy will be the sum insured or market value prior to illness whichever less is. The indemnity is limited to 75% of Sum Insured in case of a Permanent Total Disability (PTD) claim.
5. The basic premium rate per annum is 4% of the Sum Insured. Long term policies are also issued with long term discounts.
6. The premium rates under the policy are concessional for covering animals under government subsidized schemes e.g. Dairy insurance.
7. Group Discounts are also available.

Insurance Coverage

The policy shall give indemnity for death due to.

a. Accident (Inclusive of fire, lightning, flood, inundation, storm, hurricane, earthquake, cyclone, tornado, tempest and famine).

b. Diseases contracted or occurring during the period of this policy.

c. Surgical Operations.

d. Riot and Strike.

The Policy can also be extended to cover PTD on payment of extra premium

i. Permanent Total Disability which, in the case of Milch Cattle result in permanent and total incapacity to conceive or yield milk.

ii. PTD which in the case of Stud Bulls results in permanent and total incapacity for breeding purpose.

iii. In case of Bullocks, Calves / Heifers and Castrated male buffaloes results in permanent and total incapacity for the purpose of use mentioned in the proposal form.

Major Exclusions

(A) Common Exclusions

i. Malicious or willful injury or neglect, overloading, unskillful treatment or use of animal for purpose other than stated in the policy without the consent of the Company in writing.

ii. Accidents occurring and /or Disease contracted prior to commencement of risk.

iii. Intentional slaughter of the animal except in cases where destruction is necessary to terminate incurable suffering on humane consideration on the basis of certificate issued by qualified Veterinarian or in cases where destruction is resorted to by the order of lawfully constituted authority.

iv. Theft and clandestine sale of the insured animal.

v. War, invasion, act of foreign enemy, hostilities (whether war be declared or not), civil war, rebellion, revolution, insurrection, mutiny, tumult, military or usurped power or any consequences thereof or attempt threat.

vi. Any accident, loss, destruction, damage or legal liability directly or indirectly caused by or contributed to by or arising from nuclear weapons.

vii. Consequential loss of whatsoever nature.

viii. Transport by air and sea.

ix. Any non-scheme claim arising due to diseases contracted within 15 days from the date of risk are not covered.

(B) Specific Exclusions

i. Pleuropneumonia in respect of Cattle in Lakhimpur and Sibasagar Districts and newly carved out districts out of these two districts of Assam.

ii. All the claims received without ear tag.

Documents to Effect Insurance Coverage

a. Proposal Form

b. Veterinary Health Certificate from a qualified Veterinarian giving the age, identification marks, health, and market value of the animal in the prescribed format.

Identification of Animal

a. All insured animals should be suitably identified by natural Identification marks and color should be clearly noted in the proposal form and Veterinarian's Report.

b. Ear tags made of suitable material are applied to the ear of the animals and the code number is entered into the Veterinary Health Certificate.

c. Photographs of animals may be insisted in case of high value animal.

Claim Procedure

- An animal will be insured for its current market price. The market price of the animal to be insured will be assessed jointly by the beneficiary and the insurance company preferably in the presence of the Veterinary officer or the BDO. The minimum value of animal should be assessed by taking Rs.3000 per liter per day yield of milk or as per the price prevailing in the local market (declared by Government) for cow and Rs.4000 per liter per day yield of milk or as prevailing in the local market (declared by Government) for buffalo.

- The market price of pack animals i.e. Horses, Donkey, Mules, Camels, Ponies and Cattle/Buffalo Male and other livestock such as Goat, Sheep, Pigs, Rabbit, Yak and Mithun are to be assessed by negotiation jointly by owner of animal and by insurance company in the presence of veterinarians. In case of dispute the price fixation would be settled by the Gram Panchayat / BDO.

- The animal insured will have to be properly and uniquely identified at the time of insurance claim. The ear tagging should, therefore, be full proof as far as possible. The traditional method of ear tagging or the recent technology of fixing microchips could be used at the time of taking the policy. The cost of fixing the identification mark will be borne by the Insurance Companies and responsibility of its maintenance will lie on the concerned beneficiaries.

- The nature and quality of tagging materials will be mutually agreed by the beneficiaries and the Insurance Company. The Veterinary Practitioners may guide the beneficiaries about the need and importance of the tags fixed for settlement of their claim so that they take proper care for maintenance of the tags. The tag already available on animal may be utilized with unique identity number subject to the condition that it is mutually agreed by farmer and agency and there shall not be any dispute in settlement of claims on account of utilization of existing tag.

- While processing an insurance proposal, one photograph of the animal with the Owner and one photograph of the animal clearly with the ear tag visible shall be taken at the time of processing the insurance documentation. In case of sale of the animal or otherwise transfer of animal from one owner to other, before expiry of the Insurance Policy, the authority of beneficiary for the remaining period of policy will have to be transferred to the new owner.
- Only four documents would be required by insurance companies for settling the claims viz. intimation with the Insurance Company, Insurance Policy paper, Claim Form and Postmortem Report.
- In case of claim becoming due, the payment of insured amount should be made within 15 days positively after submission of requisite documents. If an Insurance company fails to settle the claim within 15 days of submission of documents, the insurance company will be liable to pay, a penalty of 12% compound interest per annum to the beneficiary.
- In the event of death of an animal, immediate intimation should be sent to the Insurers and the following requirements should be furnished:
    a. Duly completed claim form.
    b. Death Certificate obtained from qualified Veterinarian on Company's form.
    c. Postmortem examination report if required by the Company.

Ear Tag applied to the animal should be surrendered. The condition of' No Tag-No claim' will be applied if the tag is not surrendered.

Claim Procedure for PTD Claim

i. A certificate from the qualified Veterinarian to be obtained.
ii. The animal will be inspected by the company's Veterinary Officer also.
iii. Complete chart of treatment, medicines used, receipts, etc., should be submitted.
iv. Admissibility of claim will be considered after two months of Veterinary Doctor / Company Doctor's report.
v. The indemnity is limited to 75% of Sum Insured.

PashuDhan Bima Yojana 2009 (IFFCO-TOKIO General Insurance Co. Ltd)

This scheme covers death of cattle due to disease or accident. It is a one year credit linked cover for farmers with cattle loans. The sum assured is the value of the loan; if the value of the cattle is higher than the loan; the farmer bears the difference as the policy only covers the loan value. The farmer has the option to opt for a higher sum insured based on the valuation of the cattle. The identification of the animal is done through a new technology, Radio Frequency Identification Devices (RFIDs). This technology consists of a microchip within a capsule. The capsule is inserted beneath the hide of the cattle behind the ear area with the help of a syringe. Since the RFID capsule is inserted beneath the skin of the animal, the risk of it falling off or being removed is mitigated. The RFID tagging process is considered less painful than plastic tags for the animal. With ear tags it was common for the milk production of animals to reduce for a few days after tagging because of the trauma of the experience. Each chip is identifiable through a unique number readable using a RFID reader. The premium has been set at (3- 5) % of the sum assured which is lower than the existing (5-7) % in the market. The insurance product is distributed through the Primary Agricultural Cooperative Societies. On an average the claim settlement takes 8 to 30 days. The multiyear policies are offered at a discounted rate. The various services like enrolment, claim processing, value added services are available at the doorstep through the companies own network of relationship executives or bimasahayaks who run the bimakendra who are accessible by a phone call from thc farmer.

Private Players in the Field of Livestock Insurance

With the privatization of insurance and awareness amongst the livestock farmers, many insurance companies have started providing insurance services to livestock farmers.

The following are the insurance companies which are undertaking livestock insurance

1. Companies working under General Insurance Corporation of India (Public Sector)

   a. The Oriental Insurance Company Limited

   b. New India Assurance Company Limited

   c. National Insurance Company Limited

   d. United India Insurance Company Limited

2. Private Companies and Banks
   a. SBI General Insurance
   b. IFFCO-Tokio General Insurance Company Limited
   c. Bajaj-Allianz Tokio General Insurance Company
   d. Future Generali Total Insurance Solutions
   e. Royal SundaramTokio General Insurance
   f. ICICI Lombard Rural Insurance
   g. TATA-AIG Rural Insurance
   h. HDFC-ERGO Rural Insurance

Premium rates of different insurance companies

Insurance Company	Premium Rate (% of Sum Insured)	
	For 01 Year	For 03 Year
	Coverage	Coverage
The New India Insurance Co. Ltd.	2.69	6.85
Oriental Insurance Co. Ltd.	4.00	10.20
National Insurance Co. Ltd.	4.00	10.20
United India Insurance Co. Ltd.	3.14	8.05
ICICI Lombard General Insurance Co.	3.86	9.00
TATA AIG General Insurance Co. Ltd.	4.25	10.59

India being a diverse country with varied climatic zones, soil cover and livestock aggregation require an effective safeguard from environmental variations, natural disasters and sudden outbreaks of fatal diseases pertaining to livestock. This can only be achieved by creating awareness among the rural livestock farmers and motivating them to insure their animals. Although the central and the state governments are taking up policies to cater the needs of the livestock owners but still reaching to the very fabric of society is a challenge. To increase the insurance coverage, the equip livestock farmers with latest knowledge about insurance, to assess their information needs pertaining to insurance and to address them seems to few decisive challenges but they can be fulfilled by better extension and advisory services.

14

Commercial Dairy Farming

Introduction

Dairy is vital to the economics of many developing countries. Animals are a source of food, more specifically protein for human diets, income, employment and possibly foreign exchange. For low income producers, dairy can serve as a store of wealth; provide draught power and organic fertilizer for crop production and a means of transport. Consumption of dairy and dairy products in developing countries, though starting from a low base, is growing rapidly. Dairying has become an important secondary source of income for millions of rural families and has assumed a most important role in providing employment and income generating opportunity. Indian Dairying is unique in more than one ways. It ranks first with its 199.1 million cattle & 105.3 million buffaloes accounting for about 51 percent of Asia's and about 19 per cent of world's bovine population. It also ranks first in milk production with a production of 121.8 million tones in 2010-11 and the demand is expected to be 180 million tones by 2020. To achieve this demand annual growth rate in milk production has to be increased from the present 2.5 % to 5%. Thus, there is a tremendous scope/potential for increasing the milk production through profitable dairy farming. Besides milk, the manure from animals provides a good source of organic matter for improving soil fertility and crop yields. The gobar gas from the dung is used as fuel for domestic purposes as also for running engines for drawing water from well. The surplus fodder and agricultural by-products are gainfully utilised for feeding the animals. Almost all draught power for farm operations and transportation is supplied by bullocks. Since agriculture is mostly seasonal, there is a possibility of finding employment throughout the year for many persons through dairy farming. Thus, dairy also provides employment throughout the year. The main beneficiaries of dairy programmes are small/marginal farmers and landless labourers. It contributes about 3.93 per cent to India's agricultural GDP, milk is a leading agricultural produce. The value of output from milk at current prices during 2009-10 has been over Rs.2, 41,177 crores which is higher than the output from paddy alone and is also higher than the value output from Wheat and sugarcane, put together. The unique feature of the system is that about 120 million rural families are engaged in milk production activities as against big specialized dairy farmers in the west.

During the post independence period, progress made in dairy sector has been spectacular. Milk production has increased more than four folds from a mere 17 million tones during 1950-51 to 121.8 million tones in 2010-11. However, the country's per capita availability is still lower than the world's daily average of about 285 gms though it has doubled from 124 gms in 1950-51 to 281gms per day in 2010-11. This impressive growth effort speaks volume about the co-coordinated efforts of large number of milk producing farmers, scientists, planners, NGO's and industry in achieving self-sufficiency in milk production. According to World Bank estimates about 75 per cent of India's population are in 5.87 million villages, cultivating over 145 million hectares of cropland. Average farm size is about 1.66 hectares. Among 70 million rural households, 42 per cent operate upto 2 hectares and 37 per cent are landless households. These landless and small farmers have in their possession 53 per cent of the animals and produce 51 per cent of the milk. Thus, small/marginal farmers and land less agricultural labourers play a very important role in milk production of the country. Dairy farming can also be taken up as a main occupation around big urban centres where the demand for milk is high. Farmers taking up dairy as their main source of income should do commercial / big scale units with more animals and adopt scientific technology for better profit.

In spite of India's position as highest producer of milk, productivity per animal is very poor. It is only about 987 kg/lactation as against world average of 2,038 kg/lactation. This low productivity is due to the gradual genetic deterioration and general neglect of animals over the centuries and consequent to the rise in the population of non-descript cows (80%) and buffaloes (50%). Besides other factors like continuing draughts in some parts of the country, chronic shortages of feed & fodder coupled with their poor nutritive value and poor fertility of dairy animals, the unawareness among the farmers about the various techno-economic aspects of dairy farming and schemes of Govt. contributing to low productivity and that leads to low income generation for farmers that makes it unprofitable activity. So, for making it profitable venture the farmer must have a thorough idea about various technical and economic aspects of the activity. In this chapter we will try to brief the techno-economic aspects of various sizes of dairy farming. To start any activity for income generation one must think about the backward and forward linkages of that activity. Backward linkages describes about the various parameters/ things needed to start the activity say for example in dairy farming cross –bred animals, availability of feed materials and water, availability of labours, connectivity with road etc and forward linkages deals about the various parameters that required after production (i.e. mainly marketing aspect of the product). After proper analysis of both the linkages then only one should think about to start the activity or not.

B. Project Profile

To get financial support from any of the nationalized or co-operative bank. It is essential to develop and submit a technically feasible and economically viable project proposal on dairy farming. Keeping this in view a techno-economic feasibility analysis had been carried out for a farm of 10 dairy crossbred cattle for five years. The various components of this project proposal as per the norms of financial institutions have been mentioned below.

C. General Information

i) Name of the Sponsoring Bank

ii) Nature and objectives of the proposed scheme.

- To establish a unit of commercial dairy farm with 10 crossbred cows.
- To rear milch cows using improved technologies for the sale of milk and Manure
- Marketing the produce by establishing direct link with the end-users and Retailers.
- To earn income at door step and step-employment through commercial dairy farming.

iii) Importance of the project

Although India stands first in milk production, but still there is great gap between requirement and supply particularly in urban area. This has also led to production of synthetic milk and adulteration to fulfill the demand. Further, people have become more conscious about the quality of milk. If milk is produced in hygienic condition, consumers are ready to pay even remunerative price. At the same time land holding per farmer has decreased drastically. In this context, opening the organized dairy farm by any farmer with financial support of any agency would be immensely useful to farmer.

iv) Details of Investment

S.No.	Items	Physical Unit	Unit Cost (Rs./ unit)	Total Cost (Rs.)
1.	Cost of Animal	10	25000.00	250000.00
2.	Transportation Cost of Animals	10	2000.00	20000.00
3.	Cost of Construction of Shed	500	300.00	150000.00
4.	Cost of Store/Cum/office	200	500.00	100000.00
5.	Equipments (Chaff Cutter, Milking Pails, Cans etc.)	10	2000.00	20000.00
6.	Insurances (6%)	10	1500.00	15000.00
7.	Total Cost			555000.00

v) Margin money (15%) Rs. 83250.00

vi) Net finance required from bank Rs. 471750.00

vii) Name and address of the branch of the financing bank.

viii) Type of firm: Individual/ Partnership/ Company/ Cooperative Society/ Others

ix) Details of borrower's profile

a) Name and address of the firm /barrower entrepreneur

a) Capability: In terms of interest, attitude and resources

c) Experience: In the relevant area.

d) Financial soundness : In terms of availability of fixed assets, property and other successful enterprises of the borrower

e) Technical/ Other special qualifications: Enclose certificates of training, etc.

x) Suitability of the climate

Northern Indian climate is characterized by high temperature and high humidity during summer and cols during winter season. There is no much influence on milk production during winter as exotic animals are well suited for temperate climate. However, adaptability of crossbred cattle in summer is little problematic. Thus milk production may decrease to some extent during the peak summer days. In this circumstance, summer management practices would certainly help in relieving the summer stress and maintenances of milk production.

xi) Location of the farm /land.

a. Name and address of the place

b. Map/ Layout of the farm: Needs to be enclosed

c. Land available for sheds, etc. 700 sq. ft.

d. Khasra No. of the land

e. Distance from mattled road (km)

f. Distance from Veterinary Hospital (km)

g. Nearest Animal Market (km)

h. Lead Bank of the area

i. Transport facility

d. Technical Aspects

i) Animal: Crossbred cows can be reared across the country both in rural and urban conditions. Crossbreds with 50-70% exotic inheritance of Holstein Friesian/ Brown Swiss / Jersey and exotic breeds have been found suitable in Northern part of India with optimum production. However, evolved strain like Karan Fries, Frieswal, and Vrindavani are also popular.

a. Proposed Strain: Crossbred cows (as mentioned above)

b. Stage of the animals: Second or third location

c. Arrangement for vaccination, deworming and health certificate will be done through local veterinary doctor.

d. Insurance: All the animals will be insured for a premium @ 6% of the value of the animals.

e. Cost of animals: Rs 25000 each

f. Description of the animal.

Strain/Breed	Utility	Body Size	Adult Weight	Confirmation
Holstein Friesian Crosses	Milk	Large	400-500 kg	White coat colour with black patches. Good wedges.
Jersey Crosses	Milk	Large	375-475 kg	Coat is normally silky brown in colour, is occasionally gray, reddish or spotted white. Its underside has a lighter colour, white its hips, head and shoulders are usually darker.
HF, Jersey and Brown Swiss Crosses (Vrindavani)	Milk	Large	400-500 kg	Prominent brown coat colour but beige, black, blue gray, red brown, yellow brown and white are also present.

Assumption

1. Animals will be purchased in two batches at an interval of 5-6 months.
2. Second/ Third lactation animals within 30 days of calving will be purchased in first year.
3. It is assumed that the expenditure on calf rearing will nullify the income realized from its sale. However, the heifers will be retained on the farm and the old animals will sold out.
4. No. of milch animals. : 10
5. Transportation cost (Rs. per milch including) : 2000
6. Civil Structures
   a. Shed (sft per milch animal along with calf) : 50
   b. Store and Office (sft) : 200
7. Lactation period (days) : 300
8. Dry period (days) : 90
9. Milk yield (lts/day) : 12
10. Fodder requirement
    a. Green fodder requirement : 25 kg/day/animal
    b. Dry fodder requirement : 4 kg/day/animal
11. Concentrate requirement
    i. Lactation : 4 kg/day/animal
    ii. Dry Period : 1.5 kg/day/animal

Purchase of Parent Stock: The parent stock can be purchased from the progressive farmers of Haryana, Punjab and western Uttar Pradesh region. The above mentioned crossbred animals are also available in IVRI, Izatnagr (U.P.) and NDRI, Karnal, Haryana. February-March and October-November are the most suitable months for purchase of animals. Apparently healthy animals with good body conformation should be purchased. Cows with good dairy characters like good mammary system, proper wedges and average body sore conditions should be maintained. Animals should be true to the characteristics mentioned above with alert look and free from any apparent disease symptoms. Ideally the animals should be vaccinated against major diseases (Anthrax, Hemorrhagic Septicemia, Black Quarter & Foot & Month Disease).

ii) Animal Status Chart

First Year	I st Batch	II nd Batch
1		
2.		
3.		
4.		
5.		
6.		
7.		
8.		
9.		
10.		
11.		
12.		
7x30x5=1050 Days	Lactation Days	9x30x5=1350 Days

Second Year		
1.	Lactating Cows -5	-do-
2.	-do-	-do-
3.	-do-	Dry
4.	-do-	-do-
5.	-do-	-do-
6.	-do-	Lactating Cows -5
7.	-do-	-do-
8.	-do-	-do-
9.	-do-	-do-
10.	-do-	-do-
11.	-do-	-do-
12.	-do-	-do-
Lactations Days	10x 30x5 = 1500 Days	9 x 30 x5 =1350 Days

Third Year		
1.	Dry	Lactating Cows -5
2.	Lactating Cows -5	-do-
3.	-do-	-do-
4.	-do-	Dry
5.	-do-	-do-
6.	-do-	-do-
7.	-do-	Lactating Cows -5
8.	-do-	-do-
9.	-do-	-do-
10.	-do-	-do-
11.	-do-	-do-
12.	Dry	-do-
Lactation Days	10x30x5=1500 Days	9x30x5 =1350 Days
Fourth Year		
1.	Dry	-do-
2.	-do-	-do-
3.	Lactating Cows -5	-do-
4.	-do-	-do-
5.	-do-	Dry
6.	-do-	-do-
7.	-do-	-do-
8.	-do-	Lactating Cows -5
9.	-do-	-do-
10.	-do-	-do-
11.	-do-	-do-
12.	-do-	-do-
Lactation Days	10 x 30 x 5 = 1500 Days	9 x 30 x 5 =1350 Days
Fifth Year		
1.	Dry	-do-
2.	-do-	-do-
3.	-do-	-do-
4.	Lactating Cows -5	-do-
5.	-do-	-do-
6.	-do-	Dry
7.	-do-	-do-
8.	-do-	-do-
9.	-do-	Lactating Cows -5
10.	-do-	-do-
11.	-do-	-do-
12.	-	-do-
Lactation Days		

B. Lactation Chart

S.No.	Particulars	Years				
		I	II	III	IV	V
i	Lactation Days					
	a) first Batch	1350	1500	1500	1350	1350
	b) Second Batch	1050	1350	1350	1350	1350
	Total	2400	2850	2850	2850	2700
ii	Dry Days					
	a) first Batch	450	300	150	300	450
	b) Second Batch	-	450	450	450	450
	Total	450	750	600	750	900

15

Economics - Model Dairy Farm

Model Project for Setting Up 10 & 20 Cow Dairy Farm (Indicative)

- The models are only indicative and in no way designed to provide exact economics. Following guidelines may be used by the interested persons to work out the details of their project, depending upon the local market and conditions.
- An interactive module considering the land availability for fodder cultivation, willingness to opt for silage bunkers, type of chaff cutter (manual or machine operated), milking machine, mister set, etc. is under preparation.
- The proposed interactive module would require preference for set of inputs and intended herd size and accordingly generate output outlining the estimated investment, cost and return.

a) 10 Crossbred Cow Farm

I. Assumptions

- The cost of land for the project is not considered.
- Inter-calving period of 390 days (300 lactating days and 90 dry days)
- Provision for silage bunker & mister set
- Change in market price of the animals assumed in following manner
  - Animals in 1st lactation: No change
  - Animals in 2nd lactation: +5%
  - Animals in 3rd lactation: -5%
  - Animals in 4th lactation: -10%
  - Animals in 5th lactation: -30%
  - Animals in 6th lactation: -50%
  - Animals in 7th lactation: -70%

- Once the young animal, reared within the herd that is ready to calve, would replace the oldest animal.
- The animals apart from 1st, 2nd or 3rd lactations are assumed to be sold off to maintain constant herd size.
- Required land is available for cultivating green fodder for animals.
- For lactating animals, total dry matter of feed and fodder is assumed to be in the range of 3.5-4 kg per 100 kg body weight.
- For dry animals, total dry matter of feed and fodder is assumed to be around 2.5 kg per 100 kg body weight.
- The project is considered as on-going and therefore, terminal values of assets are not considered.
- Male calves are assumed to be sold off.
- Price assumptions are on average basis and would vary region to region
- Provision for any taxation has not been made
- Of total 10 cows purchased
    - 5 cows are of 1st lactation having yield of 15 litres/ day, costing [1] 60,000/ animal
    - 3 cows are of 2nd lactation having yield of 18 litres/ day, costing [1] 63,000/ animal
    - 2 cows are of 3rd lactation having yield of 17 litres/ day, costing [1] 60,000/ animal
- Of 10 animals, 5 are assumed to be purchased at the beginning of the project and rest after 6 months
- Provision for manual chaff cutter
- No milking machine

II. PROJECT DETAILS (INDICATIVE) for 10 COW FARM

i) **Pre-requisite for the project**	square feet
Land requirement for cattle shed, storage and silage bunker	2325

ii) Project cost

Item	Amount (Rs)
Cattle shed for adult animals	420,000
Cattle shed for calves	140,000
Cattle shed for heifers	245,000
Silage bunker	37,500
Construction for storage area	233,340
Animals	623,000
Equipments	16,000
Contingency	34,300
Total Project cost	**1,749,140**

b) 20 Crossbred Cow Farm

I) Assumptions

- The cost of land for the project is not considered.
- Inter-calving period of 390 days (300 lactating days and 90 dry days)
- Provision for silage bunker & mister set
- Change in market price of the animals assumed in following manner
  - Animals in 1st lactation: No change
  - Animals in 2nd lactation: +5%
  - Animals in 3rd lactation: -5%
  - Animals in 4th lactation: -10%
  - Animals in 5th lactation: -30%
  - Animals in 6th lactation: -50%
  - Animals in 7th lactation: -70%
- Once the young animal, reared within the herd that is ready to calve, would replace the oldest animal.
- The animals apart from 1st, 2nd or 3rd lactations are assumed to be sold off to maintain constant herd size.
- Required land is available for cultivating green fodder for animals.
- For lactating animals, total dry matter of feed and fodder is assumed to be in the range of 3.5-4 kg per 100 kg body weight.

iii) Fixed cost (Rs)

Item	Year 1	Year 2	Year 3	Year 4	Year 5	Year 6	Year 7
Depreciation of cattle shed	103,834	103,834	103,834	103,834	103,834	103,834	103,834
Depreciation of equipment	1,600	1,600	1,600	1,600	1,600	1,600	1,600
Relative change in value of herd	-9,000	-63,000	-15,000	18,000	72,000	0	0
Interest on capital investment	209,897	209,897	209,897	209,897	209,897	209,897	209,897
Total fixed cost	**306,331**	**252,331**	**300,331**	**333,331**	**387,331**	**315,331**	**315,331**

iv) Variable cost (Rs)

Item	Year 1	Year 2	Year 3	Year 4	Year 5	Year 6	Year 7
Green fodder cultivation	48,000	48,000	48,000	48,000	48,000	48,000	48,000
Green fodder cost	0	0	0	0	0	0	0
Dry fodder cost	143,904	210,240	245,280	280,320	280,320	280,320	280,320
Concentrate cost	171,976	240,576	261,016	281,456	281,456	281,456	281,456
Mineral mixture cost	15,282	21,564	23,754	25,944	25,944	25,944	25,944
Labour charges	60,000	60,000	60,000	60,000	60,000	60,000	60,000
Insurance charges	24,120	24,120	24,120	24,120	24,120	24,120	24,120
Veterinary & breeding expenses	15,000	15,000	15,000	15,000	15,000	15,000	15,000
Electricity & water charges	15,000	15,000	15,000	15,000	15,000	15,000	15,000
Transportation cost for milk sale	1,000	1,000	1,000	1,000	1,000	1,000	1,000
Minor repair of building/ equipments	5,000	5,000	5,000	5,000	5,000	5,000	5,000
Interest on working capital	6,866	7,331	7,520	7,710	7,710	7,710	7,710
Total variable cost	**506,148**	**647,831**	**705,690**	**763,550**	**763,550**	**763,550**	**763,550**

v) Income (Rs)

Item	Year 1	Year 2	Year 3	Year 4	Year 5	Year 6	Year 7
Milk	854,120	1,200,420	1,109,160	1,031,940	1,067,040	1,165,320	1,165,320
Gunny bags	2,460	3,440	3,730	4,020	4,020	4,020	4,020
Sale of animals	2,000	2,000	2,000	62,000	134,000	122,000	224,000
Sale of dung/ manure	12,600	16,800	16,800	16,800	16,800	16,800	16,800
Total receipt	**871,180**	**1,222,660**	**1,131,690**	**1,114,760**	**1,221,860**	**1,308,140**	**1,410,140**
PBDIT (Operating Profit) (Rs)	365,032	574,829	426,000	351,210	458,310	544,590	646,590
Net Profit (Rs)	**58,701**	**322,498**	**125,669**	**17,879**	**70,979**	**229,259**	**331,259**
IRR	18.4%						
ROI	21.9%						

- For dry animals, total dry matter of feed and fodder is assumed to be around 2.5 kg per 100 kg body weight.
- The project is considered as on-going and therefore, terminal values of assets are not considered.
- Male calves are assumed to be sold off.
- Price assumptions are on average basis and would vary region to region
- Provision for any taxation has not been made
- Of total 20 cows purchased
  - 10 cows are of 1st lactation having yield of 15 litres/ day, costing[1] 60,000/ animal
  - 6 cows are of 2nd lactation having yield of 18 litres/ day, costing[1] 63,000/ animal
  - 4 cows are of 3rd lactation having yield of 17 litres/ day, costing[1] 60,000/ animal
- Of 20 animals, 10 are assumed to be purchased at the beginning of the project and rest after 6 months
- Provision for machine operated chaff cutter
- Provision of milking machine

I. Project Details (Indicative) for 20 Cow Farm

Pre-requisite for the project	square feet
Land requirement for cattle shed, storage and silage bunker	4150

Project cost

Item	Amount (Rs)
Cattle shed for adult animals	840,000
Cattle shed for calves	280,000
Cattle shed for heifers	490,000
Silage bunker	75,000
Construction for storage area	233,340
Animals	1,246,000
Equipments	106,000
Contingency	65,410
Total Project cost	3,335,750

Fixed cost (Rs)

Item	Year 1	Year 2	Year 3	Year 4	Year 5	Year 6	Year 7
Depreciation of cattle shed	184,334	184,334	184,334	184,334	184,334	184,334	184,334
Depreciation of equipment	10,600	10,600	10,600	10,600	10,600	10,600	10,600
Relative change in value of herd	-18,000	-126,000	-12,000	57,000	114,000	0	0
Interest on capital investment	400,290	400,290	400,290	400,290	400,290	400,290	400,290
Total fixed cost	**577,224**	**469,224**	**583,224**	**652,224**	**709,224**	**595,224**	**595,224**

Variable cost (Rs)

Item	**Year 1**	**Year 2**	**Year 3**	**Year 4**	**Year 5**	**Year 6**	**Year 7**
Green fodder cultivation	93,000	93,000	93,000	93,000	93,000	93,000	93,000
Green fodder cost	0	0	0	0	0	0	0
Dry fodder cost	287,808	438,000	525,600	595,680	595,680	595,680	595,680
Concentrate cost	343,952	491,330	542,430	583,310	583,310	583,310	583,310
Mineral mixture cost	30,564	44,220	49,695	54,075	54,075	54,075	54,075
Labour charges	120,000	120,000	120,000	120,000	120,000	120,000	120,000
Insurance charges	48,240	48,240	48,240	48,240	48,240	48,240	48,240
Veterinary & breeding expenses	30,000	30,000	30,000	30,000	30,000	30,000	30,000
Electricity & water charges	30,000	30,000	30,000	30,000	30,000	30,000	30,000
Transportation cost for milk sale	2,000	2,000	2,000	2,000	2,000	2,000	2,000
Minor repair of building/ equipments	10,000	10,000	10,000	10,000	10,000	10,000	10,000
Interest on working capital	13,553	14,576	15,050	15,429	15,429	15,429	15,429
Total variable cost	**1,009,117**	**1,321,366**	**1,466,015**	**1,581,734**	**1,581,734**	**1,581,734**	**1,581,734**

Income (Rs)

Item	Year 1	Year 2	Year 3	Year 4	Year 5	Year 6	Year 7
Milk	1,708,240	2,400,413	2,217,925	2,070,531	2,168,794	2,323,206	2,323,206
Gunny bags	4,910	7,020	7,750	8,330	8,330	8,330	8,330
Sale of animals	4,500	4,500	4,500	166,500	322,500	355,500	511,500
Sale of dung/ manure	25,200	33,600	33,600	33,600	33,600	33,600	33,600
Total receipt	**1,742,850**	**2,445,533**	**2,263,775**	**2,278,961**	**2,533,224**	**2,720,636**	**2,876,636**
PBDIT (Operating Profit) (Rs)	733,733	1,124,166	797,760	697,227	951,489	1,138,902	1,294,902
Net Profit (Rs)	**156,509**	**654,942**	**214,536**	**45,003**	**242,265**	543,678	699,678
IRR	19.8%						
ROI	23.4%						

A. Project Cost	Rs.
Cost of milch animals including transportation cost	330000
Cost of construction of shed for adult animals	60000
Cost of construction of shed for calves	20000
Cost of chaff cutter	50000
Cost of equipment	10000
Capital cost	**470000**
Cost of concentrate feed for first batch for first month	4800
Cost of fodder cultivation in 2 acres	9000
Insurance of first batch of milch animals	16000
Recurring cost	29800
Total cost	499800
or say	500000
Margin (15%)	75000
Bank Loan	425000

16

Model Unit Cost and Economics of a 10 Buffalo Unit

Assumptions

- Freshly calved animals in 1st or 2nd lactation are purchased in two batches of five animals each at an interval of 5 to 6 months.
- Cost of rearing calves not considered as it will be nullified by their sale value or retention value.
- Fodder cultivation considered in two acres and working capital for one crop / season considered. Two crops considered per year.
- Manure is utilized for fodder cultivation.

Feeding Schedule Per Day

	Lactation			Dry	
	Price (Rs.)	Qty. (kg)	Cost Per Day (Rs.)	Qty. (kg)	Cost Per Day (Rs.)
Concentrate Feed	8.00	4	32.00	1	8.00
Green Fodder	Home grown	25	0.00	20	0.00
Dry Fodder	1.50	4	6.00	5	7.50
Total			38.00		15.50

Lactation Chart

Years	1	2	3	4	5	6	7
Lactation Days	2100	2425	2425	2425	2200	2425	2425
Dry Days	625	1225	1225	1425	1450	1225	1075
Gunny Bags available for sale	171	208	208	196	195	200	195

C. Economics

Particulars	Years						
	1	2	3	4	5	6	7
Sale of Milk	277200	320100	320100	293700	290400	320100	320100
Sale of Gunny bags	1710	2080	2080	1960	1950	2000	1950
Total	**278910**	**322180**	**322180**	**295660**	**292350**	**322100**	**322050**
Cost of feeding during lactation	79800	92150	92150	84550	83600	92150	92150
Cost of feeding during dry period	9690	18990	18990	22090	22480	18990	16660
Cost of fodder cultivation	18000	18000	18000	18000	18000	18000	18000
Veterinary aid and breeding charges	2500	2500	2500	2500	2500	2500	2500
Labour charges	36000	36000	36000	36000	36000	36000	36000
Electricity and misc. charges	750	1500	1500	1500	1500	1500	1500
Insurance charges	16000	16000	16000	16000	16000	16000	16000
Total	**162740**	**185140**	**185140**	**180640**	**180080**	**185140**	**182810**
Surplus	145970	137040	137040	115020	112270	136960	139240

D. Calculation of BCR and IRR

	1	2	3	4	5	6	7
Capital Costs	470000						
Recurring Cost	162740	185140	185140	180640	180080	185140	182810
Total Costs	632740	185140	185140	180640	180080	185140	182810
Benefit	278910	322180	322180	295660	292350	322100	322050
Net Benefit	-353830	137040	137040	115020	112270	136960	139240
PW Costs @ 15%	1153513						
PW Benefits @ 15%	1272701						
NPW	119187.8						
B.C. Ratio	1.10 : 1						
I.R.R. (%)	28.66						

E. Repayment schedule

Year	Loan Outstanding	Gross Surplus	Interest	Principal Total	Repayment	Surplus
1	425000	145970	51000	51200	102200	43770
2	373800	137040	44856	51044	95900	41140
3	322756	137040	38731	57169	95900	41140
4	265587	115020	31870	48630	80500	34520
5	216957	112270	26035	52565	78600	33670
6	164392	136960	19727	76173	95900	41060
7	88219	139240	10586	88219	98805	40435

Techno economic parameters

Type of Animal	Graded Murrah Buffalo
No. of Animals	10
Cost of Animal (Rs./animal)	32000
Transportation Cost/Animal	1000
Average Milk Yield (litre/day)	8
Floor space (sqft) per adult animal	60
Floor space (sqft) per calf	20
Cost of construction per sqft (Rs.)	100
Cost of chaff cutter (power operated) (Rs.)	50000
Cost of equipment per animal (Rs.)	1000
Cost of fodder cultivation (Rs./acre/season)	4500
Insurance premium (% per annum)	5
Veterinary aid/animal/ year (Rs.)	250
Cost of concentrate feed (Rs./kg)	8
Cost of dry fodder (Rs./kg)	1.50

Contd.

No. of labourers	1
Salary of labourer per month (Rs.)	3000
Cost of electricity and water/animal/year (Rs.)	150
Margin (%)	15
Rate of interest (%)	12
Repayment period (years)	7
Selling price of milk/litre (Rs./kg)	16.50
Sale price of gunny bags (Rs. per bag)	10
Lactation days	270
Dry days	150

Model Unit Cost and Economics of a 10 Buffalo Unit

A. Project Cost	**Rs.**
Cost of milch animals including transportation cost	330000
Cost of construction of shed for adult animals	60000
Cost of construction of shed for calves	20000
Cost of chaff cutter	50000
Cost of equipment	10000
Capital cost	**470000**
Cost of concentrate feed for first batch for first month	4800
Cost of fodder cultivation in 2 acres	9000
Insurance of first batch of milch animals	16000
Recurring cost	29800
Total cost	**499800**
or say	**500000**
Margin (15%)	**75000**
Bank Loan	**425000**

B. Techno economic parameters

Type of Animal	Graded Murrah Buffalo
No. of Animals	10
Cost of Animal (Rs./animal)	32000
Transportation Cost/Animal	1000
Average Milk Yield (litre/day)	8
Floor space (sqft) per adult animal	60
Floor space (sqft) per calf	20
Cost of construction per sqft (Rs.)	100
Cost of chaff cutter (power operated) (Rs.)	50000
Cost of equipment per animal (Rs.)	1000
Cost of fodder cultivation (Rs./acre/season)	4500
Insurance premium (% per annum)	5

Contd.

Veterinary aid/animal/ year (Rs.)	250
Cost of concentrate feed (Rs./kg)	8
Cost of dry fodder (Rs./kg)	1.50
No. of labourers	1
Salary of labourer per month (Rs.)	3000
Cost of electricity and water/animal/year (Rs.)	150
Margin (%)	15
Rate of interest (%)	12
Repayment period (years)	7
Selling price of milk/litre (Rs./kg)	16.50
Sale price of gunny bags (Rs. per bag)	10
Lactation days	270
Dry days	150

Assumptions

- Freshly calved animals in 1st or 2nd lactation are purchased in two batches of five animals each at an interval of 5 to 6 months.
- Cost of rearing calves not considered as it will be nullified by their sale value or retention value.
- Fodder cultivation considered in two acres and working capital for one crop / season considered. Two crops considered per year.
- Manure is utilised for fodder cultivation.

Feeding Schedule Per Day

	Lactation			Dry	
	Price (Rs.)	Qty. (kg)	Cost Per Day(Rs.)	Qty. (kg)	Cost Per Day(Rs.)
Concentrate Feed	8.00	4	32.00	1	8.00
Green Fodder	Home grown	25	0.00	20	0.00
Dry Fodder	1.50	4	6.00	5	7.50
Total			38.00		15.50

Lactation Chart

Years	1	2	3	4	5	6	7
Lactation Days	2100	2425	2425	2425	2200	2425	2425
Dry Days	625	1225	1225	1425	1450	1225	1075
Gunny Bags available for sale	171	208	208	196	195	200	195

C. Economics

Particulars	Years						
	1	2	3	4	5	6	7
Sale of Milk	277200	320100	320100	293700	290400	320100	320100
Sale of Gunny bags	1710	2080	2080	1960	1950	2000	1950
Total	**278910**	**322180**	**322180**	**295660**	**292350**	**322100**	**322050**
Cost of feeding during lactation	79800	92150	92150	84550	83600	92150	92150
Cost of feeding during dry period	9690	18990	18990	22090	22480	18990	16660
Cost of fodder cultivation	18000	18000	18000	18000	18000	18000	18000
Veterinary aid and breeding charges	2500	2500	2500	2500	2500	2500	2500
Labour charges	36000	36000	36000	36000	36000	36000	36000
Electricity and misc. charges	750	1500	1500	1500	1500	1500	1500
Insurance charges	16000	16000	16000	16000	16000	16000	16000
Total	**162740**	**185140**	**185140**	**180640**	**180080**	**185140**	**182810**
Surplus	**145970**	**137040**	**137040**	**115020**	**112270**	**136960**	**139240**

D. Calculation of BCR and IRR0

	1	2	3	4	5	6	7
Capital Costs	470000						
Recurring Cost	162740	185140	185140	180640	180080	185140	182810
Total Costs	632740	185140	185140	180640	180080	185140	182810
Benefit	278910	322180	322180	295660	292350	322100	322050
Net Benefit	-353830	137040	137040	115020	112270	136960	139240
PW Costs @ 15%	1153513						
PW Benefits @ 15%	1272701						
NPW	119187.8						
B.C. Ratio	1.10 : 1						
I.R.R. (%)	28.66						

E. Repayment schedule

Year	Loan Outstanding	Gross Surplus	Interest	Principal	Total Repayment	Surplus
1	425000	145970	51000	51200	102200	43770
2	373800	137040	44856	51044	95900	41140
3	322756	137040	38731	57169	95900	41140
4	265587	115020	31870	48630	80500	34520
5	216957	112270	26035	52565	78600	33670
6	164392	136960	19727	76173	95900	41060
7	88219	139240	10586	88219	98805	40435

17

Techno-Economic Study of Dairy Farm (10+10 Cross-bred Unit)

Name of the Owner	: XYZ
Financing Bank	: ABC
Project profile	: Dairy unit [(10+10) CB Jersey cow]
Project Cost	: Rs.9, 71,800/=
Bank Loan	: Rs.7, 80,000/= (80.3%)
Margin Money (It may vary)	: Rs.1, 91,800/= (19.7%)
Subsidy	: As per Govt. norms

Interest Rate: Provisional Interest rate @ 15.75% p.a. has been taken for evaluation of the project report. However, the exact interest rate will be decided by the sanctioning authority on the date of sanction.

Disbursement of loan: Funds for fodder cultivation and civil construction should be disbursed first. Development of sheds and fodder plots should be completed within 3 months from first disbursement. Then disbursement of 1st Batch cow (10 animals) will be done. Last disbursement for 2nd Batch cows (10 animals) should be done after 5-6 months of purchase of 1st batch cows.

Insurance: The animals and other assets (sheds, equipment) **must be insured**. Wherever necessary, Risk / Mortality fund may be considered in lieu of dairy insurance.

Repayment of loan: The loan will be repaid in **6 years** (monthly installments) starting from 6th month onwards (moratorium period of 6months).

Techno-Economic Feasibility: The project should be examined techno-economically. The different worksheets attached with this report for a ready reference. The financial viability has also been examined by discounted cash flow which shows I.R.R – 47.09%, NPW – Rs.4.81 lacs, BCR – 1.17:1.00 and Average D.S.C.R. – 1.00:2.32. In light of the above analysis, we may say that the project is technically feasible and financially viable.

Detailed Project Cost

I) Capital cost

S.No.	Particulars		Unit cost	Total (in Rs.)
i.	Land development & fencing		LS	15000
ii.	Cow shed * (20 cows)	40 sqf/ cow	@Rs. 180/sqf	144000
iii.	Shed for heifer * (10)	30 sqf/ animal	@Rs. 180/sqf	54000
iv.	Shed for calves * (20 calves)	20 sqf/ calf	@Rs. 180/sqf	72000
v.	Shed for sick animal	100 sqf/ calf	@Rs. 180/sqf	18000
vi.	Office cum Store room	150 sqf	@Rs. 200/sqf	30000
vii.	Electrification & Fans (8)		LS	30000
viii.	Equipments		@Rs.500/cow	10000
ix.	Chaff cutter	2	@Rs.5000/unit	10000
x.	Water supply system		LS	40000
xi.	Cistern for Azolla culture	2 nos	@Rs.4000/cistern	8000
xii.	Cost of cows	20	@Rs.20000/cow	400000
xiii.	Transportation cost	20	@Rs.500/cow	10000
xiv.	Insurance	20	@ 5%	20000
A	**Sub total**			**Rs. 861000**

* The sheds for animal will be of concrete flooring, Asbestos roofing, with half brick wall & wire mesh for proper ventilation.

II) Recurring Cost (for three months for 1st Batch):-

i.	Feed cost for first batch	@Rs.77/cow/day	69300
ii.	Labour (2)	@Rs.2000/man	12000
iii.	Vety. Aid @ Rs.1200/animal / year		3000
iv.	Electricity charges @ Rs.500/ month		1500
v.	Fodder cultivation for one year (4 acres)	@Rs.5000/acre	20000
vi.	Azolla cultivation for one year	LS	5000
B	**Sub total**		**Rs.110800**
C	**Total Project cost**		**Rs.971800**

III) Techno Economic Assumptions

i. Lactation period – 280 days

ii. Dry period – 120 days

iii. Days in year taken as – 360 days

iv. The unit will take 3 months (90 days) for completion of construction of sheds.

v. Lactation period lapsed with seller – 30days

vi. Average milk production - 10 litters per cow per day during lactation period

vii. Selling price of milk - Rs.17 / litter

viii. Selling price of manure - Rs.400 / cow / year

ix. Price of Concentrate feed - Rs.12/kg

x. Total 2 no of Labourer will be appointed in the farm with a salary of Rs.2000/man/month.

xi. Concentrate feed during dry period (body maintenance) 2.00 Kg. per animal

xii. Concentrate feed during lactation period [2.00 Kg. + (0.4X10)] = 6.00 Kg. per animal

xiii. Price of green fodder - Rs.0.40/kg (the applicant will grow in her own farm)

xiv. Additional 3 acres of land will be taken on lease @Rs.8000/acre/year for fodder cultivation.

xv. Price of dry fodder - Rs.1.00/kg

xvi. Selling price of gunny bags - Rs.15 / bag (50 kg capacity)

xvii. Male Female ratio (Calf) - 1:1 (10+10)

xviii. Profit from sale of 10 male calves is Rs.0/ animal after deduction of cost incurred on their rearing.

xix. Mortality during heifer raring - 20%

xx. Heifer sold 8 nos /year.

xxi. Profit from sale of heifer is Rs.8000/ animal after deduction of cost incurred on their rearing.

IV) Feeding cost / day (for one animal)

	Particulars	Rate	LP (Rs.)	DP (Rs.)
a.	Green fodder @25kg during lactation & @ 20kg during dry period	To be produced from own farm	0.00	0.00
b.	Dry fodder @5kg & 6kg during LP & DP respectively	@Rs.100/Qt.	5.00	6.00
c.	Concentrate feed @6.00kg & 2.00kg during LP & DP respectively	@Rs.12/kg	72.00	24.00
	Total		**Rs.77.00**	**Rs.30.00**

V) Milk flow chart

Year	1st batch (single animal)		2nd batch (single animal)		Total (2 animal)		Total (20 animal)		Total Milk production	Total sale value
	LP	DP	LP	DP	LP	DP	LP	DP	@10 lt. /cow	@Rs.17/lt.
1st	250	20	90	0	340	20	3400	200	34000 ltrs	Rs.578000
2nd	260	100	240	120	500	220	5000	2200	50000 ltrs	Rs.850000
3rd	240	120	240	120	480	240	4800	2400	48000 ltrs	Rs.816000
4th	240	120	240	120	480	240	4800	2400	48000 ltrs	Rs.816000
5th	240	120	280	80	520	200	5200	2000	52000 ltrs	Rs.884000
6th	240	120	280	80	520	200	5200	2000	52000 ltrs	Rs.884000

VI) Calculation for Depreciations

(Rupees)

Particulars	Cost	%	1st Year	2nd Year	3rd Year	4th Year	5th Year	6th Year	Cl. value
Cow shed	144000	10%	14400	12960	11664	10498	9448	8503	76528
Shed for heifer	54000	10%	5400	4860	4374	3937	3543	3189	28698
Shed for calves	72000	10%	7200	6480	5832	5249	4724	4252	38264
Sick animal shed	18000	10%	1800	1620	1458	1312	1181	1063	9566
Office-godown	30000	10%	3000	2700	2430	2187	1968	1771	15943
Azolla cistern	8000	10%	800	720	648	583	525	472	4252
Elect. & Fans	30000	15%	4500	3825	3251	2764	2349	1997	11314
Equipments	10000	15%	1500	1275	1084	921	783	666	3771
Chaff cutter	10000	15%	1500	1275	1084	921	783	666	3771
Water supply	40000	15%	6000	5100	4335	3685	3132	2662	15086
Total	416000		46100	40815	36160	32057	28436	25241	207193

VII) Year wise Income – Expenditure Analysis

Income (Rupees)

S.No.	Particulars	1ST YR.	2ND YR.	3RD YR.	4TH YR.	5TH YR.	6TH YR.
i	Sale of milk	578000	850000	816000	816000	884000	884000
ii	Sale of manure	4000	8000	8000	8000	8000	8000
iv	Profit from sale of heifers	0	64000	64000	64000	64000	64000
v	Sale of gunny bags	6240	10320	10080	10080	10560	10560
A.	Total income	588240	932320	898080	898080	966560	966560

Expenditure

i	Feed	267800	451000	441600	441600	460400	460400
ii	Insurance	20000	20000	20000	20000	20000	20000
iii	Vety. Aid & breeding	12000	24000	24000	24000	24000	24000
iv	Labour charge	36000	48000	48000	48000	48000	48000
v	Energy charge	4500	6000	6000	6000	6000	6000
vi	Fodder cultivation	20000	20000	20000	20000	20000	20000
vii	Lease amount of fodder plots	24000	24000	24000	24000	24000	24000
viii	Azolla cultivation	5000	5000	5000	5000	5000	5000
B.	Total Expenditure	389300	598000	588600	588600	607400	607400
C.	Gross profit (A-B)	198940	334320	309480	309480	359160	359160
D.	Depreciation	46100	40815	36160	32057	28436	25241
E.	Earning before Interest (C-D)	152840	293505	273320	277423	330724	333919
F.	Interest on loan	87043	71147	59826	47601	31947	11951
G.	Earning before tax (E-F)	65797	222358	213494	229822	298777	321968
H.	Provision for tax	Nil	Nil	Nil	Nil	Nil	Nil
I.	Net Income (G-H)	65797	222358	213494	229822	298777	321968
J.	Cash Accruals (I+F+D)	198940	334320	309480	309480	359160	359160
K.	Repayment	99400	142800	132000	132000	150000	149314
L.	DSCR (J/K)	1:2.00	1:2.34	1:2.34	1:2.34	1:2.39	1:2.41

VIII) Repayment Schedule:

(Rupees)

Month.	Investment	Promoter's contribution	DISB.	Loan amount	Subsidy provision	Interest (15.75%)	Principal	Interest	Instal lment	Total during the year	Outstanding
							<<<<<<REPAYMENT>>>>>>				
0	456000	186000	270000	270000	284000	—	—	—	—	—	270000
1	—	—	—	270000	—	3544	—	—	—	—	273544
2	—	—	—	273544	—	3590	—	—	—	—	277134
3	—	—	—	277134	—	3637	—	—	—	—	280771
4	300800	5800	295000	575771	—	7557	—	—	—	—	583328
5	—	—	—	583328	—	7656	—	—	—	—	590985
6	—	—	—	590985	—	7757	6443	7757	14200	—	584541
7	—	—	—	584541	—	7672	6528	7672	14200	—	578013
8	—	—	—	578013	—	7586	6614	7586	14200	—	571400
9	—	—	—	571400	—	7500	6700	7500	14200	—	564699
10	215000	0	215000	779699	—	10234	3966	10234	14200	—	775733
11	—	—	—	775733	—	10181	4019	10181	14200	—	771714
12	—	—	—	771714	Received	10129	4071	10129	14200	99400	767643
13	—	—	—	767643	—	6348	5552	6348	11900	—	762091
14	—	—	—	762091	—	6275	5625	6275	11900	—	756466
15	—	—	—	756466	—	6201	5699	6201	11900	—	750767
16	—	—	—	750767	—	6126	5774	6126	11900	—	744993
17	—	—	—	744993	—	6051	5849	6051	11900	—	739144
18	—	—	—	739144	—	5974	5926	5974	11900	—	733218
19	—	—	—	733218	—	5896	6004	5896	11900	—	727214
20	—	—	—	727214	—	5817	6083	5817	11900	—	721131
21	—	—	—	721131	—	5737	6163	5737	11900	—	714968
22	—	—	—	714968	—	5656	6244	5656	11900	—	708725
23	—	—	—	708725	—	5575	6325	5575	11900	—	702399

Contd.

Month.	Investment	Promoter's contribution	DISB.	Loan amount	Subsidy provision	Interest (15.75%)	Principal	Interest	Instal lment	Total during the year	Outstanding
24	—	—	—	702399	—	5491	6409	5491	11900	142800	695991
25	—	—	—	695991	—	5407	5593	5407	11000	—	690398
26	—	—	—	690398	—	5334	5666	5334	11000	—	684732
27	—	—	—	684732	—	5260	5740	5260	11000	—	678992
28	—	—	—	678992	—	5184	5816	5184	11000	—	673176
29	—	—	—	673176	—	5108	5892	5108	11000	—	667284
30	—	—	—	667284	—	5031	5969	5031	11000	—	661314
31	—	—	—	661314	—	4952	6048	4952	11000	—	655267
32	—	—	—	655267	—	4873	6127	4873	11000	—	649140
33	—	—	—	649140	—	4792	6208	4792	11000	—	642932
34	—	—	—	642932	—	4711	6289	4711	11000	—	636643
35	—	—	—	636643	—	4628	6372	4628	11000	—	630271
36	—	—	—	630271	—	4545	6455	4545	11000	132000	623816
37	—	—	—	623816	—	4460	6540	4460	11000	—	617276
38	—	—	—	617276	—	4374	6626	4374	11000	—	610651
39	—	—	—	610651	—	4287	6713	4287	11000	—	603938
40	—	—	—	603938	—	4199	6801	4199	11000	—	597137
41	—	—	—	597137	—	4110	6890	4110	11000	—	590247
42	—	—	—	590247	—	4019	6981	4019	11000	—	583266
43	—	—	—	583266	—	3928	7072	3928	11000	—	576194
44	—	—	—	576194	—	3835	7165	3835	11000	—	569029
45	—	—	—	569029	—	3741	7259	3741	11000	—	561770
46	—	—	—	561770	—	3646	7354	3646	11000	—	554416
47	—	—	—	554416	—	3549	7451	3549	11000	—	546965
48	—	—	—	546965	—	3451	7549	3451	11000	132000	539417
49	—	—	—	539417	—	3352	9148	3352	12500	—	530269
50	—	—	—	530269	—	3232	9268	3232	12500	—	521001
51	—	—	—	521001	—	3111	9389	3111	12500	—	511612

Contd.

Month.	Investment	Promoter's contribution	DISB.	Loan amount	Subsidy provision	Interest (15.75%)	Principal	Interest	Instal lment	Total during the year	Outstanding
52	—	—	—	511612	—	2987	9513	2987	12500	—	502099
53	—	—	—	502099	—	2863	9637	2863	12500	—	492462
54	—	—	—	492462	—	2736	9764	2736	12500	—	482698
55	—	—	—	482698	—	2608	9892	2608	12500	—	472806
56	—	—	—	472806	—	2478	10022	2478	12500	—	462784
57	—	—	—	462784	—	2347	10153	2347	12500	—	452631
58	—	—	—	452631	—	2213	10287	2213	12500	—	442344
59	—	—	—	442344	—	2078	10422	2078	12500	—	431922
60	—	—	—	431922	—	1941	10559	1941	12500	150000	421364
61	—	—	—	421364	—	1803	10697	1803	12500	—	410667
62	—	—	—	410667	—	1662	10838	1662	12500	—	399829
63	—	—	—	399829	—	1520	10980	1520	12500	—	388849
64	—	—	—	388849	—	1376	11124	1376	12500	—	377725
65	—	—	—	377725	—	1230	11270	1230	12500	—	366456
66	—	—	—	366456	—	1082	11418	1082	12500	—	355038
67	—	—	—	355038	—	932	11568	932	12500	—	343470
68	—	—	—	343470	—	781	11719	781	12500	—	331751
69	—	—	—	331751	—	627	11873	627	12500	—	319877
70	—	—	—	319877	—	471	12029	471	12500	—	307848
71	—	—	—	307848	—	313	12187	313	12500	—	295661
72	—	—	—	295661	Adjusted	153	11661	153	11814	149314	NIL

X) Financial analysis of all resources

(Rs. in Thousands)

Yr	Fixed cost	Var. cost	Total cost	Total benefit	Net benefit	DF 15%	PWB 15%	PWC 15%	PWNB 15%	DF 50%	PWNB 50%
1.	861	389	1250	588	(662)	0.869	510.97	1086.25	(575.28)	0.667	(441.55)
2.		598	598	932	334	0.756	704.59	452.09	252.50	0.444	148.30
3.		589	589	898	309	0.658	590.88	387.56	203.32	0.296	91.46
4.		589	589	898	309	0.572	513.66	336.91	176.75	0.197	60.87
5.		607	607	967	360	0.497	480.60	301.68	178.92	0.132	47.52
6.		607	607	1174	567	0.432	507.17	262.22	244.94	0.088	49.90
						Σ	**3307.87**	**2826.71**	**481.16**		**(43.51)**

i. Benefit cost ratio (BCR) : 1.17:1

ii. NPW : Rs.4.81 lacs

iii. IRR (Internal Rate of Return) : 47.09%

IRR = Lower Discountrate + Differencein both thediscounting rate X NPW at lower discount rate / Absolute difference between theNPWs at both the discount rate

XI) Net Surplus & Debt Service Coverage Ratio (DSCR)

(Rupees)

Year	Income	Repayment	Net Surplus	DSCR
1	198940	99400	99540	1:2.00
2	334320	142800	191520	1:2.34
3	309480	132000	177480	1:2.34
4	309480	132000	177480	1:2.34
5	359160	150000	209160	1:2.39
6	359160	149314	209846	1:2.41
			Average Gross DSCR:	1:2.32

18

Techno – Economic Study of Dairy Farm (5+5 Crossbred UNIT)

Name of the proprietor : XYZ

Address : ABC

Financing Bank : PNB

Project profile : Dairy Farm (5+5 cows)

Project Cost : Rs.4, 99,000/=

Bank Loan : Rs.4, 00,000/= (80.16%)

Margin Money : Rs.99,000/= (19.84%)

Subsidy : Rs.1, 15,300/=

Interest Rate : Provisional Interest rate @ 14.50% p.a. has been taken for evaluation of the project report. However, the sanctioning authority may consider the exact rate of interest applicable, on the date of sanction. Development of farm should be completed within 3 months from first disbursement.

Repayment of loan : A five-year repayment programme has been drawn with six months moratorium period, the installments will be monthly starting from 6th month onwards. The applicant has to make tie-up with the local MPCS and the repayment should be routed through the MPCS.

Techno-Economic Feasibility: The proposal is examined techno-economically and the different worksheets attached with this report. The financial viability has also been examined by discounted cash flow which shows I.R.R – 31.58%, NPW – Rs.111760, BCR – 1.09:1.00 and Average Gross D.S.C.R. – 1.00:2.00. In light of the above study, the project may be considered technically feasible and financially viable.

I) Detail Project Cost

Capital cost:-

	Particulars		Unit cost	Total (in Rs.)
i.	Cow shed (10 cows)	40 sqf/ cow	@Rs. 180/sqf	72000
ii.	Shed for heifer (5)	30 sqf/heifer	@Rs. 180/sqf	27000
iii.	Shed for calves (10 calves)	20 sqf/ calf	@Rs. 180/sqf	36000
iv.	Sick animal shed	100 sqf	@Rs. 180/sqf	18000
v.	Store room	150 sqf	@Rs. 200/sqf	30000
vi.	Electrification		LS	10000
vii.	Ceiling Fan	5	LS	7500
viii.	Equipments		@Rs.500/cow	5000
ix.	Fodder cultivation	2.0 acre	@Rs.5000/acre	10000
x.	Water supply system		LS	30000
xi.	Cost of cows	10	@Rs.20000/cow	200000
xii.	Transportation cost	10 cows	@Rs.500/cow	5000
xiii.	Insurance	10	@ 5.5%	11000
A	**Sub- total**			**Rs.461500**

Working capital (for three months for 1st Batch):-

i	Feed cost for first batch	@Rs.77/cow/day	34500
ii	Vety. aid @ Rs.1200/animal / year		1500
iii	Electricity charges @ Rs.500/ month		1500
B	**Sub total**		**Rs. 37500**
C	**Total Project cost**		**Rs.499000**
	Margin (19.70%)		**Rs.99000**
	Bank Loan		**Rs.400000**

Techno Economic Assumptions

i. Lactation period – 280days

ii. Dry period – 120days

iii. Days in year taken as – 360days

iv. The farmer will take 3 months (90 days) for completion of construction of sheds.

v. Lactation period lapsed with seller – 30days

vi. Average milk production - 10 litters per cow per day during lactation period

vii. Selling price of milk - Rs.16 / litter

viii. Selling price of manure - Rs.500 / cow / year

ix. Price of Concentrate feed - Rs.12/kg

x. Price of dry fodder - Rs.1.00/kg

xi. Selling price of gunny bags - Rs.15 / bag (50 kg)

xii. Male Female ratio (Calf) - 1:1 (5+5)

xiii. Profit from sale of 3 male calves is Rs.0/ animal after deduction of cost incurred on their rearing.

xiv. Heifer sold 5 nos. /year.

xv. Profit from sale of heifer is Rs.8000/ animal after deduction of cost incurred on their rearing.

Feeding cost / day (for one animal)

	Particulars	Rate	LP (Rs.)	DP (Rs.)
a	Green fodder @25kg during lactation & @ 20kg during dry period	To be produced from own farm	0.00	0.00
b	Dry fodder @5kg & 6kg during LP & DP respectively	@Rs.100/Qt.	5.00	6.00
c	Concentrate feed @6.00kg & 2.00kg during LP & DP respectively	@Rs.12/kg	72.00	24.00
	Total		**Rs.77.00**	**Rs.30.00**

Milk flow chart

Year	1st batch (single animal)		2nd batch(single animal)		(2 animal)		Total(10 animal)		Total Milk production	Total sale value
	LP	DP	LP	DP	LP	DP	LP	DP	@10 lt. /cow	@Rs.16/lt.
1st	250	20	90	—	340	20	1700	100	17000 ltr	Rs.272000
2nd	260	100	240	120	500	220	2500	1100	25000 ltr	Rs.400000
3rd	240	120	240	120	480	240	2400	1200	24000 ltr	Rs.384000
4th	240	120	240	120	480	240	2400	1200	24000 ltr	Rs.384000
5th	240	120	280	80	520	200	2600	1000	26000 ltr	Rs.416000

Year wise Income – Expenditure Analysis (Rupees)

Particulars		1st YR.	2nd YR.	3rd YR.	4th YR.	5th YR.
Income						
i	Sale of milk	272000	400000	384000	384000	416000
ii	Sale of manure	2500	5000	5000	5000	5000
iii	Sale of gunny bags	3120	5160	5040	5040	5280
iv	Sale of heifer	0	40000	40000	40000	40000
A	Total	277620	450160	434040	434040	466280
Expenditure						
i	Feed	133900	225500	220800	220800	230200
ii	Insurance	11000	11000	11000	11000	11000
iii	Veterinary aid	9000	12000	12000	12000	12000
iv	Electricity	6000	6000	6000	6000	6000
v	Fodder cultivation	10000	10000	10000	10000	10000
B	Total	169900	264500	259800	259800	269200
C	Gross Profit (A-B)	107720	185660	174240	174240	197080
D	Interest on loan	44077	36221	27885	18720	7345
E	Net Profit (C-D)	63643	149439	146355	155520	189735
F	Cash Accrual (E+D)	107720	185660	174240	174240	197080
G	Repayment	53900	92400	87000	87000	98646
H	DSCR (G:F)	1:2.00	1:2.01	1:2.00	1:2.00	1:2.00

Repayment Schedule:

(Rupees)

Month.	Investment	margin	DISB.	Loan amount	Subsidy provision	Interest (14.50%)	Principal	Interest	Installment	Total during the year	Outstanding
							<<<<<<REPAYMENT>>>>>>				
0	245500	55500	190000	190000	115300	—	—	—	—	—	190000
1	—	—	—	190000	—	2296	—	—	—	—	192296
2	—	—	—	192296	—	2324	—	—	—	—	194619
3	—	—	—	194619	—	2352	—	—	—	—	196971
4	145500	30500	115000	311971	—	3770	—	—	—	—	315741
5	—	—	—	315741	—	3815	—	—	—	—	319556
6	—	—	—	319556	—	3861	3839	3861	7700	—	315717
7	—	—	—	315717	—	3815	3885	3815	7700	—	311832
8	—	—	—	311832	—	3768	3932	3768	7700	—	307900
9	—	—	—	307900	—	3720	3980	3720	7700	—	303921
10	108000	13000	95000	398921	—	4820	2880	4820	7700	—	396041
11	—	—	—	396041	—	4785	2915	4785	7700	—	393126
12	—	—	—	393126	Recd.	4750	2950	4750	7700	53900	390177
13	—	—	—	390177	—	3321	4379	3321	7700	—	385798
14	—	—	—	385798	—	3269	4431	3269	7700	—	381367
15	—	—	—	381367	—	3215	4485	3215	7700	—	376882
16	—	—	—	376882	—	3161	4539	3161	7700	—	372342
17	—	—	—	372342	—	3106	4594	3106	7700	—	367748
18	—	—	—	367748	—	3050	4650	3050	7700	—	363099
19	—	—	—	363099	—	2994	4706	2994	7700	—	358393
20	—	—	—	358393	—	2937	4763	2937	7700	—	353630

Month.	Investment	margin	DISB.	Loan amount	Subsidy provision	Interest (14.50%)	Principal	Interest	Installment	Total during the year	Outstanding
21	—	—	—	353630	—	2880	4820	2880	7700	—	348810
22	—	—	—	348810	—	2822	4878	2822	7700	—	343932
23	—	—	—	343932	—	2763	4937	2763	7700	—	338994
24	—	—	—	338994	—	2703	4997	2703	7700	92400	333997
25	—	—	—	333997	—	2643	4607	2643	7250	—	329390
26	—	—	—	329390	—	2587	4663	2587	7250	—	324727
27	—	—	—	324727	—	2531	4719	2531	7250	—	320007
28	—	—	—	320007	—	2474	4776	2474	7250	—	315231
29	—	—	—	315231	—	2416	4834	2416	7250	—	310397
30	—	—	—	310397	—	2357	4893	2357	7250	—	305504
31	—	—	—	305504	—	2298	4952	2298	7250	—	300552
32	—	—	—	300552	—	2238	5012	2238	7250	—	295541
33	—	—	—	295541	—	2178	5072	2178	7250	—	290469
34	—	—	—	290469	—	2117	5133	2117	7250	—	285335
35	—	—	—	285335	—	2055	5195	2055	7250	—	280140
36	—	—	—	280140	—	1992	5258	1992	7250	87000	274882
37	—	—	—	274882	—	1928	5322	1928	7250	—	269560
38	—	—	—	269560	—	1864	5386	1864	7250	—	264174
39	—	—	—	264174	—	1799	5451	1799	7250	—	258723
40	—	—	—	258723	—	1733	5517	1733	7250	—	253206
41	—	—	—	253206	—	1666	5584	1666	7250	—	247622
42	—	—	—	247622	—	1599	5651	1599	7250	—	241971
43	—	—	—	241971	—	1531	5719	1531	7250	—	236252
44	—	—	—	236252	—	1462	5788	1462	7250	—	230463

Month.	Investment	margin	DISB.	Loan amount	Subsidy provision	Interest (14.50%)	Principal	Interest	Installment	Total during the year	Outstanding
45	—	—	—	230463	—	1392	5858	1392	7250	—	224605
46	—	—	—	224605	—	1321	5929	1321	7250	—	218676
47	—	—	—	218676	—	1249	6001	1249	7250	—	212675
48	—	—	—	212675	—	1177	6073	1177	7250	87000	206601
49	—	—	—	206601	—	1103	7097	1103	8200	—	199505
50	—	—	—	199505	—	1017	7183	1017	8200	—	192322
51	—	—	—	192322	—	931	7269	931	8200	—	185053
52	—	—	—	185053	—	843	7357	843	8200	—	177696
53	—	—	—	177696	—	754	7446	754	8200	—	170250
54	—	—	—	170250	—	664	7536	664	8200	—	162714
55	—	—	—	162714	—	573	7627	573	8200	—	155087
56	—	—	—	155087	—	481	7719	481	8200	—	147367
57	—	—	—	147367	—	387	7813	387	8200	—	139555
58	—	—	—	139555	—	293	7907	293	8200	—	131648
59	—	—	—	131648	—	198	8002	198	8200	—	123645
60	—	—	—	123645	Adj.	101	8345	101	8446	98646	NIL

Net Surplus & Debt Service Coverage Ratio (DSCR)

(Rupees)

Year	Income	Repayment	Net Surplus	DSCR
1	107720	53900	53820	1:2.00
2	185660	92400	93260	1:2.01
3	174240	87000	87240	1:2.00
4	174240	87000	87240	1:2.00
5	197080	98646	98434	1:2.00
			Average Gross DSCR	1:2.00

Financial analysis of all resources

(Rupees in 000)

Yr	Fixed cost	Var. cost	Total cost	Total ben.	Net ben.	DF 15%	PWB 15%	PWC 15%	PWNB 15%	DF 50%	PWNB 50%
0	246	0	246	0	(246)	1.000	0.00	246.00	(246.00)	1.000	(246.00)
1	216	170	386	278	(108)	0.869	241.58	335.43	(93.85)	0.667	(72.04)
2		265	265	450	185	0.756	340.20	200.34	139.86	0.444	82.14
3		260	260	434	174	0.657	285.14	170.82	114.32	0.296	51.50
4		260	260	434	174	0.572	248.25	148.72	99.53	0.197	34.28
5		269	269	466	197	0.497	231.60	133.69	97.91	0.132	26.00
						Σ	**1346.77**	**1235.01**	**111.76**		**(124.11)**

i. Benefit cost ratio (BCR) : 1.09
ii. IRR : 31.58%
iii. PWNB : Rs.111760/-

C) Scheme for Financing (1+1) CB Jersey Cows to General Farmers

Project Cost-

Capital cost:-

	Particulars		Unit cost	Total (in Rs.)
i.	Cow shed (2 cows)	40 sqf/ cow	@Rs. 180/sqf	14400
ii.	Shed for heifer (1)	30 sqf/heifer	@Rs. 180/sqf	5400
iii.	Shed for calves (2 calves)	20 sqf/ calf	@Rs. 180/sqf	7200
iv.	Electrification		LS	2000
v.	Ceiling Fan	1	LS	1500
vi.	Equipments		@Rs.500/cow	1000
vii.	Fodder cultivation	0.4 acre	@Rs.5000/acre	2000
viii.	Water supply system		LS	15000
ix.	Cost of cows	2	@Rs.20000/cow	40000
x.	Transportation cost	2 cows	@Rs.500/cow	1000
xi.	Insurance	2	@ 5.5%	2200
A.	**Sub total**			**Rs.91700**

Working capital (for three months for 1st Batch)

i.	Feed cost for first batch	@Rs.77/cow/day	6930
ii.	Vety. aid @ Rs.1200/animal / year		300
iii.	Electricity charges @ Rs.200/ month		600
B.	**Sub total**		**Rs. 7830**
C.	**Total Project cost**		**Rs.99530**
	Margin (19.6%)		**Rs.19530**
	Bank Loan		**Rs.80000**

- Rate of interest : @ 13.25% per annum
- Repayment period : 60 months including six months grace
- Repayment schedule : Monthly starting from 6th month onwards
- Subsidy : Rs.22900/=

Techno Economic Assumptions

i. Lactation period – 280 days

ii. Dry period – 120 days

iii. Days in year taken as – 360 days

iv. The farmer will take 3 months (90 days) for completion of construction of sheds.

v. Lactation period lapsed with seller – 30 days

vi. Average milk production - 10 litters per cow per day during lactation period

vii. Selling price of milk - Rs.16 / litter

viii. Selling price of manure - Rs.500 / cow / year

ix. Price of Concentrate feed - Rs.12/kg

x. Price of dry fodder - Rs.1.00/kg

xi. Selling price of gunny bags - Rs.15 / bag (50 kg)

xii. Male Female ratio (Calf) - 1:1 (1+1)

xiii. Profit from sale of 1 male calves is Rs.0/ animal after deduction of cost incurred on their rearing.

xiv. Heifer sold 1 no. /year.

xv. Profit from sale of heifer is Rs.8000/ animal after deduction of cost incurred on their rearing.

Feeding cost / day (for one animal)

Particulars	Rate	LP (Rs.)	DP (Rs.)
a. Green fodder @25kg during lactation & @ 20kg during dry period	To be produced from own farm	0.00	0.00
b. Dry fodder @5kg & 6kg during LP & DP respectively	@Rs.100/Qt.	5.00	6.00
c. Concentrate feed @6.00kg & 2.00kg during LP & DP respectively	@Rs.12/kg	72.00	24.00
Total		**Rs.77.00**	**Rs.30.00**

Milk flow chart

Year	1st batch (single animal)		2nd batch (single animal)		Total (2 animal)		Total Milk production	Total sale value
	LP	DP	LP	DP	LP	DP	@10 lt. /cow	@Rs.16/lt.
1st	250	20	90	—	340	20	3400 ltrs	Rs.54400
2nd	260	100	240	120	500	220	5000 ltrs	Rs.80000
3rd	240	120	240	120	480	240	4800 ltrs	Rs.76800
4th	240	120	240	120	480	240	4800 ltrs	Rs.76800
5th	240	120	280	80	520	200	5200 ltrs	Rs.83200

Yearwise Income – Expenditure Analysis (Rupees)

Particulars	1st YR.	2nd YR.	3rd YR.	4th YR.	5th YR.
Income					
i. Sale of milk	54400	80000	76800	76800	83200
ii. Sale of manure	500	1000	1000	1000	1000
iii. Sale of gunny bags	624	1032	1008	1008	1056
iv. Sale of heifer	0	8000	8000	8000	8000
A. Total	55524	90032	86808	86808	93256
Expenditure					
i. Feed	26780	45100	44160	44160	46040
ii. Insurance	2200	2200	2200	2200	2200
iii. Veterinary aid	1800	2400	2400	2400	2400
iv. Electricity	2400	2400	2400	2400	2400
v. Fodder cultivation	2000	2000	2000	2000	2000
B. Total	35180	54100	53160	53160	55040
C. Gross Profit (A-B)	20344	35932	33648	33648	38216
D. Interest on loan	8037	6593	5045	3373	1321
E. Net Profit (C-D)	12307	29339	28603	30275	36895
F. Cash Accrual (E+D)	20344	35932	33648	33648	38216
G. Repayment	10220	18120	16920	16920	19288
H. DSCR (G:F)	1:1.99	1:1.98	1:1.99	1:1.99	1:1.98

Net Surplus & Debt Service Coverage Ratio (DSCR)

(Rupees)

Year	Income	Repayment	Net Surplus	DSCR
1.	20344	10220	10124	1:1.99
2.	35932	18120	17812	1:1.98
3.	33648	16920	16728	1:1.99
4.	33648	16920	16728	1:1.99
5.	38216	19288	18928	1:1.98
			Average Gross DSCR	1:1.99

Financial analysis of all resources

(Rupees in 000)

Yr	Fixed cost	Var. cost	Total cost	Total ben.	Net ben.	DF 15%	PWB 15%	PWC 15%	PWNB 15%	DF 50%	PWNB 50%
0	49	0	49	0	(49)	1.000	0.00	49.00	(49.00)	1.000	(49.00)
1	43	35	78	56	(22)	0.869	48.66	67.78	(19.12)	0.667	(14.67)
2		54	54	90	36	0.756	68.04	40.82	27.22	0.444	15.98
3		53	53	87	34	0.657	57.16	34.82	22.34	0.296	10.06
4		53	53	87	34	0.572	49.76	30.32	19.45	0.197	6.70
5		55	55	93	38	0.497	46.22	27.34	18.89	0.132	5.02
						“	**269.85**	**250.08**	**19.77**		**(25.91)**

Repayment Schedule:

(Rupees)

Month.	Investment	margin	DISB.	Loan amount	Subsidy provision	Interest (13.25%)	Principal	Interest	Installment	Total during the year	Outstanding
							<<<<<<REPAYMENT>>>>>>				
0	48500	8500	40000	40000	22900	—	—	—	—	—	40000
1	—	—	—	40000	—	442	—	—	—	—	40442
2	—	—	—	40442	—	447	—	—	—	—	40888
3	—	—	—	40888	—	451	—	—	—	—	41340
4	29430	9430	20000	61340	—	677	—	—	—	—	62017
5	—	—	—	62017	—	685	—	—	—	—	62702
6	—	—	—	62702	—	692	768	692	1460	—	61934
7	—	—	—	61934	—	684	776	684	1460	—	61158
8	—	—	—	61158	—	675	785	675	1460	—	60373
9	—	—	—	60373	—	667	793	667	1460	—	59580
10	21600	1600	20000	79580	—	879	581	879	1460	—	78999
11	—	—	—	78999	—	872	588	872	1460	—	78411
12	—	—	—	78411	Recd.	866	594	866	1460	10220	77817
13	—	—	—	77817	—	606	904	606	1510	—	76913
14	—	—	—	76913	—	596	914	596	1510	—	75999
15	—	—	—	75999	—	586	924	586	1510	—	75076
16	—	—	—	75076	—	576	934	576	1510	—	74142
17	—	—	—	74142	—	566	944	566	1510	—	73198
18	—	—	—	73198	—	555	955	555	1510	—	72243
19	—	—	—	72243	—	545	965	545	1510	—	71278
20	—	—	—	71278	—	534	976	534	1510	—	70302

Month.	Investment	margin	DISB.	Loan amount	Subsidy provision	Interest (13.25%)	Principal	Interest	Installment	Total during the year	Outstanding
21	—	—	—	70302	—	523	987	523	1510	—	69315
22	—	—	—	69315	—	513	997	513	1510	—	68318
23	—	—	—	68318	—	501	1009	501	1510	—	67309
24	—	—	—	67309	—	490	1020	490	1510	18120	66290
25	—	—	—	66290	—	479	931	479	1410	—	65359
26	—	—	—	65359	—	469	941	469	1410	—	64418
27	—	—	—	64418	—	458	952	458	1410	—	63466
28	—	—	—	63466	—	448	962	448	1410	—	62504
29	—	—	—	62504	—	437	973	437	1410	—	61531
30	—	—	—	61531	—	427	983	427	1410	—	60548
31	—	—	—	60548	—	416	994	416	1410	—	59553
32	—	—	—	59553	—	405	1005	405	1410	—	58548
33	—	—	—	58548	—	394	1016	394	1410	—	57532
34	—	—	—	57532	—	382	1028	382	1410	—	56504
35	—	—	—	56504	—	371	1039	371	1410	—	55465
36	—	—	—	55465	—	360	1050	360	1410	16920	54415
37	—	—	—	54415	—	348	1062	348	1410	—	53353
38	—	—	—	53353	—	336	1074	336	1410	—	52279
39	—	—	—	52279	—	324	1086	324	1410	—	51193
40	—	—	—	51193	—	312	1098	312	1410	—	50096
41	—	—	—	50096	—	300	1110	300	1410	—	48986
42	—	—	—	48986	—	288	1122	288	1410	—	47864
43	—	—	—	47864	—	276	1134	276	1410	—	46730
44	—	—	—	46730	—	263	1147	263	1410	—	45583

Month.	Investment	margin	DISB.	Loan amount	Subsidy provision	Interest (13.25%)	Principal	Interest	Installment	Total during the year	Outstanding
45	—	—	—	45583	—	250	1160	250	1410	—	44423
46	—	—	—	44423	—	238	1172	238	1410	—	43251
47	—	—	—	43251	—	225	1185	225	1410	—	42066
48	—	—	—	42066	—	212	1198	212	1410	16920	40867
49	—	—	—	40867	—	198	1402	198	1600	—	39466
50	—	—	—	39466	—	183	1417	183	1600	—	38049
51	—	—	—	38049	—	167	1433	167	1600	—	36616
52	—	—	—	36616	—	151	1449	151	1600	—	35167
53	—	—	—	35167	—	135	1465	135	1600	—	33703
54	—	—	—	33703	—	119	1481	119	1600	—	32222
55	—	—	—	32222	—	103	1497	103	1600	—	30725
56	—	—	—	30725	—	86	1514	86	1600	—	29211
57	—	—	—	29211	—	70	1530	70	1600	—	27681
58	—	—	—	27681	—	53	1547	53	1600	—	26134
59	—	—	—	26134	—	36	1564	36	1600	—	24570
60	—	—	—	24570	Adj.	18	1670	18	1688	19288	NIL

i. Benefit cost ratio (BCR) : 1.08
ii. Average DSCR : 1:1.99
iii. IRR : 30.15%
iv. PWNB : Rs.19770/-

Section B: Dairy Husbandry Information & Practices for Dairy Entrepreneurs

19

Breeds of Dairy Cattle and Buffaloes

A) Selection of Dairy Cattle

Proper selection is the first and the most important step to be adopted in dairying. Records are the basis of selection and hence proper identification of animals and record keeping is essential. Cross-breed animals with exotic inheritance of about 50 percent are preferable.

Bringing animals from different agro-climatic conditions causes problems due to non-adjustment in many cases. In case, purchase becomes absolutely essential it should be from similar environmental conditions as far as possible.

General selection procedures for dairy breeds

Selecting a calf in calf show, a cow in cattle show by judging is an art. A dairy farmer should build up his own herd by breeding his own herd. Following guidelines will be useful for selection of a dairy cow.

- Whenever an animal is purchased from cattle fair, it should be selected based upon its breed characters and milk producing ability.
- History sheet or pedigree sheet which is generally maintained in organized farms reveals the complete history of animal.
- The maximum yields by dairy cows are noticed during the first five lactations. So generally selection should be carried out during First or Second lactation and that too are month after calving.
- There successive complete milking has to be done and an average of it will give a fair idea regarding production by a particular animal.
- A cow should allow anybody to milk, and should be docile.
- It is better to purchase the animals during the months of October and November.
- Maximum yield is noticed till 90 days after calving.

Breed characteristics of high yielding dairy cows

- Attractive individuality with feminity, vigor, harmonious blending of all parts, impressive style and carriage.
- Animal should have wedge shaped appearance of the body.
- It should have bright **eyes** with lean neck.
- The udder should be well attached to the abdomen.
- The skin of the udder should have a good network of blood vessels.
- All four quarters of the udder should be well demarcated with well placed teats.

Selecting breeds for Commercial Dairy Farm – Suggestions

- Under Indian condition a commercial dairy farm should consist of minimum 20 animals (10 cows, 10 buffaloes) this strength can easily go up to 100 animals in proportion of 50:50 or 40:60. After this however, you need to review your strength and market potential before you chose to go for expansion.
- Middle class health-Conscious Indian families prefer low fat milk for consumption as liquid milk. It is always better to go for a commercial farm of mixed type. (Cross breed, cows and buffaloes kept in separate rows under one shed).
- Conduct a thorough study of the immediate market where you are planning to market your milk You can mix milk from both type of animals and sold as per need of the market. Hotels and some general customers (can be around 30%) prefer pure buffalo milk. Hospitals, sanitariums prefer cow's milk.

Selection of cow breeds for commercial farm

- Good quality cows are available in the market and it cost around Rs.2500 to Rs.3000 per liter of milk production per day. (E.g. Cost of a cow producing 10 liter of Milk per day will be between Rs.25000 to Rs.30,000).
- If proper care is given, cows breed regularly giving one calf every 13-14 month interval.
- They are more docile and can be handled easily. Good milk yielding cross breeds (Holstein and Jersey crosses) has well adapted to Indian climate.
- The fat percentage of cow's milk varies from 3-5.5% and is lower than Buffaloes.

b) Economic Characters in Dairy Cattle and Buffalo

The various economic characters in Dairy Cattle and Buffalo management are:

1. Lactation yield
2. Lactation period
3. Persistency of yield
4. Age at first calving
5. Service period
6. Dry period
7. Inter calving period
8. Reproductive efficiency
9. Efficiency of feed utilization
10. Disease resistance.

1. **Lactation yield:** The lactation yield in a lactation period is known as lactation yield. 'The lactation yield in Indian breeds is very low compared to exotic breeds. Normally in dairy cattle 30 - 40 % increase in milk production from first lactation to maturity is observed. After 3 or 4 lactation the production starts declining.

   After parturition the milk yield per day will be increased and reaches peak within 2-4 weeks after calving. This yield is known as peak yield. The maintenance of peak yield for more time is importance for better milk production.

2. **Lactation period:** The length of milk producing period after calving is known as lactation period. The optimum lactation period is 305 days. The milk production will be less, if this period is shortened. Indian breeds will have less lactation period, but in some breeds this period is more with very little milk production.

3. **Persistency of Milk Yield:** During lactation period the animal reaches maximum milk yield per day within 2-4 weeks which is called peak yield. For high level of lactation yield, this peak yield should be maintained for longer period as far as possible. The maintenance of peak yield for long period is known as persistency, slow decrease in dairy milk yield after reaching peak yield in necessary. High persistency is necessary to maintain high level of milk production.

4. **Age at first calving:** The desirable age at first calving in Indian breeds is 3 years, 2 years in cross breed cattle and 3½ years in Buffaloes. Prolonged age at first calving will have high production in the first lactation but the life time production will be decreased due to less no. of calvings. If the age at first calving is below optimum, the calves born are weak, difficulty in calving and less milk production in first lactation.

5. **Service period:** It is the period between date of calving and date of successful conception. For cattle the optimum service period is 60-90 days. If the service period is too prolonged the calving interval prolonged, less number of calves will be obtained in her life time and ultimately less life time production. If the service period is too short, the animal will become weak and persistency of milk production is poor due to immediate pregnancy.

6. **Dry period:** It is the period from the date of drying (stop of milk production) to next calving. The animal should be given rest period to compensate for growth of fetus. A minimum of 2 - 2½ months dry period should be allowed. If suitable dry period is not given, or too low dry period, the animals suffer from stress and in next lactation, the milk production drops substantially and also it gives weak calves. On the other hand if the dry period given is too high, it may not have that much effect on increasing milk yield in the next lactation, but it decrease the production in the present lactation.

7. **Inter-calving period:** This is the period between two successive calvings. It is more, profitable to have one calf yearly in cattle and at least one calf for every 15 months in buffaloes. If the calving interval is more, the total no. of carvings in the life time will be decreased and also total life production of milk decrease.

8. **Reproductive Efficiency:** The reproductive efficiency means the more number of calves during life time, so that total life time production is increased. The reproduction or breeding efficiency is determined by the combined effect of hereditary and environment. Several measures of breeding efficiency like number of services per conception, calving interval days from first breeding to conception are useful.

9. **Efficiency of Feed Utilization and Conversion into Milk:** The animal should utilize the feed efficiently to convert into the milk.

10. **Disease Resistance:** Indian breeds are more resistant to majority of disease compared to exotic cattle. Cross breeding helps to get this character.

C) Breeds

Breeds of Indigenous Cattle

SAHIWAL

Sahiwal is a breed of Zebu cattle which primarily is used in dairy production. Sahiwal originated from the Sahiwal district of Punjab province in Pakistan. They produce the most milk of all zebu breeds, followed by the very similar Red Sindhi and Butana breeds.

The Sahiwal originated in the dry Punjab region i.e. central and southern regions, which lies along the Indian-Pakistani border. They were once kept in large herds by professional herdsmen called "Junglies". With the introduction of irrigation systems to the region they began to be kept in smaller numbers by the farmers of the region, who used them as draught and dairy animals. Today, Sahiwal is one of the best dairy breeds in India and Pakistan. Due to their heat tolerance and high milk production they have been exported to other Asian countries as well as Africa and the Caribbean.

General Information

1. **Species:** Cattle
2. **Synonyms**: Lambi Bar, Lola, Montgomery, Multani and Teli.
3. **Habitat:** Sahiwal cattle lives in parts of districts Sahiwal, Okara, Pakpattan, Multan, and Faisalabad in Punjab, Pakistan and Ferozepur belt of Punjab, India especially the Fazilka and Abohar towns, Rohtak, Karnal, Hissar, Gurgaon district of Haryana, and the Union Territory of Delhi and in West Uttar Pradesh.
4. **Breeding tract:** Ferozepur and Amritsar districts of Punjab, Sri Ganganagar district if Rajasthan, pedigree herds are also maintained at Uttar Pradesh, Delhi, Bihar, Madhya Pradesh.
5. **Soil and Climate:** The area is sandy, except along the river banks (Sutlej and Ravi) and portions watered by the canals where silt has accumulated. Sandy loam and loam soils are predominant. The whole area is undulating plain. A very large portion of the land is under canal irrigation. The average rainfall of the area is about 25 to 30 cm with an average number of 23 rainy days from April to October and 8 rainy days during the rest of the year. The heat of the summer is severe; the maximum temperature may go as high as 48°C. Winters are mild and -pleasant.
6. **Main utility:** Milk for food.

7. **Origin:** Sahiwal area of Montgomery district of Punjab, Pakistan.
8. **Distribution:** The contribution of the Sahiwal breed to adaptability is well documented in Kenya, Jamaica, Guyana, Burundi, Somalia, Sierra Leone, Nigeria and several ecological zones of Africa. Due to its unique characteristics, Sahiwal breed is exported to wide list of countries and regions. The Sahiwal breed arrived in Australia via New Guinea in the early 1950s. In Australia, the Sahiwal breed was initially selected as a dual-purpose breed. It played a valuable role in the development of the two Australian tropical dairy breeds, the Australian Milking Zebu and the Australian Friesian Sahiwal.

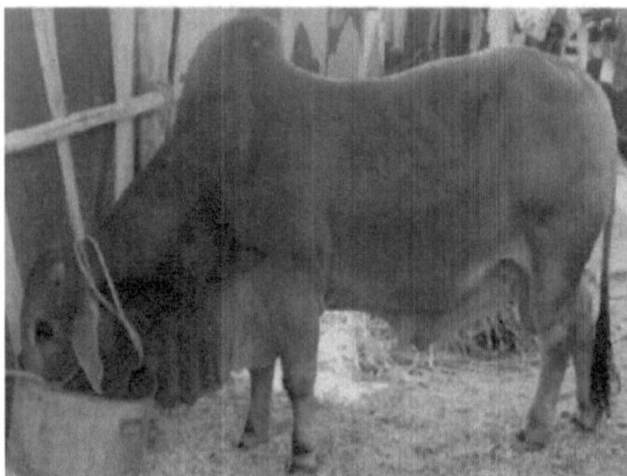

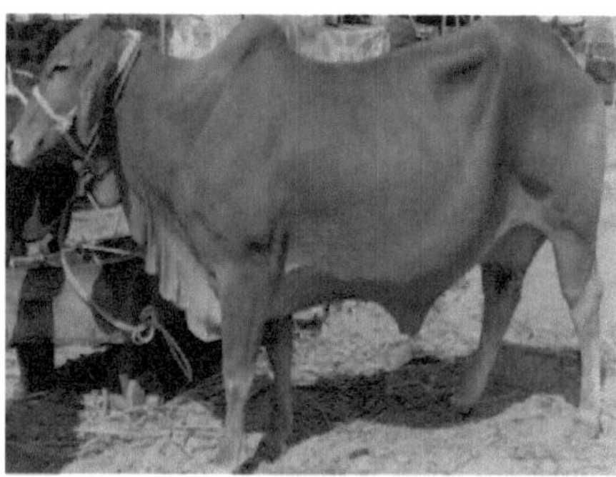

Sahiwal Bull Sahiwal Cattle

Phenotypic traits

1. **Color:** Brownish red color, shades may vary from a mahogany red brown to more greyish red. Extremities in bulls are darker than rest of body color.Occasionally there are white patches.
2. **Number of Horns:** 2
3. **Shape of Horns:** Horns are stumpy and short to medium running outwards, upwards and then inwards.
4. **Visible characteristics:** Pale red color, short horns and loose skin (Lola).

	Male	Female
5. Height (Avg. cm)	170	124
6. Body length (Avg. cm)	150	131
7. Heart Girth (Avg. cm)	190	164
8. Weight (Avg. Kg)	540	327
9. Birth Weight (Avg. Kg)	22.4	20.7
10. Length (Avg. cm)	166	140

Physical Characteristics

1. **Body:** This breed is medium-sized, and has a fleshy body.
2. **Color:** Females have reddish dun color; males may have a darker color around the orbit, neck, and hindquarters.
3. **Horns:** Males have stumpy horns; females are often dehorned.
4. **Ears:** Ears are medium-sized and drooping.
5. **Muzzle and eyes:** The distinguishing feature between Sahiwal and Red Sindhi is the muzzle. Red Sindhi has dark color muzzle whereas Sahiwal has lighter color muzzle. Sahiwal has also whitish ring along the eye. Muzzle and eye-lashes are of lighter color.
6. **Skin:** Skin is loose and fine with a voluminous dewlap and sheath.
7. **Hump:** The hump in the male is massive and falls on one side, but in the female it is nominal.
8. **Tail:** The tail ends in a black switch reaching almost ground.
9. **Udder:** The udder is large and strong and occasionally has white patches.
10. This is tick resistant breed because its skin naturally keeps on shivering.
11. This breed involved in development of new cattle breed Jamaica Hope.

Management

1. **Management System:** Semi-Intensive
2. **Mobility:** Stationary
3. **Feeding of adults:** Grazing, Fodder and Concentrate
4. **Housing:** kept loose in open area, housing not required for adults, bush enclosures for calves.
5. **Feeding system:** Animals are let loose for grazing, seldom stall fed.
6. **Feeds to be fed:** Berseem, oats and mustard are the green fodder in rabi; and sorghum, pearl millet and cluster bean in kharif. Commercial feed can be fed anytime of the year. . Milking cows are provided supplementary feeding in the form of cotton seed, barley and oil cake. Feed is given in soaked form at the time of milking. Calves are reared on whole milk up to 1 month of age after which some green fodder is also fed. Calves are allowed to suck 1-2 teats up to 6 months of age.
7. **Feeding of concentrates:** 1kg/2kg milk at the time of milking.

8. **Feeding of roughages:** 1/10th of body weight per day.
9. **Milking:** should be done twice a day, however thrice a day milking gives higher milk yield.
10. **Milking practice:** full hand milking should be done. Avoid knuckling.
11. **Milk let down time:** 4-5 minutes.

Performance traits

	Average	Minimum	Maximum
Age at first calving (Avg. months)	41.7	30	50
Calving interval (months)	15.6	13	18
Lactation length (days)	-	282	305
Milk yield per lactation (kg)	2325	1600	2750
Milk fat (%)	4.9	4.8	5.1
Daily lactation in peak period (kg)	8.33	6.23	32.3 (Record)
Dry period (days)	59	55	69

- **Peculiarity of the breed:** It is tick-resistant, heat-tolerant and noted for its high resistance to parasites, both internal and external, ease of calving, drought resistant, bloat tolerant, good temperament.
- **Research highlights:** All the productive and reproductive traits were affected by herd, year, season of calving and parity. The phenotypic correlations among various performance traits have also been reported. Phenotypic deterioration in milk yield was noted over the years.

Major problems associated with health of Sahiwal cattle

Being indigenous, Sahiwal is very hardy and disease resistant breed. However, the production performance decreases when the animal is exposed to environmental and dietary stressors. Therefore, management of the cattle is utmost important in prolonging and promoting the health status.

Price range

Rs. 30,000/- to Rs. 1,50,000/- (tentative)

For further details please see the following link

http://210.212.93.85/agris/breed.aspx

Can be purchased from

1. **Gupta Dairy Farm**: Address; plot No. 41-42, Govind Colony, near water tank, Doon Valley College Road, Jundla Gate, Karnal-132001, Haryana. Phone no. 09416031427.

   Website: www.guptadairyfarm.com, email: guptadairyfarm@gmail.com
2. **Khurana Dairy Farm**, Rohtak, Haryana. Mobile Number : +91-9215450001 / 9215430001 / 9215450003
3. **Model Dairy Farm:** Mr. Prateek Vaish (VP-Operations). Address: Naramau, GT Road, near ALIMCO, Kanpur-209217, UP.
4. **Khalsa Dairy Farm,** Karnal, Haryana. Owner: Sham Singh, Mobile No. **09896603975.**
5. **Chopra Dairy Farm,** Nawashahr, Ludhiana, Punjab, Mobile No. **09592454093.**

RED SINDHI

Red Sindhi cattle are the most popular of all Zebu dairy breeds. The breed originated in the Sindh province of Pakistan, they are widely kept for milk production across Pakistan, India, Bangladesh, Sri Lanka, and other countries. They have been used for crossbreeding with temperate (European) origin dairy breeds in many countries to combine their tropical adaptations (heat tolerance, tick resistance, disease resistance, fertility at higher temperatures, etc.) with the higher milk production found in temperate regions. It has been crossed with Jerseys in many places, including India, the United States, Australia, Sri Lanka, etc.

General Information

1. **Species:** Cattle
2. **Synonyms:** Malir (Baluchistan), Red Karachi and Sindhi.
3. **Habitat:** Found in Sindh Pradesh of Pakistan& Orissa, Bengal, Bihar, Jharkhand, Chattisgarh, Rajasthan & Punjab states of India.
4. **Breeding tract:** The original breeding tract is in Pakistan but some organized herds are available in Orissa, Tamil Nadu, Bihar, Kerala and Assam states of India.
5. **Soil and Climate:** The soil varies from loam through sandy loam to sandy. Annual rainfall ranges from 25 to 30 cm and a large proportion of this precipitation is during the months from July to October.

6. **Main utility:** Milk for food, crossbreds are used for meat.
7. **Origin:** Red Sindhi is considered to have originated from Las Bela cattle found in the state of Bela, Baluchistan. **Originated in Karachi and Hyderabad (Pakistan)** regions of undivided India and also reared in certain organized farms in our country.
8. **Distribution:** Pakistan, India, Bangladesh, Sri Lanka.

Phenotypic traits

1. **Color:** This breed has **distinctly red color**. Red shades vary from dark red to dim yellow. Though patches of white are seen on dewlap and sometime on forehead, no large white patches are present on the body. In bulls, color is dark on the shoulders and thighs.
2. **Number of Horns:** 2
3. **Shape of Horns:** Horns are thick at the base and emerge laterally and curve upward.
4. **Visible characteristics**: Dark to pale red color. Horns are thick at the base and emerge laterally and curve upward. Hump is well developed in males.

		Male	Female
5.	Height (Avg. cm)	130	120
6.	Body length (Avg. cm)	140	140
7.	Heart Girth (Avg. cm)	180	140
8.	Weight (Avg. Kg)	450	320
9.	Birth Weight (Avg. Kg)	22.5	21.4
10.	Length (Avg. cm)	147	129

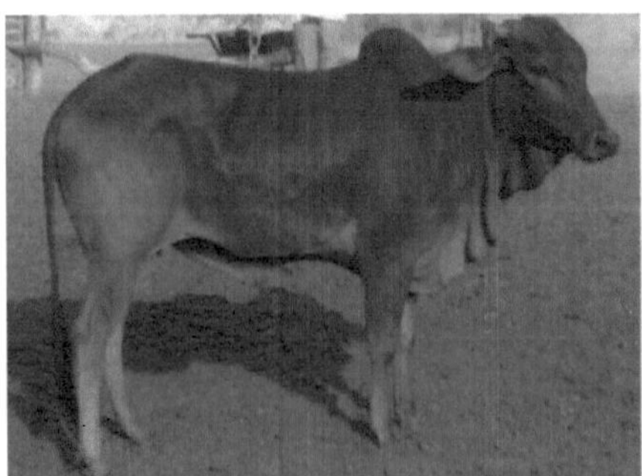

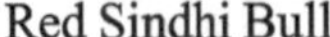

Red Sindhi Bull

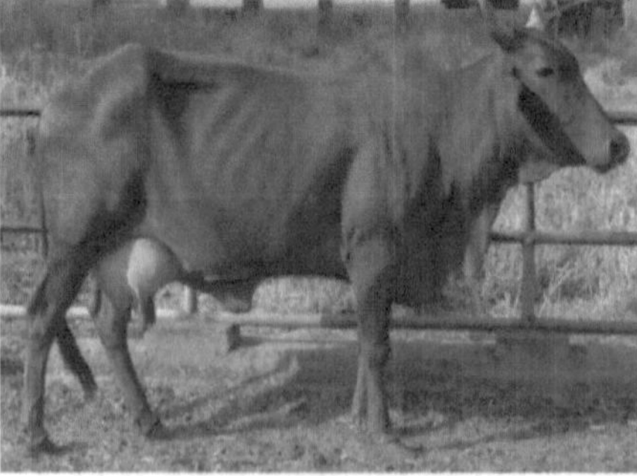

Red Sindhi Cattle

Physical Characteristics

1. **Body Color: Dark Red:** The bull, as a rule, runs to a much darker red than the cow, its extremities being almost black when full grown.
2. **Body Size:** Medium size well proportionate compact body confirmation.
3. **Forehead: Mild bulging forehead:** A white marking on the forehead with a little sprinkling of white along the dewlap and underneath the barrel is generally permitted. Forehead is broad between eyes and flat or slightly protruding, carrying a short crop of hair.
4. **Horns:** About 12-14" in size & grow upward & backwards.
5. **Temperament:** The Sindhi cow is particularly docile and is a distinctive dairy animal.
6. **Face:** Face is of medium length and is clear-cut, gradually tapering into a square, and has a well-developed black muzzle with wide nostrils and muscular lips.
7. **Eyes**: Eyes are fairly large, clear and well set apart with eyebrows rather light.
8. **Ears:** Ears are of medium size, fine clean-cut and are carried at an angle. Generally, the skin inside is colored butter yellow with a dark fringe along the edge.
9. **Dewlap:** Dewlap is rather abundant both in males and females but thin and hangs well in nice folds, with a soft mellow feel.
10. **Udder:** Capacious & Pendulous.
11. **Hump:** Hump is medium-sized but well developed in bull, slopping gradually forward but with an abrupt fall at the back.

Difference between Red Sindhi and Tharparkar

They are distinguished from the other dairy breed of Sindh, Tharparkar or White Sindhi, both by color and form, the Red Sindhi is smaller, rounder, with a more typical dairy form, and with short, curved horns, while the Tharparkar are taller with a shape more typical of Zebu draft breeds, and with longer, lyre shaped horns.

Management

1. **Management System:** Intensive
2. **Mobility:** Stationary

3. **Feeding of adults:** Fodder and Concentrate
4. **Housing:** Well developed housing for organized herds.
5. **Feeding system:** Stall feeding.
6. **Feeds to be fed:** Berseem, oats and mustard are the green fodder in rabi; and sorghum, pearl millet and cluster bean in kharif. Commercial feed can be fed anytime of the year. . Milking cows are provided supplementary feeding in the form of cotton seed, barley and oil cake. Feed is given in soaked form at the time of milking. Calves are reared on whole milk up to 1 month of age after which some green fodder is also fed. Calves are allowed to suck 1-2 teats up to 6 months of age.
7. **Feeding of concentrates:** 1kg/2kg milk at the time of milking.
8. **Feeding of roughages**: 1/10th of body weight per day.
9. **Milking:** should be done twice a day, however thrice a day milking gives higher milk yield.
10. **Milking practice:** full hand milking should be done. Avoid knuckling.
11. **Milk let down time:** 4-5 minutes.

Performance traits

	Average	Minimum	Maximum
Age at first calving (Avg. months)	43.54	31.97	51.32
Calving interval (months)	14.57	12.5	18.09
Lactation length (days)	-	260	305
Milk yield per lactation (kg)	1840	1100	2600
Milk fat (%)	4.5	4	5.2
Daily lactation in peak period (kg)	7.87	4.32	13.66
Dry period (days)	86	69	125

- **Peculiarity of the breed**

They have been used for crossbreeding with temperate (European) origin dairy breeds in many countries to combine their tropical adaptations (heat tolerance, tick resistance, disease resistance, fertility at higher temperatures, etc.) with the higher milk production found in temperate regions. It has been crossed with Jerseys in many places, including India, the United States, Australia, Sri Lanka, etc.

- **Research highlights**

Due to various tropical characteristics, the cattle prove to be an excellent choice for cross breeding with Jersey, Brown Swiss, Ayershire, for meat and milk production.

Major problems associated with health of Red Sindhi cattle

Being indigenous Red Sindhi is very hardy and disease resistant breed. However, the production performance decreases when the animal is exposed to environmental and dietary stressors. Therefore, management of the cattle is utmost important in prolonging and promoting the health status.

Price range

Rs. 30,000/- to Rs. 1,40,000/- (tentative)

Free Sale of Red Sindhi bulls

In Gauriakarma, in Hazaribagh in the Indian state of Jharkhand, a farm was established to maintain the germplasm of Red Sindhi cattle. Here, bulls are given free of cost to the villagers of the state. This government cattle farm is single farm of Jharkhand having Red Sindhi cow. The area of this was earlier about 2750 acres of land but due to transfer of land to other organization the area of this farm is reduced. Presently this farm is pride of Jharkhand. Dr. Niraj Kumar Verma is manager of this farm. This farm has a target to keep 350 cows.

Can be purchased from

1. **Gupta Dairy Farm:** Address; plot No. 41-42, Govind Colony, near water tank, Doon Valley College Road, Jundla Gate, Karnal-132001, Haryana. Phone no. 09416031427.

   Website: www.guptadairyfarm.com, email: guptadairyfarm@gmail.com

2. **Khurana Dairy Farm**: Rohtak, Haryana. Mobile Number : +91-9215450001 / 9215430001 / 9215450003

3. **Model Dairy Farm:** Mr. Prateek Vaish (VP-Operations). Address: Naramau, GT Road, near ALIMCO, Kanpur-209217, UP.

4. **Khalsa Dairy Farm**: Karnal, Haryana. Owner: Sham Singh, Mobile No. **09896603975.**

5. **Chopra Dairy Farm:** Nawashahr, Ludhiana, Punjab, Mobile No. **09592454093.**

HARIANA

Hariana is one of the most important breeds of cattle in India known all over the country as a first class dual purpose breed. The Hariana cattle are produced more or less in pure form in certain parts of Punjab, Rajasthan and Uttar Pradesh. The Hariana, a *Bos indicus* breed used for draft purposes in northern India where they are found. They are well suited to fast road work, being able to pull a one ton load at 2 miles per hour and cover 20 miles a day. While females are kept primarily for breeding of oxen, they are also milked. Hariana cattle are proportionately built and are compact. The bulls are good workers. The breed belongs to the shorthorn type of zebu and is grey or white.

General Information

1. **Species:** Cattle
2. **Synonyms:** Hansi, Haryanvi, Hissari.
3. **Habitat**: This is a medium heavy type of dual-purpose breed found in Rohtak, Karnal, Hissar, Gurgaon district of Haryana, and the Union Territory of Delhi and in West Uttar Pradesh.
4. **Breeding tract:** It is bred particularly in the districts of Rohtak, Hissar, Jind, Karnal, Gurgaon, and Karnal of Haryana State and the Union Territory of Delhi.
5. **Soil and Climate:** The soil, in general, is firm clay. In Rohtak district it is mostly light-colored alluvial loam, and in Hissar, soft loam with reddish tinge, interspersed with sand and clay. In some areas, sand hills are present. All soils give excellent crop returns when irrigated. The climate of Haryana State is relatively dry, average annual rainfall being about 46 cm. Rain usually occur during the months of July, August and September. During the summer months, day temperatures may go as high as 46°C, whereas in winters (December, January and February) the minimum and maximum temperatures may approximately be 5° and 24°C respectively.
6. **Main utility:** Food - Milk; Work - Draught and Transport
7. **Origin:** It was originated from Rohtak, Hisar, Jind and Gurgaon districts of Haryana.
8. **Distribution:** In India, the cattle is present in northern as well southern parts of the country like Orissa, Tamil Nadu and Andhra Pradesh.

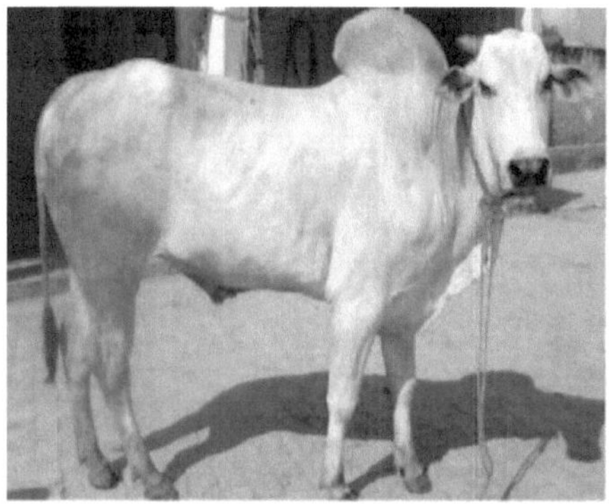
Hariana Bull

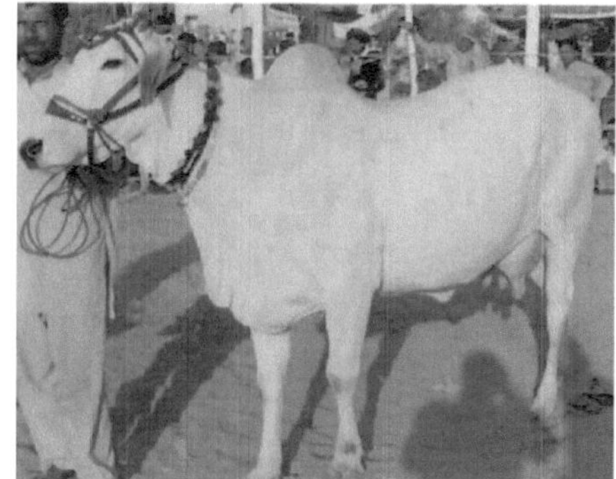
Hariana Cattle

Phenotypic traits

1. **Color:** The popular color is white or light grey. In some of the males, the head, neck, hump and quarters are dark grey. This color changes to white after castration.
2. **Number of Horns:** 2
3. **Shape of Horns:** Horns are small in size, arched, tapers upward.
4. **Visible characteristics:** White color, long and narrow face, well marked bony prominence at the centre of poll and small horns.

	Male	Female
5. Height (Avg. cm)	138.43	136.1
6. Body length (Avg. cm)	141.02	139.2
7. Heart Girth (Avg. cm)	173.96	169.8
8. Weight (Avg. Kg)	499	325
9. Birth Weight (Avg. Kg)	23.3	21.7
10. Length (Avg. cm)	153	137

Physical Characteristics

1. **Body Color:** whitish to grayish white.
2. **Body Size:** Medium size well proportionate compact body confirmation.
3. **Forehead:** The long and narrow face with flat forehead and a well-marked bony prominence at the centre of the poll are the indications of purity of breed.
4. **Horns:** Horns are fine and rather short or of moderate length. Generally they are 10 to 23 cm in length and thinner in females than in males. They are more or less horizontal when short, and as they grow longer they curve upwards and inwards.

5. **Temperament:** The animal need to be trained at early age for draught purposes.
6. **Face:** Face is long and narrow with a flat or slightly convex forehead. The muzzle is black and nostrils are wide.
7. **Ears:** Ears are small, active and slightly pendulous.
8. **Dewlap:** Dewlap is small, thin and free from fleshy folds, but fairly large in bulls. Chest is well developed with a wide brisket.
9. **Udder:** Udder is capacious and extends well forward with a well-developed milk vein. The teats are medium sized and proportionate in size; the fore-teats being longer than the hind ones.
10. **Hump:** Hump is large in males but decreases after castration. It is medium sized in females.

Points for Disqualification

Markedly sloping rump, loose sheath, coarse tail, color other than white or grey, white hair at switch of tail, long tail with switch nearly touching ground (distance less than 15 cm from ground), a typical horn, concave or' bulging forehead, and white eyelashes are the points for disqualification in Hariana breed.

Management

1. **Management System:** Semi-Intensive
2. **Mobility:** Stationary
3. **Feeding of adults:** Grazing, Fodder and Concentrate
4. **Housing:** No special requirement of housing. The cattle are let loose for grazing in an open pasture. The working bulls are kept tied with basic housing facilities.
5. **Feeding system:** Grazing, Stall feeding for working bulls.
6. **Feeds to be fed:** Animals are allowed to graze on crop residues, grasses, weeds,etc. Calves are not weaned. Since Hariana cows are mainly reared for producing bullocks, greater attention is paid to rearing of male calves than of female calves. High yielding cows, bullocks and young males given green fodder and concentrate in addition to grazing.
7. **Feeding of concentrates:** 2kg/day for working bullocks, 1kg/2kg milk at the time of milking.
8. **Feeding of roughages:** 1/10th of body weight per day.

9. **Milking:** should be done twice a day, however thrice a day milking gives higher milk yield.
10. **Milking practice:** full hand milking should be done. Avoid knuckling.
11. **Milk let down time:** 4-5 minutes.
12. **Draughtability:** Hariana bulls are known for their draughtability and traction power. Bullocks are only harnessed in the cooler hours during morning and evening. Males are castrated at 3 years of age.

Performance traits

	Average	Minimum	Maximum
Age at first calving (Avg. months)	51.3	40	61
Calving interval (months)	15.88	13	18
Lactation length (days)	-	230	251
Milk yield per lactation (kg)	997	693	1745
Milk fat (%)	4.5	4.3	5.3
Daily lactation in peak period (kg)	3.67	1.32	6.95
Dry period (days)	124	112	158

- **Peculiarity of the breed**

The main focus is given on the production of calves by using artificial insemination due to their ability of fast road transport and fast ploughing.

Major problems associated with health of Hariana cattle

Being indigenous breed of cattle the problems faced are very less as compared to exotic breed. The breed is resistant to parasitic infestation, heat stress and possesses many desirable characters.

Price range

Rs. 15,000/- to Rs. 70,000/- (tentative)

Can be purchased from

1. **Gupta Dairy Farm:** Address; plot No. 41-42, Govind Colony, near water tank, Doon Valley College Road, Jundla Gate, Karnal-132001, Haryana. Phone no. 09416031427.

   Website: www.guptadairyfarm.com, email: guptadairyfarm@gmail.com
2. **Khurana Dairy Farm,** Rohtak, Haryana. Mobile Number : +91-9215450001 / 9215430001 / 9215450003
3. **Model Dairy Farm:** Mr. Prateek Vaish (VP-Operations). Address: Naramau, GT Road, near ALIMCO, Kanpur-209217, UP.
4. Hariana Breeding Herd, Haringhata, near Kolkata, West Bengal.

GIR

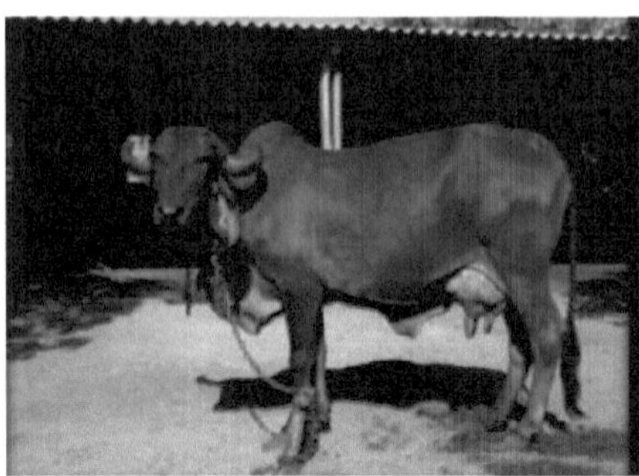
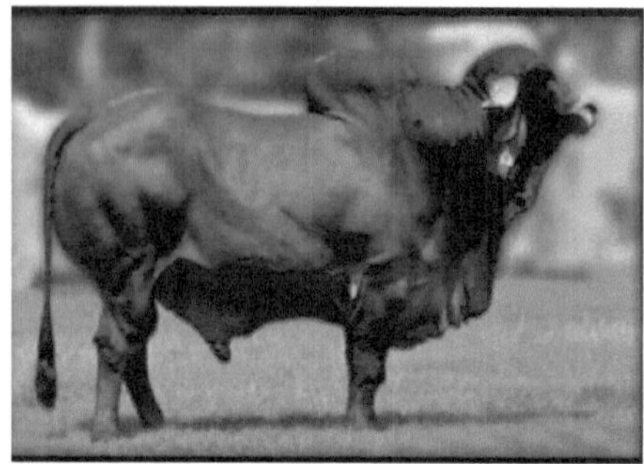

- Gir is one of the best milkers among indigenous cattle.
- The breed is also known as "Bhodali", "Desan", "Gujarati", "Kathiawari", "Sorthi", and "Surati".
- The breeding tract of the breed includes Amreli, Bhavnagar, Junagadh and Rajkot districts of Gujarat and is named after the Gir forest, the geographical area of origin of the breed.
- Bullocks can drag heavy loads on all kinds of soils, be it sandy, black or rocky.
- This is a world-renowned breed known for its tolerance to stress conditions. Having faced scarcity situations for a numbers of years, it has the capacity for yielding more milk with less feeding and is resistant to various tropical diseases.
- Due to their special qualities, animals of this breed have been imported by countries like Brazil, USA, Venezuela and Mexico, and are being bred there successfully.
- The animals are of red colour. Many animals have white spots. Variants with different sheds of red are also available.
- The animals have typically dome shaped fore head and long ears.
- Reported Average Milk production is 2110 lit per lactation. Animals with as high as 5000 litre can also be found in organized farms.

For further details please see the following link

http://210.212.93.85/agris/breed.aspx

RATHI

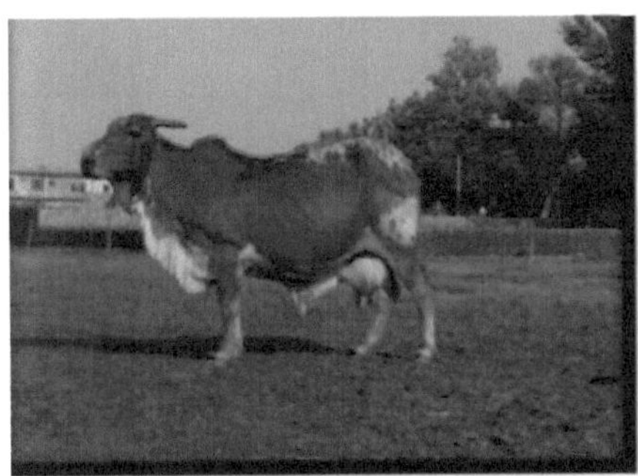

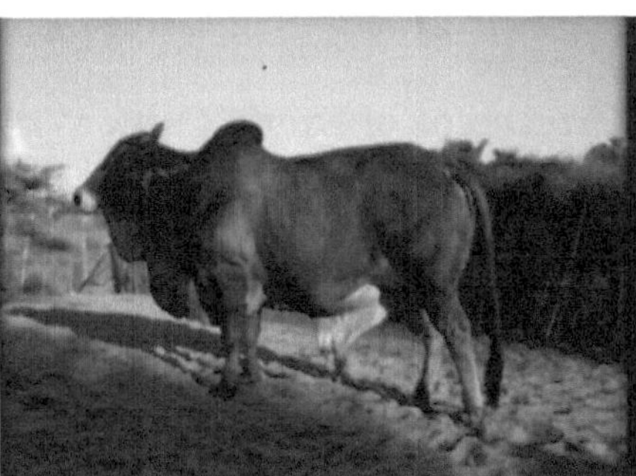

- Rathi is an important milch breed of cattle found in the arid regions of Rajasthan. This breed functions as a major livelihood source for the farmers in this region.
- It takes its name from a pastoral tribe called Raths who are Muslims of Rajput extraction and lead a nomadic life.
- Rathi animals are particularly concentrated in Loonkaransar tehsil of Bikaner district, which is also known as Rathi tract.
- The Breeding tract of this breed lies in the heart of Thar Desert consisting of Bikaner, Ganganagar and Jaisalmer districts of Rajasthan.
- Rathi cattle are thought to have evolved from intermixing of Sahiwal, Red Sindhi, Tharparkar and Dhanni breeds with a preponderance of Sahiwal blood.
- The animals are usually brown with white patches all over the body, but animals having completely brown or black coat with white patches are also seen.
- The ecosystem in its native tract is fragile and the lands are less fertile with very low productivity. Scorching summer (50 degree C), chilly winter (2 degree C), dry monsoon (less than 200 mm rainfall in a year) and dust storms are the characteristics of the region.
- Rathi cows are efficient and good milkers.
- The cows on an average produce 1560 Kg of milk. The lactation milk yield ranges from 1062 to 2810 Kg. Selected cows have produced around 4800 Kg at farmer's doorstep.

For further details please see the following link

http://210.212.93.85/agris/breed.aspx

Crossbreds of Exotic Cattle With Indigenous Cattle

HOLSTEIN FRIESIAN CROSS

The HF crosses are more suitable for cooler climatic regions like hilly areas as they are less tolerant to heat. Have less resistance to tropical diseases than Jersey crosses. Although the milk yield is higher in HF crosses but fat per cent is less than Jersey crosses.

General Information

1. **Species:** Cattle
2. **Synonyms:** HF Cross.
3. **Habitat:** Temperate countries but the crosses have been well adapted to tropical countries like India, Pakistan, Sri Lanka, Bangladesh, and other countries of Indian Subcontinent.
4. **Breeding tract:** In India, the Central Government had come out with different policies time to time to upgrade the local cattle for increased milk production. So every state through its Animal Husbandry Departments, upgrade local cattle by using HF semen.
5. **Main utility:** Milk for food.
6. **Origin:** Different states of India.
7. **Distribution:** Almost entire country.

Phenotypic traits

1. **Color:** usually black and white but color also depends on the breed color with which HF is crossed.
2. **Number of horns:** 2
3. **Visible characteristics:** Patches of sharp black and white colors, large udder, wedge shaped conformation from rear view, highly developed milk vein.

Different HF Crosses are as

1. Frieswal

a. Cross between HF and Sahiwal.
b. 3/8th to 5/8th exotic inheritance.

c. Done at Military Dairy Farms at Allahabad.

d. Age at first calving: 36.2 months

e. Calving Interval: 432 days

f. First lactation milk yield: 2538 kg

g. Mortality to first calving: 4%

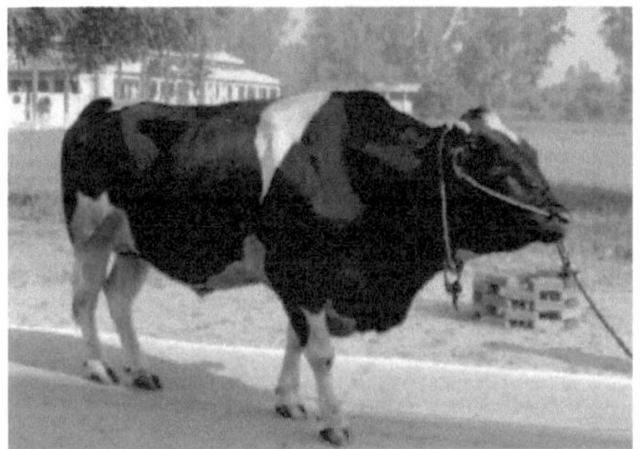

Frieswal Bull

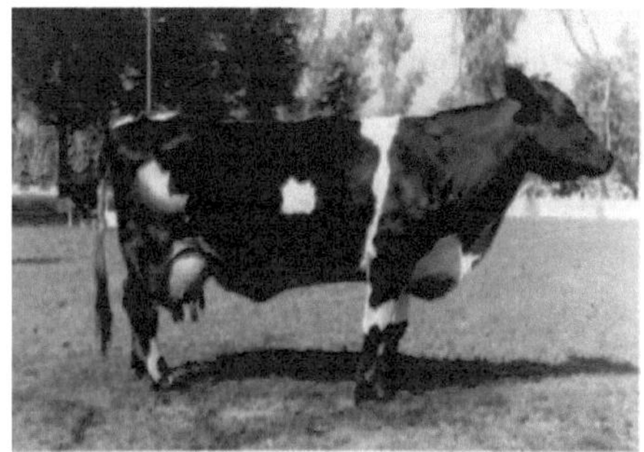

Frieswal Cow

2. HF and Red Dane cross with Red Sindhi

a. Done at Military Dairy Farm, Bangalore.

b. ½ Red Dane + 1/4th HF + 1/4th Red Sindhi.

c. Age at first calving: 28.1 months

d. First lactation milk yield: 2093 kg

e. Lactation length: 320 days

f. First calving interval: 422 days

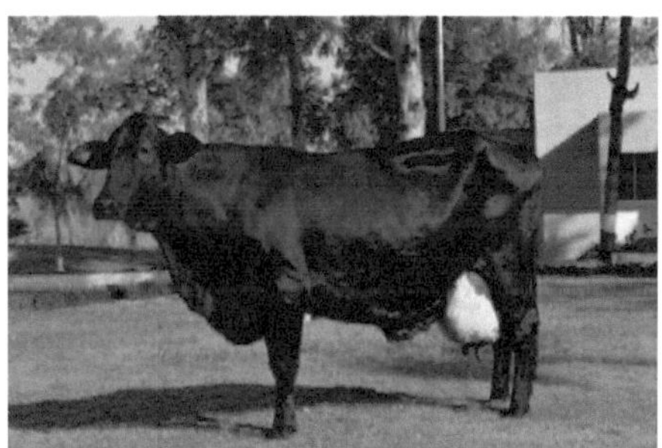

HF & Red Sindhi Cross

3. Karan Fries

a. Cross done at National Dairy Research Institute, Karnal.

b. Cross between HF and Tharparkar.

c. ½ HF and ½ Tharparkar.

d. Age at first calving: 28.5 months

e. First lactation milk yield: 3392 kg (305 days)

f. Calving interval: 363 days

g. Calf Mortality: 6%

4. HF cross with Jersey and Tharparkar

a. Age at first calving: 31.6 months

b. First lactation milk yield: 2283 kg

c. Calving interval: 460 days

d. Calf Mortality: 8.4%

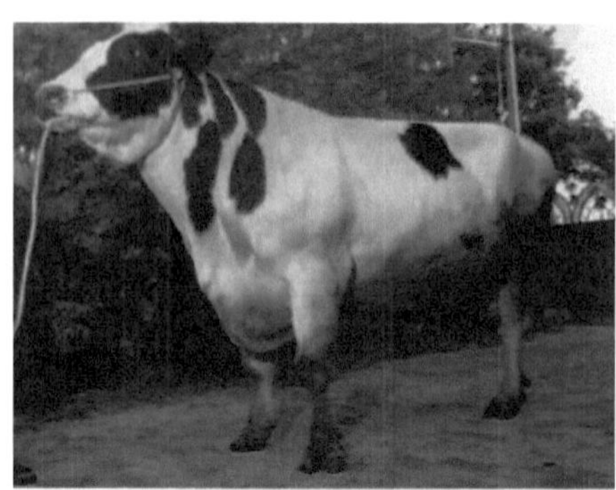

HF & Tharparkar Cross

5. HF and Hariana

a. Done at Government Livestock Farm, Hissar, Haryana.

b. ½ HF and ½ Hariana.

c. Age at first calving: 1158 days

d. First lactation milk yield: 2002 kg

e. Calving interval: 438 days

f. Lactation length: 305 days

6. HF and Non descript Desi Cattle:

a. Done at Haringhata Cattle Breeding Farm, Kolkata, West Bengal.

b. First lactation milk yield: **2080 kg**

Management

1. **Management System:** Intensive
2. **Mobility:** Stationary
3. **Feeding of adults:** Fodder and Concentrate
4. **Housing:** Well developed housing for organized herds.
5. **Feeding system:** Stall feeding.
6. **Feeds to be fed:** Berseem, oats and mustard are the green fodder in rabi; and sorghum, pearl millet and cluster bean in kharif. Commercial feed can be fed anytime of the year. Milking cows are provided supplementry feeding in the form of cotton seed, barley and oil cake. Feed is given in soaked form at the time of milking. Calves are reared on whole milk up to 1 month of age after which some green fodder is also fed. Calves are allowed to suck 1-2 teats up to 6 months of age

7. **Feeding of concentrates:** 1kg/2kg milk at the time of milking.
8. **Feeding of roughages:** 1/10th of body weight per day.
9. **Milking:** should be done 2-3 times a day.
10. **Milking practice:** full hand milking should be done. Avoid knuckling.
11. **Milk let down time:** 4-5 minutes.

- **Benefits of cross breeding**
  1. More milk production.
  2. Efficient feed conversion ratio (FCR).
  3. Economical dairy.
  4. Better reproductive traits.
  5. Continuity in production.

- **Major problems associated with health of HF Cross**
  1. **Mastitis:** Being very high yielding cattle, the risk of mastitis is always present.
  2. **Calcium Deficiency:** The cattle should be supplied with Calcium and Phosphorous supplements to maintain the health of animal.
  3. **Genital Diseases:** The risk of genital diseases like pyometra, metritis, is always present and should be taken care of.
  4. **Milk Fever** due to deficiency of Calcium.
  5. Parasitic infestations.

Price range

Upto Rs. 1, 40, 000/- (tentative)

Can be purchased from

1. **Gupta Dairy Farm:** Address; plot No. 41-42, Govind Colony, near water tank, Doon Valley College Road, Jundla Gate, Karnal-132001, Haryana. Phone no. 09416031427.

   Website: www.guptadairyfarm.com, email: guptadairyfarm@gmail.com
2. **Khurana Dairy Farm**, Rohtak, Haryana. Mobile Number : +91-9215450001 / 9215430001 / 9215450003

3. **Model Dairy Farm**: Mr. Prateek Vaish (VP-Operations). Address: Naramau, GT Road, near ALIMCO, Kanpur-209217, UP.
4. **Karnal Livestock Sales. Contact Details:** Dabas House, 17-E, Session Road, Karnal - 132001, Haryana, India, Mr. Anand Parkash Dabas (Proprietor).
5. **Anand Cows Sales and Dealership.** Contact Details: K. Subramanyam Raju, S/O K. Narayana Raju, Kothaindlu, Punganur(P&T), Chittoor - 517247, Andhra Pradesh, India. Mobile : +918497009383.
6. **Sachdeva Dairy Farm:** Mr. Anil Sachdeva, 940/31, Buffalo Market,Behind Durga Bhavan Mandir,, Rohtak, Haryana, India – 124001. Mobile : +91-9896146700 Website: http://www.sachdevadairyfarm.com

   Webpage: http://www.exportersindia.com/sachdevadairyfarm/

Jersey Cross

Jersey crosses are produced by upgrading/ cross breeding the non-descript / Indigenous breeds of cows with Jersey semen. Jersey crosses are suitable dairy animals for tropical plains of our country. They are medium sized, have better heat tolerance than other exotic crosses and well adapted to our climate. Depending on the milk production potential of our indigenous cows, the **Jersey** crosses may show 2 to 3 fold increase in milk yield in the first generation.

General Information

1. **Species:** Cattle.
2. **Habitat:** Temperate countries but the crosses have been well adapted to tropical countries like India, Pakistan, Sri Lanka, Bangladesh, and other countries of Indian Subcontinent.
3. **Breeding tract:** In India, the Central Government had come out with different policies time to time to upgrade the local cattle for increased milk production. So every state through its Animal Husbandry Departments, upgrade local cattle by using Jersey semen.
4. **Main utility:** Milk for food.
5. **Origin:** Different states of India.
6. **Distribution:** Almost entire country.

Phenotypic traits

1. **Color:** usually fawn color with individual breed variability.
2. **Visible characteristics:** Patches of fawn color, large udder, wedge shaped conformation from rear view, highly developed milk vein.

Different Jersey Crosses are as

1. Taylor

a. Cross of Jersey and Shorthorn with local breeds of Patna, Bihar.

b. Crosses of *Bos taurus* bulls (Shorthorn and Channel Island bulls from the United Kingdom) with local cows by Mr. Taylor.

c. Their coat color is red, gray or black and they do not possess a hump.

d. No published records on the performance of this breed are available.

e. The breed is almost extinct.

2. Jersind

a. Indigenous breeds viz. Kankrej, Gir, Hariana, Sahiwal and Red Sindhi were crossed to Holstein Friesian, Brown-Swiss, Jersey and Guernsey at the Agricultural Institute, Naini, Allahabad.

b. The results of crossbreeding suggested that Red Sindhi x Jersey crosses had the most desirable traits for Indian conditions.

c. These included, small body size, better adaptability and high fat percentage. The Jersey crossbreeds between 3/8 and 5/8 have been interbred and named as 'Jersindh'.

d. Similarly, 3/8-5/8 Brown-Swiss x Red Sindhi crosses have been interbred and named as 'Brown-Sind'.

e. Jersindh crosses gave milk yield between 1557 and 1861 kg in first lactation. The breed has shown deterioration over the years mainly because of small numbers and being confined to the Institute farm.

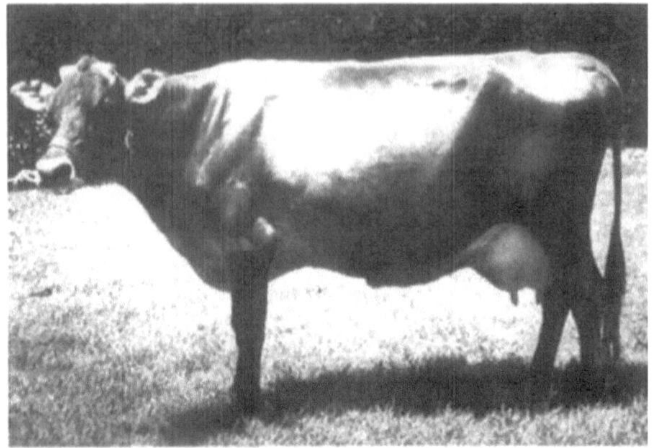

Jersind

3. Jerthar

a. Cross done at Bangalore.
b. Cross between Jersey and Tharparkar.
c. ½ Jersey and ½ Tharparkar.
d. Age at first calving: 27.8 months
e. First lactation milk yield: 2714 kg (305 days)
f. Calving interval: 384 days
g. Calf Mortality: 2.4%

4. HF cross with Jersey and Tharparkar

a. Age at first calving: 31.6 months
b. First lactation milk yield: 2283 kg
c. Calving interval: 460 days
d. Calf Mortality: 8.4%

5.Jersey and Hariana

a. Done at Haringhata Cattle Breeding Farm, Kolkata, West Bengal.
b. ½ Jersey and ½ Hariana.
c. Age at first calving: 31.7 months
d. First lactation milk yield: 1679 kg
e. Calving interval: 434 days

f. Lactation length: 305 days

g. Milk per day of calving interval: 4.51kg

6. Jersey and Non descript Desi Cattle

a. Done at Haringhata Cattle Breeding Farm, Kolkata, West Bengal.

b. First lactation milk yield: 1269 kg

c. Age at first calving: 35.6 months.

d. First lactation length: 327 days.

e. Calving interval: 433 days.

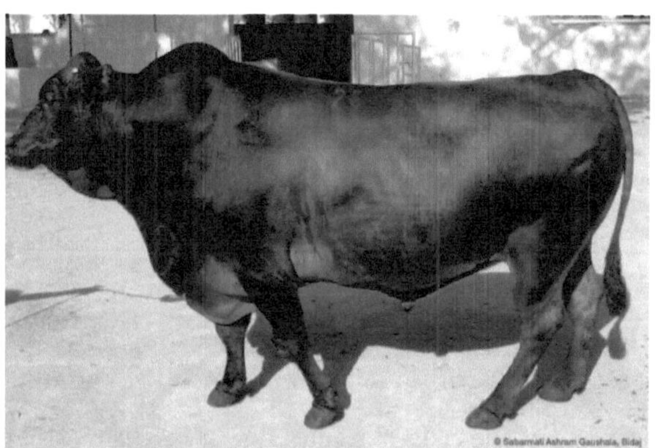

Jersey & Sahiwal Cross for beef purposes

Management

1. **Management System:** Intensive
2. **Mobility:** Stationary
3. **Feeding of adults:** Fodder and Concentrate
4. **Housing:** Well developed housing for organized herds.
5. **Feeding system:** Stall feeding.
6. **Feeds to be fed:** Berseem, oats and mustard are the green fodder in rabi; and sorghum, pearl millet and cluster bean in kharif. Commercial feed can be fed anytime of the year. Milking cows are provided supplementry feeding in the form of cotton seed, barley and oil cake. Feed is given in soaked form at the time of milking. Calves are reared on whole milk up to 1 month of age after which some green fodder is also fed. Calves are allowed to suck 1-2 teats up to 6 months of age.

7. **Feeding of concentrates:** 1kg/2kg milk at the time of milking.
8. **Feeding of roughages:** 1/10th of body weight per day.
9. **Milking:** should be done 2-3 times a day.
10. **Milking practice:** full hand milking should be done. Avoid knuckling.
11. **Milk let down time:** 4-5 minutes.

Benefits of cross breeding:

1. More milk production.
2. Efficient feed conversion ratio (FCR).
3. Economical dairy.
4. Better reproductive traits.
5. Continuity in production.

Major problems associated with health of Jersey Cross

1. **Mastitis:** Being very high yielding cattle, the risk of mastitis is always present.
2. **Calcium Deficiency:** The cattle should be supplied with Calcium and Phosphorous supplements to maintain the health of animal.
3. **Genital Diseases:** The risk of genital diseases like pyometra, metritis, is always present and should be taken care of.
4. **Milk Fever** due to deficiency of Calcium.
5. Parasitic infestations.

Price range:

Upto Rs. 1,40,000/- (tentative)

Can be purchased from

1. **Gupta Dairy Farm:** Address; plot No. 41-42, Govind Colony, near water tank, Doon Valley College Road, Jundla Gate, Karnal-132001, Haryana. Phone no. 09416031427.

   Website: www.guptadairyfarm.com, email: guptadairyfarm@gmail.com
2. **Khurana Dairy Farm,** Rohtak, Haryana. Mobile Number : +91-9215450001 / 9215430001 / 9215450003
3. **Model Dairy Farm:** Mr. Prateek Vaish (VP-Operations). Address: Naramau, GT Road, near ALIMCO, Kanpur-209217, UP.

4. **Karnal Livestock Sales:** Dabas House, 17-E, Session Road, Karnal - 132001, Haryana, India, Mr. Anand Parkash Dabas (Proprietor).
5. **Anand Cows Sales and Dealership**: K. Subramanyam Raju, S/O K. Narayana Raju, Kothaindlu, Punganur(P&T), Chittoor - 517247 Andhra Pradesh, India. Mobile : +918497009383.
6. **Sachdeva Dairy Farm**: Mr. Anil Sachdeva, 940/31, Buffalo Market,Behind Durga Bhavan Mandir,, Rohtak, Haryana, India – 124001.
   Mobile : +91-9896146700 Website: http://www.sachdevadairyfarm.com
   Webpage: http://www.exportersindia.com/sachdevadairyfarm/

BROWN SWISS CROSS

Brown Swiss crosses are produced by upgrading the local cattle with Brown Swiss semen. Brown Swiss being a heavier breed is suitable for grading up of the non-descript cattle of our country. The breed stands in second place next to HF in milk production and this capacity of the breed is harnessed to full extent by cross breeding of the native cattle. The crosses so produced shows better survivability with sharp rise in milk production.

General Information

1. **Species:** Cattle.
2. **Habitat:** Temperate countries but the crosses have been well adapted to tropical countries like India, Pakistan, Sri Lanka, Bangladesh, and other countries of Indian Subcontinent.
3. **Breeding tract:** In India, the Central Government had come out with different policies time to time to upgrade the local cattle for increased milk production. So every state through its Animal Husbandry Departments, upgrade local cattle by using Jersey semen.
4. **Main utility:** Milk for food.
5. **Origin:** Different states of India.
6. **Distribution:** Almost entire country.

Phenotypic traits

1. **Color:** usually grayish brown color with individual breed variability.
2. **Number of horns:** 2
3. **Visible characteristics:** grayish brown to dull black color, large udder, wedge shape conformation from rear view, highly developed milk vein.

Different Brown Swiss Crosses are as

1. Sunandini

a. Cross of Brown Swiss with non-descript cattle of Munar, Kerala.

b. Under an Indo-Swiss Project in Kerala which started in 1963, local non-descript cows were crossed with Brown-Swiss bulls.

c. The crosses with 50 per cent, 75 per cent and 62.5 per cent Brown-Swiss inheritance were produced.

d. The crossbreeds with 62.5 per cent Brown-Swiss inheritance were mated, followed by selection to synthesise a new breed named 'Sunandini'.

e. Sunandini animals under field conditions give a lactation yield of 1351 kg in 305 days.

f. Sunandini bulls are being progeny tested for milk using performance recording under field conditions. A total 323 Sunandini bulls have been evaluated and 42 bulls declared proven.

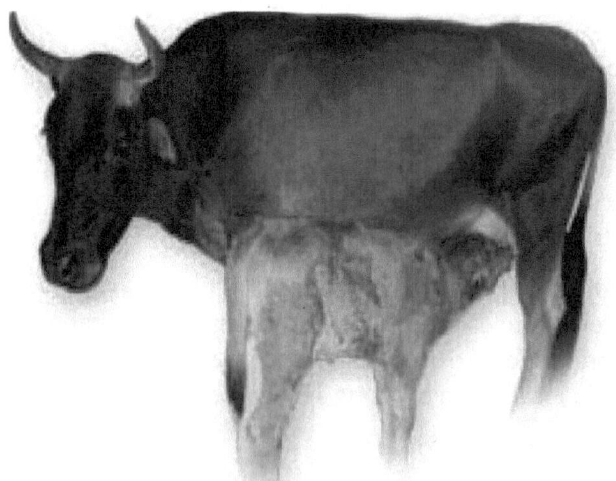

Sunandini cow and calf India

2. Karan Swiss

a. Karan Swiss evolved from crossing American Brown Swiss bulls with Sahiwal and Red Sindhi cows at the National Dairy Research Institute (NDRI), Karnal, India.

b. Brown-Swiss inheritance is around 50 per cent.

c. The color of the breed is red dun.

d. It resembles Sahiwal in its body size and general appearance, and the dewlap is pendulous as in the case of Sahiwal.

e. The hump is almost non-existent, the barrel is long and deep, the naval flap is from tight to slightly loose.

f. Eyes are full, ears small, oblong and hairy from the inside.

g. The neck is of medium size.

h. The legs are proportionate in size and well set apart.

i. The udder is of good size, wide, deep and long. The udder is mostly bowl shaped; teats are cylindrical pointed or round and are of medium size. The milk veins are well developed and tortuous.

j. The males have powerful shoulders.

k. The average age at first calving was 32 months.

l. The first lactation yield was 2564.7 kg with 4.2 to 4.4 per cent fat.

m. The total milk yield based on pooled lactations was 3257.3 kg with an overall calving interval of 395.5 days.

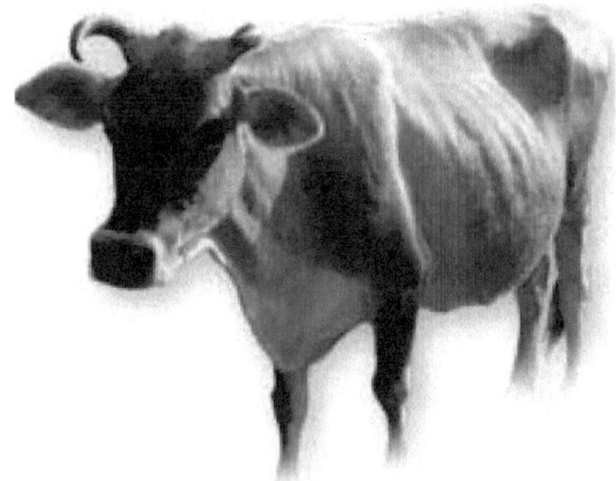

Karan Swiss heifer India

3. Brown Swiss cross with Tharparkar

a. Age at first calving: 30.5 months

b. First lactation milk yield: 2755 kg

c. Calving interval: 409 days

d. Calf Mortality: 7.7%

4. Brown Swiss and Hariana

a. Done at Haringhata Cattle Breeding Farm, Kolkata, West Bengal.
b. ½ Brown Swiss and ½ Hariana.
c. Age at first calving: 36 months
d. First lactation milk yield: 1717 kg
e. Calving interval: 449 days
f. Lactation length: 300 days

Management

1. **Management System:** Intensive
2. **Mobility:** Stationary
3. **Feeding of adults:** Fodder and Concentrate
4. **Housing:** Well developed housing for organized herds.
5. **Feeding system:** Stall feeding.
6. **Feeds to be fed**: Berseem, oats and mustard are the green fodder in rabi; and sorghum, pearl millet and cluster bean in kharif. Commercial feed can be fed anytime of the year. Milking cows are provided supplementry feeding in the form of cotton seed, barley and oil cake. Feed is given in soaked form at the time of milking. Calves are reared on whole milk up to 1 month of age after which some green fodder is also fed. Calves are allowed to suck 1-2 teats up to 6 months of age
7. **Feeding of concentrates:** 1kg/2kg milk at the time of milking.
8. **Feeding of roughages:** $1/10^{th}$ of body weight per day.
9. Milking: should be done 2-3 times a day.
10. **Milking practice:** full hand milking should be done. Avoid knuckling.
11. **Milk let down time:** 4-5 minutes.

Benefits of cross breeding

1. More milk production.
2. Efficient feed conversion ratio (FCR).
3. Economical dairy.
4. Better reproductive traits.
5. Continuity in production.

Major problems associated with health of Jersey Cross

1. **Mastitis:** Being very high yielding cattle, the risk of mastitis is always present.
2. **Calcium Deficiency:** The cattle should be supplied with Calcium and Phosphorous supplements to maintain the health of animal.
3. **Genital Diseases:** The risk of genital diseases like pyometra, metritis, is always present and should be taken care of.
4. **Milk Fever** due to deficiency of Calcium.
5. Parasitic infestations.

Price range

Upto Rs. 1,40,000/- (tentative)

Can be purchased from:

1. **Gupta Dairy Farm**: Address; plot No. 41-42, Govind Colony, near water tank, Doon Valley College Road, Jundla Gate, Karnal-132001, Haryana. Phone no. 09416031427.

   Website: www.guptadairyfarm.com, email: guptadairyfarm@gmail.com
2. **Khurana Dairy Farm,** Rohtak, Haryana.
   Mobile Number : +91-9215450001 / 9215430001 / 9215450003
3. **Model Dairy Farm**: Mr. Prateek Vaish (VP-Operations). Address: Naramau, GT Road, near ALIMCO, Kanpur-209217, UP.
4. **Karnal Livestock Sales. Contact Details:** Dabas House, 17-E, Session Road, Karnal - 132001, Haryana, India, Mr. Anand Parkash Dabas (Proprietor).
5. **Anand Cows Sales and Dealership.** K. Subramanyam Raju, S/o K. Narayana Raju, Kothaindlu, Punganur(P&T), Chittoor - 517247, Andhra Pradesh, India. Mobile : +918497009383.
6. **Sachdeva Dairy Farm:** Mr. Anil Sachdeva, 940/31, Buffalo Market, Behind Durga Bhavan Mandir,, Rohtak, Haryana, India – 124001. Mobile : +91-9896146700 Website: http://www.sachdevadairyfarm.com

   Webpage: http://www.exportersindia.com/sachdevadairyfarm

Exotic Breeds of Cattle

Holstein Friesian

Holstein Friesians (often shortened as Friesians in Europe and Holsteins in North America) are a breed of cattle known today as the world's highest-production dairy animals. Originating in Europe, Friesians were bred in what is now the Netherlands and more specifically in the two northern provinces of North Holland and Friesland, and Northern Germany, more specifically what is now Schleswig-Holstein, Germany. The animals were the regional cattle of the Frisians and the Saxons. The Dutch and German breeders bred and oversaw the development of the breed with the goal of obtaining animals that could best use grass, the area's most abundant resource. Over the centuries, the result was a high-producing, black-and-white dairy cow. It is black and white due to artificial selection by the breeders.

General Information

1. **Species:** Cattle
2. **Synonyms:** HF, Black & White Cattle.
3. **Habitat:** Countries lying in the temperate zone like UK, USA, Holland, Germany and Canada.
4. **Breeding tract:** However, the breed is bred only in temperate zones but in India breeding is largely confined to organized herds only whereby standard management and housing conditions are required for dwelling of the cattle. Areas of Punjab, Haryana, Tamil Nadu, Karnataka, Uttar Pradesh and Delhi have some private farms dealing with breeding of HF.
5. **Main utility:** Milk for food, Meat in South Europe only.
6. **Origin:** Europe (Netherlands).
7. **Distribution:** Europe, North America, South Asia, Japan.

Phenotypic traits:

1. **Color:** Sharp Black and white.
2. **Number of horns:** 2 (mostly polled cattle is found).
3. **Visible characteristics:** Patches of sharp black and white colors, large udder, wedge shaped conformation from rear view, highly developed milk vein.

		Male	Female
4.	Height (Avg. cm)	139	147
5.	Body length (Avg. cm)	156	160
6.	Heart Girth (Avg. cm)	190	198
7.	Weight (Avg. Kg)	1000	675
8.	Birth Weight (Avg. Kg)	42	40
9.	Length (Avg. cm)	163	165

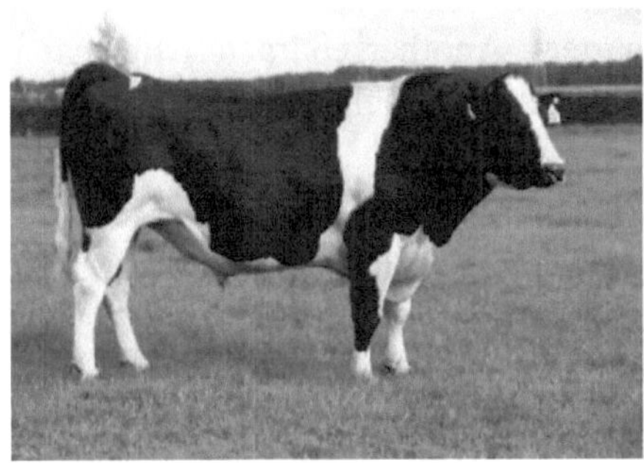

HF Bull

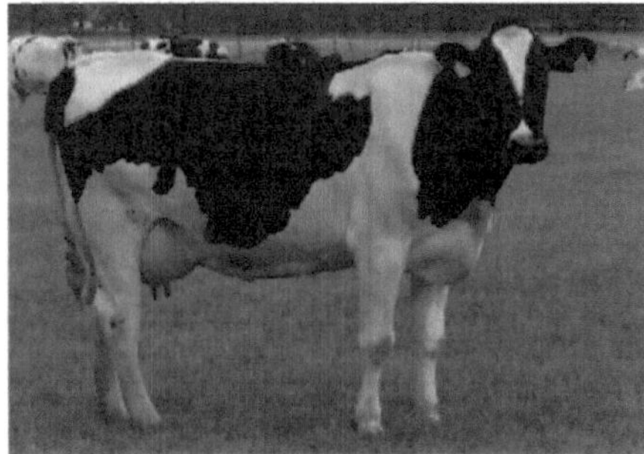

HF Cattle

Physical Characteristics

1. **Body Color:** All Holsteins are black-and-white. This color pattern always is patchy, with big black, rounded patches over the animal's body.
2. **Body Size:** Large size well proportionate compact body confirmation. Holsteins are a dairy breed. Dairy cattle are always thinner and more angular than beef cattle. Holsteins, like all dairy breeds, have more angle over the hips, tail-head and shoulders than beef breeds.
3. **Head:** A Holstein cow's head is quite long. The long nose bridge gives this look, and is quite unmistakable when comparing to other dairy breeds like Jersey.
4. **Horns:** Mostly Holsteins are horned breeds but they are polled early in life.
5. **Temperament:** Docile and is a distinctive dairy animal.
6. **Face:** Face is elongated and is clear-cut, gradually tapering into a square.
7. **Ears:** Ears are of medium size.
8. **Dewlap:** slight.
9. **Udder:** Capacious & Pendulous, Massive in size with prominent milk vein.

10. **Hump:** Absent.
11. **Withers:** Round.

Funnel butts

Holsteins have what are called "funnel-butts;" this means that, from the pin bones (of the hips) to the hocks, the hind quarters form a funnel-type angle from the pelvis to the legs; this is quite evident when looking at an animal from the side. Being "funnel-butted" means that these animals, as was mentioned before, lack muscling over the hind quarters. Another characteristic that is typical of all dairy breeds is the huge udder between their back legs.

Highest Milk Producing Cattle

Holstein-Friesians are the highest-quantity producing dairy cow in the world, and are thus far more commonly sought-after and used in commercial dairy operations across the world. It is known that Holsteins are capable of producing as much as 50 gallons (189.3 L) of milk per day! Holsteins are actually the largest dairy breed used in dairy operations, a little bigger than Brown Swiss, and more so than Jersey, Ayrshire, Guernsey, Randall and Canadian breeds. A mature cow can weigh around and over 700 Kg.

Management

1. **Management System:** Intensive
2. **Mobility:** Stationary
3. **Feeding of adults**: Fodder and Concentrate
4. **Housing:** Well developed housing for organized herds.
5. **Feeding system:** Stall feeding.
6. **Feeds to be fed:** Berseem, oats and mustard are the green fodder in rabi; and sorghum, pearl millet and cluster bean in kharif. Commercial feed can be fed anytime of the year. . Milking cows are provided supplementry feeding in the form of cotton seed, barley and oil cake. Feed is given in soaked form at the time of milking. Calves are reared on whole milk up to 1 month of age after which some green fodder is also fed. Calves are allowed to suck 1-2 teats up to 6 months of age. The adult cattle is also fed silage for better milk production.
7. **Feeding of concentrates:** 1kg/2kg milk at the time of milking.
8. **Feeding of roughages:** 1/10th of body weight per day.

9. **Milking:** should be done 2-3 times a day, however thrice a day milking gives higher milk yield.
10. **Milking practice:** full hand milking should be done. Avoid knuckling. Machine milking is generally practiced.
11. **Milk let down time:** 4-5 minutes.

Performance traits

	Average	Minimum	Maximum
Age at first calving (Avg. months)	36	31	41
Calving interval (months)	12.4	11.2	14
Lactation length (days)	305 (standardized)	-	-
Milk yield per lactation (kg)	6150	5876	28800 (record)
Milk fat (%)	3.5	3.1	3.7
Daily lactation in peak period (kg)	22.1	20.7	94.09 (record)
Dry period (days)	60	55	70

- **Peculiarity of the breed**

1. The world record for milk production was set by a Holstein cow in 2010 when "Ever-Green-View My 1326-ET", a cow from Wisconsin, produced 72,170 pounds of milk in a year.
2. Black and white Holstein cows have claimed Supreme Champion honors, the highest recognition given for elite phenotypic characteristics, at the world's largest dairy cattle exhibition, the World Dairy Expo (held each fall in Madison, Wis.) 32 times in the past 42 years.
3. A Holstein's spots are like a fingerprint or a snowflake. No two cows have exactly the same pattern of spots.

- **Research highlights**

1. **Use of milk production hormone, recombinant bST:** A study in February 1999 determined the "response to bST over a 305-day lactation equaled 894 kg of milk, 27 kg of fat, and 31 kg of protein". Monsanto Company estimates a figure of about 1.5 million of 9 million dairy cows are being treated with bST, or about 17% of cows nationally.
2. **Greater use of three-times-per-day milking:** In a study performed in Florida between 1984 and 1992 using 4293 Holstein lactation records from eight herds, 48% of cows were milked three times a day. The practice was responsible for extra 17.3% milk, 12.3% fat and 8.8% protein. Three-times-a-day milking has become a common in recent years. Twice-a-day milking is the most common milking schedule of dairy cattle.

In Europe, Australia, and New Zealand, milking at 10- to 14-hour intervals is common.

- **Major problems associated with health of HF Cattle**
  1. **Mastitis:** Being very high yielding cattle, the risk of mastitis is always present.
  2. **Calcium Deficiency:** The cattle should be supplied with Calcium and Phosphorous supplements to maintain the health of animal.
  3. **Genital Diseases:** The risk of genital diseases like pyometra, metritis, is always present and should be taken care of.
  4. **Milk fever**

Price range

Rs. 1,40,000/- to Rs. 3,50,000/- (tentative)

Can be purchased from

1. **Gupta Dairy Farm:** Address; plot No. 41-42, Govind Colony, near water tank, Doon Valley College Road, Jundla Gate, Karnal-132001, Haryana Phone no. 09416031427.

   Website: www.guptadairyfarm.com, email: guptadairyfarm@gmail.com
2. **Khurana Dairy Farm**, Rohtak, Haryana
   Mobile Number : +91-9215450001 / 9215430001 / 9215450003
3. **Model Dairy Farm:** Mr. Prateek Vaish (VP-Operations). Address: Naramau, GT Road, near ALIMCO, Kanpur-209217, UP.
4. **Karnal Livestock Sales. Contact Details:** Dabas House, 17-E, Session Road, Karnal - 132001, Haryana, India, Mr. Anand Parkash Dabas (Proprietor).
5. **Anand Cows Sales and Dealership.** Contact Details: K. Subramanyam Raju, S/O K. Narayana Raju, Kothaindlu, Punganur(P&T), Chittoor - 517247, Andhra Pradesh, India. Mobile : +918497009383.
6. **Sachdeva Dairy Farm:** Mr. Anil Sachdeva, 940/31, Buffalo Market,Behind Durga Bhavan Mandir,, Rohtak, Haryana, India – 124001. Mobile : +91-9896146700 Website: http://www.sachdevadairyfarm.com

   Webpage: http://www.exportersindia.com/sachdevadairyfarm/

Jersey

Jerseys are a small breed that is fawn brown in color. Because of their color and the shape of their eyes, they are often described as "deer like." They originated on the Isle of Jersey in Great Britain. The Jersey's milk is rich and high in butter fat, so it is usually considered the best-tasting milk. It is also known for the lower maintenance costs attending its lower bodyweight, as well as its genial disposition.

General Information

1. **Species:** Cattle
2. **Synonyms:** Dairy Queen, Farmer's Jersey.
3. **Habitat:** The Jersey can now be found across the world with a large population in Countries such as Australia, Canada, Denmark, New Zealand, South Africa, USA, and Zimbabwe, as well as in the UK.
4. **Breeding tract:** However, the breed is bred only in temperate zones but in India breeding is largely confined to organized herds only whereby standard management and housing conditions are required for dwelling of the cattle. Areas of Punjab, Haryana, Tamil Nadu, Karnataka, Uttar Pradesh and Delhi have some private farms dealing with breeding of Jersey.
5. **Main utility:** Milk for food.
6. **Origin:** The Jersey breed originated on the Island of Jersey, a small British island in the English Channel off the coast of France.
7. **Distribution:** Europe, North America, Southern Parts of Africa, South Asia.

Phenotypic traits

1. **Color: Fawn**, ranging from light fawn to tan. Saddle is tan in color.
2. **Number of horns:** 2 (mostly polled cattle is found).
3. **Visible characteristics:** Tan saddle, capacious udder, stout and angular body, lighter coloration around their noses and eyes, and on the inside of each leg.

		Male	Female
4.	Height (Avg. cm)	137	133
5.	Body length (Avg. cm)	150	139
6.	Heart Girth (Avg. cm)	189	180
7.	Weight (Avg. Kg)	600	580
8.	Birth Weight (Avg. Kg)	38	35
9.	Length (Avg. cm)	152	141

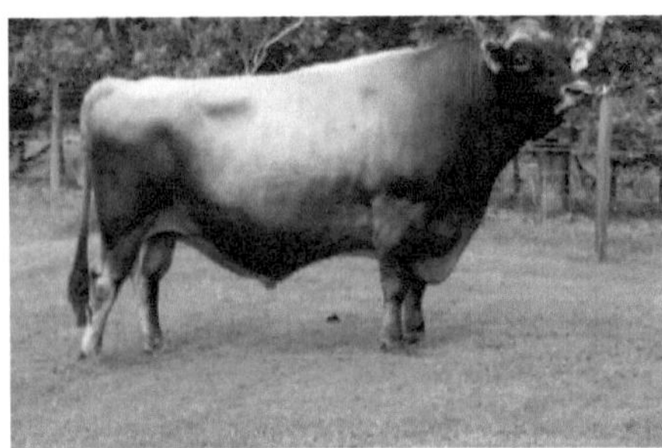

Jersey Bull

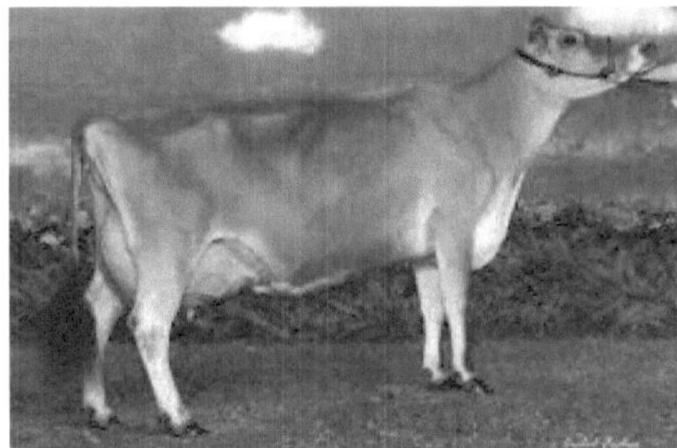

Jersey Cattle

Physical Characteristics

1. **Body Color:** Generally fawn, ranges from brown to tan. Light fawn is generally found in most of the Jersey cattle. A lot of fawn-colored mature cattle have a darker face from just below their poll or just above their eye-brows to just before their noses.
2. **Body Size:** Shorter and stout body. Jerseys look to be more finer-boned and bodied than most any beef breed or even Holsteins. Just like Holsteins, though, Jerseys are quite angular in body type because they are selected to be a milk-producer and not a beef-producer.
3. **Head:** Jersey cows are very feminine looking animals, with a finer, more feminine head.
4. **Horns:** Jerseys are a naturally horned breed, though there are genetics for polled cattle as well.
5. **Temperament:** Docile and is a distinctive dairy animal. The bulls are very aggressive.
6. **Face:** small face as compared to bodily characteristics.
7. **Ears:** Ears are of small size.
8. **Dewlap:** slight.
9. **Udder:** Capacious & Pendulous, Massive in size with prominent milk vein.

10. **Hump:** Absent.
11. **Withers:** Round.

Breed helpful in raising economy of the farm

The Jersey cow is quite small, ranging from only 400–500 kilograms (880–1,100 lb). The main factor contributing to the popularity of the breed has been their greater economy of production, due to:

1. The ability to carry a larger number of effective milking cows per unit area due to lower body weight, hence lower maintenance requirements, and superior grazing ability.
2. Calving ease and a relatively lower rate of dystocia, leading to their popularity in crossbreeding with other dairy and even beef breeds to reduce calving related injuries.
3. High fertility.
4. High butterfat conditions, 4.84% butterfat and 3.95% protein, and the ability to thrive on locally produced food. Bulls are also small, ranging from 540 to 820 kg (1200 to 1800 pounds), and are notoriously aggressive.
5. Castrated males can be trained into fine oxen which, due to their small size and gentle nature, make them popular with young teamsters. Jersey oxen are not as strong as larger breeds however and are generally out of favor among competitive teamsters.

Jersey versus Guernsey

Jerseys are not to be confused with Guernseys. Though both names sound the same, they are two entirely different dairy cattle. Guernseys neither have the fawn coloration nor have dark eyes, nose, hooves and tail switch that Jerseys have, and are brown in color than fawn, and have more white on them than a typical Jersey would.

Management

1. **Management System:** Intensive
2. **Mobility:** Stationary
3. **Feeding of adults:** Fodder and Concentrate
4. **Housing:** Well developed housing for organized herds.
5. **Feeding system:** Stall feeding, grazing.
6. **Feeds to be fed:** Berseem, oats and mustard are the green fodder in

rabi; and sorghum, pearl millet and cluster bean in kharif. Commercial feed can be fed anytime of the year. . Milking cows are provided supplementry feeding in the form of cotton seed, barley and oil cake. Feed is given in soaked form at the time of milking. Calves are reared on whole milk up to 1 month of age after which some green fodder is also fed. Calves are allowed to suck 1-2 teats up to 6 months of age. The adult cattle is also fed silage for better milk production.

7. **Feeding of concentrates:** 1kg/2kg milk at the time of milking.
8. **Feeding of roughages:** 1/10th of body weight per day.
9. **Milking:** should be done 2-3 times a day, however thrice a day milking gives higher milk yield.
10. **Milking practice:** full hand milking should be done. Avoid knuckling. Machine milking is generally practiced.
11. **Milk let down time:** 4-5 minutes.

Performance traits

	Average	Minimum	Maximum
Age at first calving (Avg. months)	28	26	30
Calving interval (months)	13	12	14
Lactation length (days)	305 (standardized)	-	-
Milk yield per lactation (kg)	5600	4500	10,550 (record)
Milk fat (%)	4.84	3.87	5.17
Daily lactation in peak period (kg)	18.3	13.6	34.5 (record)
Dry period (days)	60	55	70

- **Peculiarity of the breed**

1. All Jerseys have dark eyes and dark pigmented skin around their eyes and their noses. They also have black hooves and a dark tail-switch. Those dark noses and dark eyes in Jersey calves make them look adorably cute, much more so than any other bovine calf of any other breed.

2. After the Holstein the Jersey is the second most popular specialist Dairy breed world-wide. Jerseys thrive under both extremes of temperature - they can grow thick coats in very cold climates, whilst suffering form much less heat stress than the other dairy breeds in hotter regions of the world.

3. Despite her small size the Jersey is renowned for its ease of calving, allowing it to be crossed with the larger beef breeds.

- **Research highlights**
  1. Jersey cow produces milk more efficiently than other breeds. This can be especially important in countries where feed may be restricted. As well as making the Jersey a profitable option in agriculturally developed countries.
  2. Many herds of Jerseys in the UK now average well over 5000kgs of milk produced per cow per year, with the best individual animals yielding around 9000kgs or higher.
  3. Jersey milk is in many ways unique. As a product it contains 18% more protein, 20% more calcium, 25% more butterfat than "average" milk.

- **Major problems associated with health of HF Cattle**
  1. **Mastitis:** Being very high yielding cattle, the risk of mastitis is always present.
  2. **Calcium Deficiency:** The cattle should be supplied with Calcium and Phosphorous supplements to maintain the health of animal.
  3. **Genital Diseases:** The risk of genital diseases like pyometra, metritis, is always present and should be taken care of.
  4. Unfortunately, they have a greater tendency towards post-parturient hypocalcaemia (or "milk fever") in dams and frail calves that require more attentive management in cold weather than other dairy breeds due to their smaller body mass and greater relative surface area.

Price range:

Rs. 80,000/- to Rs. 2,50,000/- (tentative)

Can be purchased from

1. **Gupta Dairy Farm:** Address; plot No. 41-42, Govind Colony, near water tank, Doon Valley College Road, Jundla Gate, Karnal-132001, Haryana. Phone no. 09416031427.

   Website: www.guptadairyfarm.com, email: guptadairyfarm@gmail.com
2. **Khurana Dairy Farm,** Rohtak, Haryana. Mobile Number : +91-9215450001 / 9215430001 / 9215450003
3. **Model Dairy Farm:** Mr. Prateek Vaish (VP-Operations). Address: Naramau, GT Road, near ALIMCO, Kanpur-209217, UP.
4. **Karnal Livestock Sales. Contact Details:** Dabas House, 17-E, Session Road, Karnal - 132001, Haryana, India, Mr. Anand Parkash Dabas (Proprietor).

5. **Anand Cows Sales and Dealership**. Contact Details: K. Subramanyam Raju, S/O K. Narayana Raju, Kothaindlu, Punganur(P&T), Chittoor - 517247, Andhra Pradesh, India. Mobile : +918497009383.
6. **Sachdeva Dairy Farm:** Mr. Anil Sachdeva, 940/31, Buffalo Market,Behind Durga Bhavan Mandir,, Rohtak, Haryana, India – 124001. Mobile : +91-9896146700 Website: http://www.sachdevadairyfarm.com

   Webpage: http://www.exportersindia.com/sachdevadairyfarm/
7. **Chaudhary Dairy Farm.** Contact Details: Mr. Arvind A Chaudhary **Address:** Chaudhary Dairy Farm, Mewad. Tal. & Dist.Mehsana, Gujarat. **Mob No:** 9898816448

Brown Swiss

Brown Swiss is a breed of dairy cattle that produces the second largest quantity of milk per annum, over 9,000 kg (20,000 lb). The milk contains on average 4% butterfat and 3.5% protein, making their milk excellent for production of cheese. The Brown Swiss is known for a long gestation period, immense size, large furry ears, and an extremely docile temperament. Regardless, the Brown Swiss is quite a resilient breed of cattle; they are hardy and capable of subsisting with little care or feed.

General Information

1. **Species:** Cattle
2. **Synonyms:** BS
3. **Habitat:** Switzerland, South Europe, US, UK, Canada.
4. **Breeding tract:** However, the breed is bred only in temperate zones but in India breeding is largely confined to organized herds only whereby standard management and housing conditions are required for dwelling of the cattle. Areas of Punjab, Haryana, Tamil Nadu, Karnataka, Uttar Pradesh and Delhi have some private farms dealing with breeding of Brown Swiss.
5. **Main utility:** Milk for food.
6. **Origin:** The Brown Swiss originated on the slopes of the Alps in Switzerland; because they were bred in this harsh climate, they are resistant to the heat, cold and many other common cattle problems.
7. **Distribution:** Europe, North America, Southern Parts of Africa, South Asia.

Phenotypic traits:

1. **Color**: Black, Grey, Dark brown, Tan or White.
2. **Number of horns:** 2
3. **Visible characteristics:** They are often noted for their big floppy ears and docile temperament.

	Male	Female
4. Height (Avg. cm)	142	137
5. Body length (Avg. cm)	155	145
6. Heart Girth (Avg. cm)	196	188
7. Weight (Avg. Kg)	780	650
8. Birth Weight (Avg. Kg)	40	39
9. Length (Avg. cm)	157	147

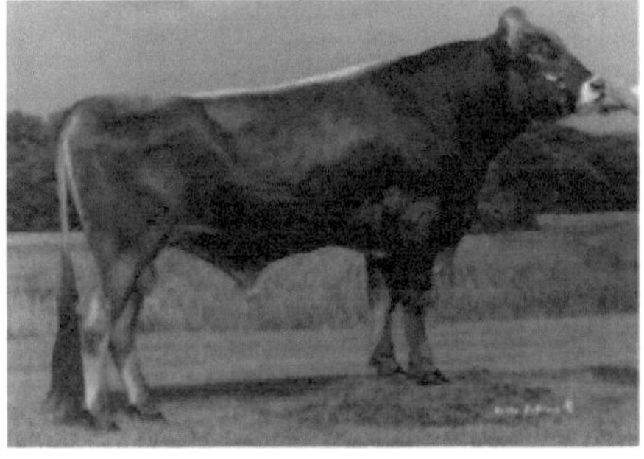

Brown Swiss bull

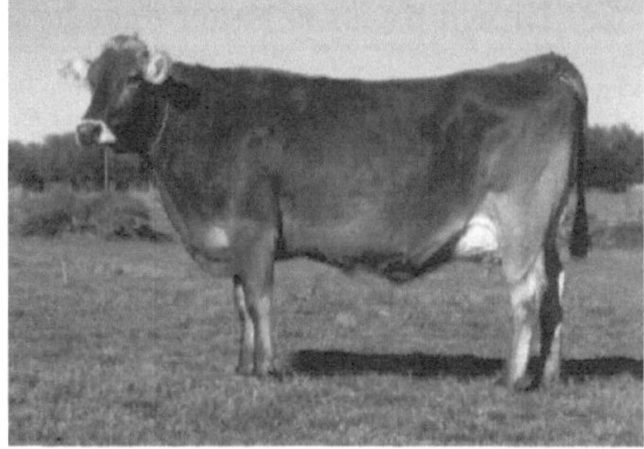

Brown Swiss Cattle

Physical Characteristics

1. **Body Color:** the color of the body varies from grayish black to brown to white. There is great variability in the color of different progenies.
2. **Body Size:** the body is angular and comparitively larger than the Jersey.
3. **Head:** Jersey cows are very feminine looking animals, with a finer, more feminine head.
4. **Horns**: Horns are present but now polled breeds are formed as a result of genetic selection.
5. **Temperament:** Docile and is a distinctive dairy animal.
6. **Face:** moderate sized face with large distinctive ears and poll.
7. **Ears:** Ears are of large size.

8. **Dewlap:** Slight.
9. **Udder:** Capacious & Pendulous, Massive in size with prominent milk vein.
10. **Hump:** Absent.
11. **Withers:** Round.

Light points in identification

Some light points are present above the eyebrows in V-shape fashion on the face which are very much helpful in identification of the cattle. These light colored areas are also present on legs.

Brown Swiss Versus Jersey

1. Coat color of Brown Swiss is Not Fawn.
2. Brown Swiss is larger than Jersey.

Management:

1. **Management System:** Intensive
2. **Mobility:** Stationary
3. **Feeding of adults**: Fodder and Concentrate
4. **Housing:** Well developed housing for organized herds.
5. **Feeding system:** Stall feeding, grazing.
6. **Feeds to be fed:** Berseem, oats and mustard are the green fodder in rabi; and sorghum, pearl millet and cluster bean in kharif. Commercial feed can be fed anytime of the year. . Milking cows are provided supplementry feeding in the form of cotton seed, barley and oil cake. Feed is given in soaked form at the time of milking. Calves are reared on whole milk up to 1 month of age after which some green fodder is also fed. Calves are allowed to suck 1-2 teats up to 6 months of age. The adult cattle is also fed silage for better milk production.
7. **Feeding of concentrates:** 1kg/2kg milk at the time of milking.
8. **Feeding of roughages:** $1/10^{th}$ of body weight per day.
9. Milking should be done 2-3 times a day, however thrice a day milking gives higher milk yield.

10. **Milking practice:** full hand milking should be done. Avoid knuckling. Machine milking is generally practiced.
11. **Milk let down time**: 4-5 minutes.

Performance traits:

	Average	Minimum	Maximum
Age at first calving (Avg. months)	32	28	35
Calving interval (months)	14	13	15
Lactation length (days)	305 (standardized)	-	-
Milk yield per lactation (kg)	5800	4700	7800
Milk fat (%)	4.10	3.87	4.76
Daily lactation in peak period (kg)	19.01	15.54	25.57
Dry period (days)	65	55	75

- **Peculiarity of the breed:**

Very hardy breed and can be raised without much attention to feeding.

- **Research highlights**

Excellent results have been seen in upgrading the local cattle in tropics with Brown Swiss blood. The cattle seem to be an excellent option for cross breeding too with other cattle like HF, Jersey. The milk production of the non-descript increase significantly when crossed with Brown Swiss.

Major problems associated with health of HF Cattle

1. **Mastitis**: Being very high yielding cattle, the risk of mastitis is always present.
2. **Calcium Deficiency**: The cattle should be supplied with Calcium and Phosphorous supplements to maintain the health of animal.
3. **Genital Diseases:** The risk of genital diseases like pyometra, metritis, is always present and should be taken care of.
4. They have a greater tendency towards post-parturient hypocalcaemia (or **"milk fever"**) in dams.

Price range:

Rs. 80,000/- to Rs. 2,50,000/- (tentative)

Can be purchased from

1. **Khurana Dairy Farm**, Rohtak, Haryan
   Mobile Number: +91-9215450001 / 9215430001 / 9215450003

2. **Model Dairy Farm**: Mr. Prateek Vaish (VP-Operations). Address: Naramau, GT Road, near ALIMCO, Kanpur-209217, UP.
3. **Karnal Livestock Sales. Contact Details**: Dabas House, 17-E, Session Road, Karnal - 132001, Haryana, India, Mr. Anand Parkash Dabas (Proprietor).
4. **Anand Cows Sales and Dealership**. Contact Details: K. Subramanyam Raju, S/O K. Narayana Raju, Kothaindlu, Punganur(P&T), Chittoor - 517247, Andhra Pradesh, India. Mobile : +918497009383.
5. **Sachdeva Dairy Farm**: Mr. Anil Sachdeva, 940/31, Buffalo Market,Behind Durga Bhavan Mandir,, Rohtak, Haryana, India – 124001. Mobile : +91-9896146700 Website: http://www.sachdevadairyfarm.com

   Webpage: http://www.exportersindia.com/sachdevadairyfarm/

Indigenous Breeds of Buffalo

Murrah

Murrah breed of buffalo, the pride of Haryana, is a milk type animal. The Murrah is the most important Indian breed of buffalo, also called as 'black gold' and is the most efficient producer of milk, not only in the India but probably in the world. Bulls of this breed are used extensively for up-grading inferior stock. She-buffaloes are used in most of the important cities for the supply of milk and ghee.

General Information

1. **Species:** Buffalo
2. **Synonyms:** Delhi, Kundi, Kali.
3. **Habitat:** Central Haryana & Delhi
4. **Breeding tract:** Hissar, Rohtak, Jind, Gurgaon Districts of Haryana, Nabha and Patiala Districts of Punjab & Delhi.
5. **Main utility:** Milk and Meat for food, Draught power for work.
6. **Origin:** India, Pakistan
7. **Distribution:** Azerbaijan, Brazil, Colombia, China, Ecuador, Guatemala, Indonesia, Laos, Malaysia, Nepal, Philippines, Sri Lanka, Viet Nam

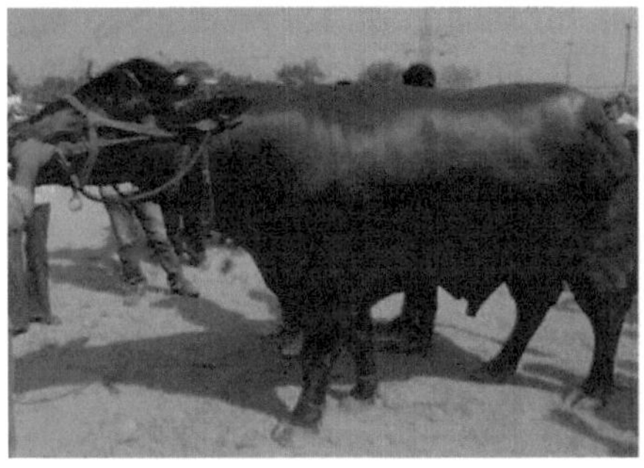

Murrah Bull

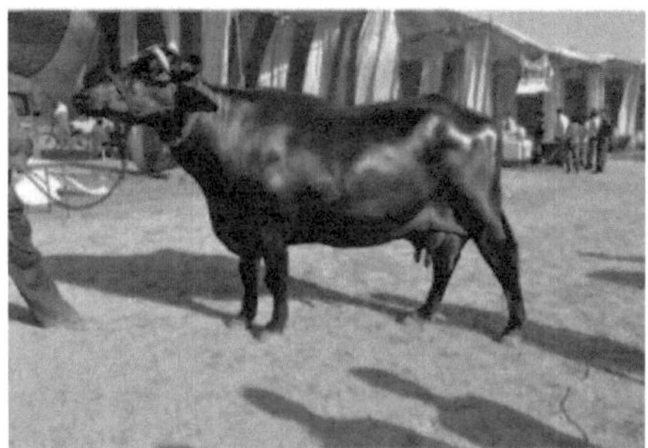

Murrah Buffalo

Phenotypic traits:

1. **Colour:** Jet black
2. **Number of Horns**: 2
3. **Shape of Horns: Tightly curved in a spiral form.** Short in size.
4. **Visible characteristics:** Jet black color, tightly curled horns.

		Male	Female
5.	Height (Avg. cm)	142	133
6.	Body length (Avg. cm)	150	148
7.	Heart Girth (Avg. cm)	220	202
8.	Weight (Avg. Kg)	567	516
9.	Birth Weight (Avg. Kg)	32	30
10.	Length (Avg. cm)	150.2	148.6

Physical Characteristics

1. **Body:** Sound built, heavy and wedge shaped.
2. **Head:** Comparatively small.
3. **Face:** Comparatively long.
4. **Neck:** Comparatively long.
5. White markings on face and leg extremities may be there, but are not generally preferred.
6. **Eyes:** Should not be walled i.e. the cornea should not have whiteness.
7. **Tail:** Long reaching up to fetlock joint with black or white switch up to 8.0 inches.

8. **Horns:** Different from other breeds of buffaloes; short, tight, turning backward and upward and finally spirally curving inward. The horns should be somewhat flattened. As the age advances the horns get loosened slightly but spiral curves increases.
9. **Limbs:** Comparatively short but strong built.
10. **Skin:** Soft, smooth with scanty hairs as compared to other buffaloes.
11. **Udder:** Fully developed, drooping.
12. **Teats:** Equally distributed over the udder but hind teats are longer than fore teats. Cylindrical forms of the teats are most common in the Murrah breed. The front teats are, on average, 5.8 cm to 6.4 cm long and their diameter is approximately 2.5 cm to 2.6 cm. Respective figures for the hind teats are 6.9 cm to 7.8 cm and 2.6 to 2.8 cm.
13. **Loin:** Broader and sliding forward.

Management

1. **Management System:** Semi-Intensive
2. **Mobility:** Stationary
3. **Feeding of adults:** Grazing Fodder and Concentrate
4. **Housing:** Buffaloes are kept in mixed type of housing system. Mostly they are tied to a tree or a pole in the open, but shelter is provided during extreme weather conditions. Houses are well ventilated and mostly made up of a pucca wall with kutcha floor.
5. **Feeding system:** Animals are stall fed, can also be let loose for grazing.
6. **Feeds to be fed:** Berseem, oats and mustard are the green fodder in rabi; and sorghum, pearl millet and cluster bean in kharif. Commercial feed can be fed anytime of the year.
7. **Feeding of concentrates:** 1kg/3kg of milk.
8. **Feeding of roughages:** 1/10th of body weight per day.
9. **Milking:** should be done twice a day, however thrice a day milking gives higher milk yield.
10. **Milking practice:** full hand milking should be done. Avoid knuckling.
11. **Milk let down time:** averages 2 minutes but may be as long as 10 minutes.

Performance traits:

	Average	Minimum	Maximum
Age at first calving (Avg. months)	43.4	39.9	54.2
Calving interval (months)	14.9	14.1	19.9
Lactation length (days)	305 (standardized)	-	-
Milk yield per lactation (kg)	1752	1003	2057
Milk fat (%)	7.3	6.9	8.3
Daily lactation in peak period (kg)	15.7	6.85	31.5 (Record)
Dry period (days)	89	75	98

- **Peculiarity of the breed**

This breed has spread to almost all parts of the world and is being bred either in pure form or is being used for grading up local buffaloes. It has been exported to many developing countries and is bred there.

- **Research highlights**

Murrah buffaloes performed well under hot semi-arid and humid climatic conditions existed in the study area.

Major problems associated with health of Murrah buffaloes

1. **Reproductive problems:** repeat breeders, anestrous, metritis.
2. **Udder problems:** poor udder development, milk let down problem, mastitis and teat defects.
3. Locomotive disorders
4. **General debility**: poor health, weakness.

Price range

High merit: upto Rs. 25 lakhs.

Low merit: upto Rs. 2 lakhs (Avg. Rs. 65,000/- to Rs. 77,000/-).

For further details please see the following links

- http://210.212.93.85/agris/breed.aspx
- http://www.buffalopedia.cirb.res.in/

Can be purchased from

1. **Gupta Dairy Farm:** Address; plot No. 41-42, Govind Colony, near water tank, Doon Valley College Road, Jundla Gate, Karnal-132001, Haryana. Phone no. 09416031427.

   Website: www.guptadairyfarm.com, email: guptadairyfarm@gmail.com

2. **Utsav Dairy Farm:** Mr. Ganda Bhai. Chaudhary
   Address: Near Talab, Punasan Road, Post Mewad, Taluka and District Mehsana-382710, Gujarat. Phone no.: 09978588952, 02762285691
3. **Model Dairy Farm:** Mr. Prateek Vaish (VP-Operations).
   Address: Naramau, GT Road, near ALIMCO, Kanpur-209217, UP.
4. **Bharathi Dairy Farm:** Nellore, Andhra Pradesh.
5. **Khurana Dairy Farm:** Rohtak, Haryana.
   Mobile Number : +91-9215450001 / 9215430001 / 9215450003

NILI - RAVI

The Nili and Ravi are two type of buffaloes found in the valley of Montgomery and Ferozepur. There is no essential difference between the two types. Although for a long time they were treated as different breeds, but closer study indicated it was distinction without a difference, and now, they are officially treated as one breed. The animals are massive, black in color, sometimes brown with white markings. The best animals are found in the riverine tracts along the Sutlej river, south-west of Pakpattan tehsil, Mailsi tehsil of Multan district and Bahawalpur state.

General Information

1. **Species:** Buffalo
2. **Synonyms:** Panch Kalyani
3. **Habitat:** Ferozepur district of Punjab
4. **Breeding tract:** Nili Ravi buffaloes are found in Fazilka, Ferozepur, Zira and Makhu tehsils of Ferozepur district; and Patti and Khemkaran tehsils of Amritsar district. **Whole tract of Sutlej is breeding tract.** Nili-Ravi buffaloes are found in almost all the districts, with major concentration in Amritsar, Gurdaspur and Ferozepur districts of Indian Punjab and in Lahore, Sheikhupura, Faizabad, Okora, Sahiwal, Multan, Bohawalpur and Bahwalnagar districts of Pakistan Punjab.
5. **Main utility:** Milk for food, Draught power for work.
6. **Origin:** India, Pakistan. The name Nili is supposed to have been derived from the blue water of river Sutlej. Ravi buffaloes are mostly bred in Pakistan around the river Ravi, after which they are named. After 1960, they were classified into one breed as Nili - Ravi
7. **Distribution:** Bangladesh, China, India, Pakistan, Philippines, Sri Lanka.

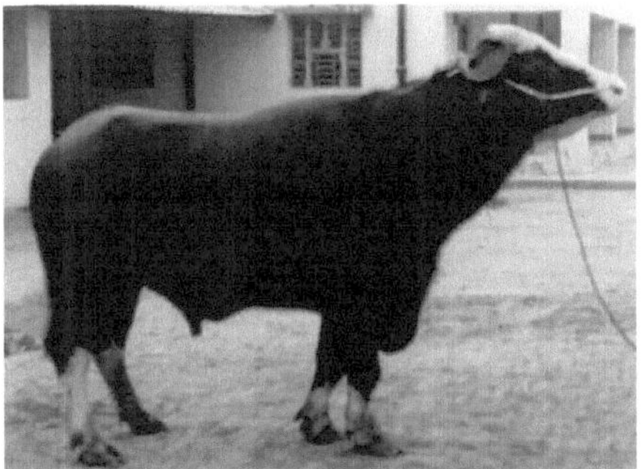
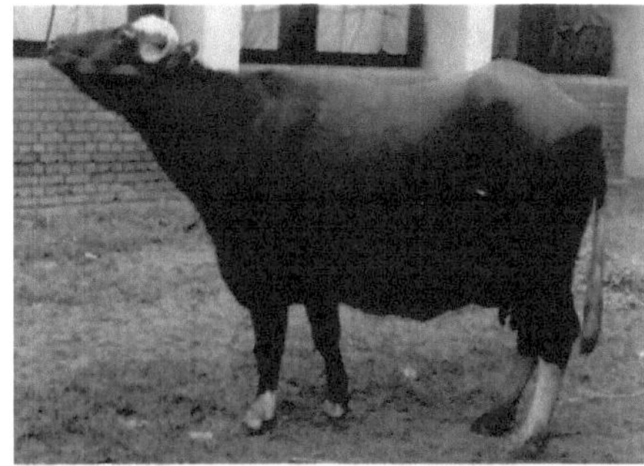

Nili-Ravi Bull and Buffalo at CIRB-Hissar

Phenotypic traits

1. **Color:** Usually black with white marking on forehead, face, muzzle, legs and tail.
2. **Number of Horns:** 2
3. **Shape of Horns:** Horns are tightly curved and circular in cross section, small in size. Horns are less curled than Murrah.
4. **Visible characteristics:** The most desired character of the buffaloes with such white markings highly desired and popularly called "Panch Kalyani").

		Male	Female
5.	Height (Avg. cm)	140	134
6.	Body length (Avg. cm)	160	165
7.	Heart Girth (Avg. cm)	230	208
8.	Weight (Avg. Kg)	567	454
9.	Birth Weight (Avg. Kg)	35	34
10.	Length (Avg. cm)	159.0	147.3

Physical Characteristics

1. **Body color:** The color is usually black but brown is not uncommon. Prominent white markings are present.
2. **Horns:** Horns are small, tightly curled but slightly less curled as compared to that of Murrah and circular in cross section.
3. **Markings:** White markings are found on hind legs, forelegs and white spots on forehead, muzzle and tail switch.

4. **Eyes:** They have usually walled eyes.
5. **Tail:** Tail is thick at the base, gradually tapers towards the end and extends below hocks with a white switch.
6. **Body:** Nili-Ravi buffaloes are large size and have deep and low set frames.
7. **Head:** The head is elongated, bulging at top and is depressed between eyes. Forehead is convex at the centre.
8. **Neck:** Neck is long and thin in females while it is thick and powerful in the males.
9. **Udder:** Udder is well shaped, capacious and extends well forward to naval flap. Pink markings are sometimes seen on udder and brisket.
10. **Teats:** Teats are long, even squarely placed.

Management

1. **Management System:** Intensive
2. **Mobility:** Stationary
3. **Feeding of adults:** Grazing Fodder and Concentrate
4. **Housing:** Farmers usually keep the animals along with them. Provisions of an open shed are made along the residential premises of the farmers and the animals are kept there. The day to day operations are carried out by the farmer in the shed only. Animal houses are usually open, made up of mud and bricks, full walled and have mud floor. Most of the farmers grow fodder for feeding to their animals.
5. **Feeding system:** Animals are stall fed.
6. **Feeds to be fed:** They are fed different kinds of roughages such as barley and wheat straw, cornstalks and sugar cane residuals. In addition, they are given concentrate mixtures. If grazing is available, they graze all day long.
7. **Feeding of concentrates:** 1kg/3kg of milk.
8. **Feeding of roughages:** $1/10^{th}$ of body weight per day.
9. **Milking:** should be done twice a day.
10. **Milking practice:** full hand milking should be done. Avoid knuckling.
11. **Milk let down time:** Averages 3 to 4 minutes.

Performance traits

	Average	Minimum	Maximum
Age at first calving (Avg. months)	45	40	53
Calving interval (months)	16	10	31
Lactation length (days)	305 (standardized)	-	-
Milk yield per lactation (kg)	1850	1586	1929
Milk fat (%)	6.8	5.1	8.0
Daily lactation in peak period (kg)	15.9	7.3	22.8
Dry period (days)	90	65	110

- **Peculiarity of the breed:** Similar to Murrah in almost all respects except for some white markings on extremities, and walled eyes.
- **Research highlights:** The season of calving had significant effect on milk yield. Buffaloes calving in spring showed the highest and those calving in summer showed the lowest milk yield. Sex of calf did not affect milk yield.
- Ravi breed is heavier than Nili buffalo, but their yields are same.

Major problems associated with health of Murrah buffaloes

1. **Reproductive problems:** repeat breeders, anestrous, metritis, reproductive inefficiency.
2. **Udder problems:** poor udder development, milk let down problem, mastitis and teat dcfccts.
3. Herd health and calf management.

Price range

From Rs. 50,000/- to Rs. 1,00,000/- (tentative).

For further details please see the following links

- http://210.212.93.85/agris/breed.aspx
- http://www.buffalopedia.cirb.res.in/

Can be purchased from

1. **Gupta Dairy Farm:** Address; plot No. 41-42, Govind Colony, near water tank, Doon Valley College Road, Jundla Gate, Karnal-132001, Haryana. Phone no. 09416031427.

   Website: www.guptadairyfarm.com, email: guptadairyfarm@gmail.com

2. **Khurana Dairy Farm**, Rohtak, Haryana
   Mobile Number : +91-9215450001 / 9215430001 / 9215450003
3. CIRB, Sub-Centre Nabha, Punjab. Contact Details: Dr. Raman Malik, Principal Scientist & Officer I/c. Ph.01765263167

BHADAWARI

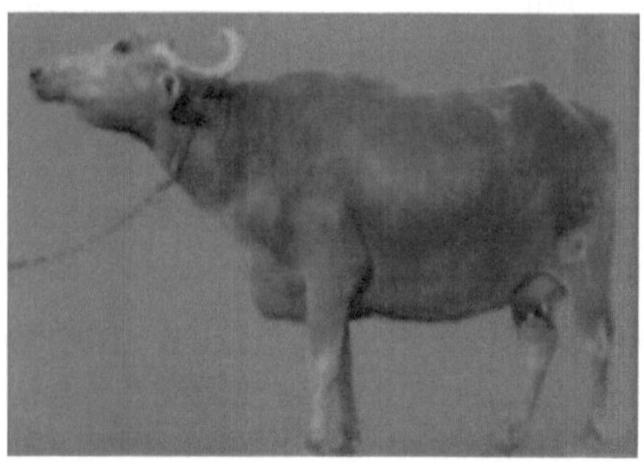

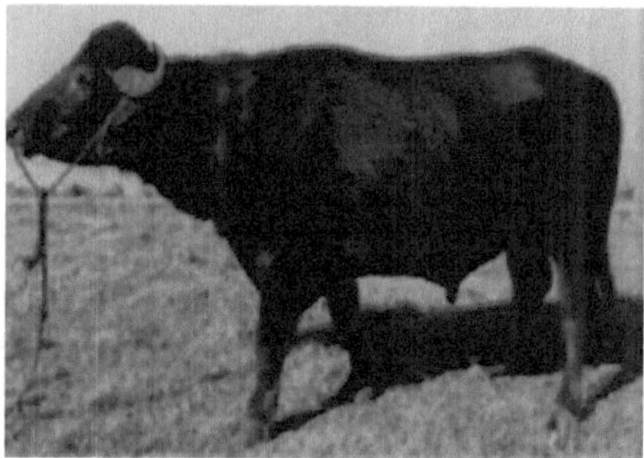

- Also known as "Etawah", Bhadawari is a dual type buffalo breed of central and northern India.
- **Breeding tract**: Bhind and Morena districts of Madhya Pradesh and Agra and Etawah districts of Uttar Pradesh. This tract is a part of former Bhadawar state, from which the name of the breed is derived.
- Bhadawari buffaloes are found in the ravines of Yamuna, Chambal and Utangan rivers spread over in Uttar Pradesh and Madhya Pradesh.
- They are blackish copper to light copper coloured with wheat straw-like colour over the legs. Two white lines, "Chevron", called as "Kanthy" in local language, are present on lower side of the neck.
- **Horns** are black curling slightly outward and downward before running parallel backward near neck and finally turning upward.
- The animals of this breed are famous for their efficient ability to utilize low quality coarse fodder available in the area.
- Though the total lactation yield is lower, fat content in the milk has been recorded as high as 13%.
- Average milk yield of the breed is 1294 Kg per lactation with an average fat % of 7.88 (Yield ranging between 540-1400 Kg per lactation and fat % from 6 to 12.8).

For further details, please follow below given links

- http://210.212.93.85/agris/breed.aspx
- http://www.buffalopedia.cirb.res.in/

JAFFARABADI

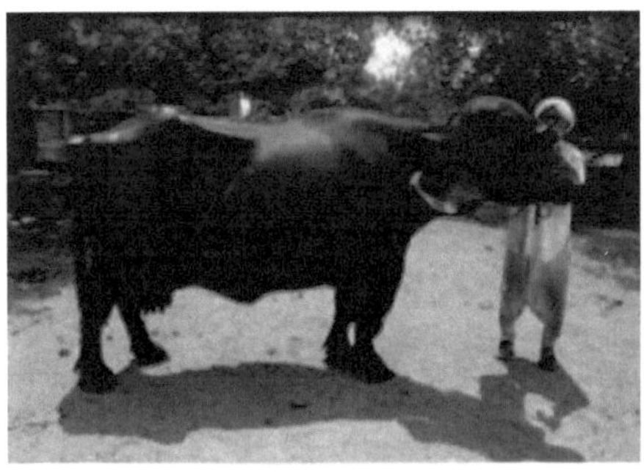

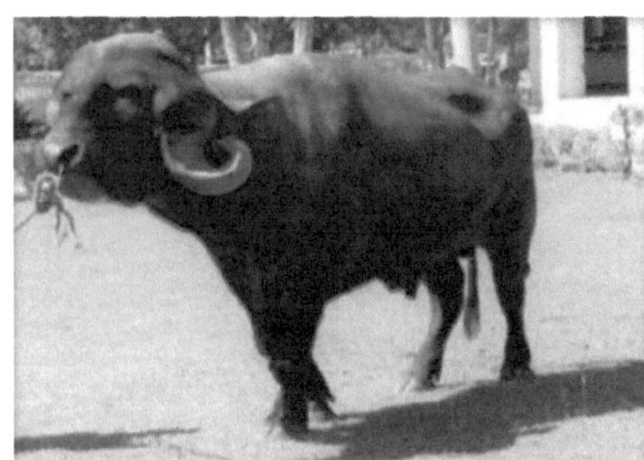

- Jaffarabadi is one of the heaviest buffalo breeds and is a native of Saurashtra region of Gujarat around Gir forest.
- It is also known as Bhavanagri, Gir or Jaffari. It is named after the town of Jaffarabad of Gujarat state.
- The breeding tract includes Amreli, Bhavnagar, Jamnagar, Junagadh, Porbandar and Rajkot districts of Gujarat state.
- The animals may weigh up to 800 Kg and mature bull may weigh up to 1 ton.
- The animal have **a** big dome shaped forehead with flat, thick, downwardly curved horns. The bulge of forehead sometimes covers eyelids also.
- Horns exhibit wide variation, but usually emerge out by compressing the head, go downward sideways, then upward and inward finally forming a ring like structure. Horn shape is peculiar in this breed. It makes eyes to look small - termed as study eye, especially in males.
- This breed is known for its ability to fight lions in Gir forest.
- The animals are generally black but some animals having white or grey tail switch are also seen.
- They are very good milkers.
- Average milk yield of the animals is 2239 Kg per lactation with a fat % of 7.7.

- The lactation yield ranges from 2150 to 2340 Kg. There are reports of animals producing more than 30 lit milk in a day and animals with fat % as high as 18% in this breed.

For further details please see the following links

- http://210.212.93.85/agris/breed.aspx
- http://www.buffalopedia.cirb.res.in/

MEHSANA

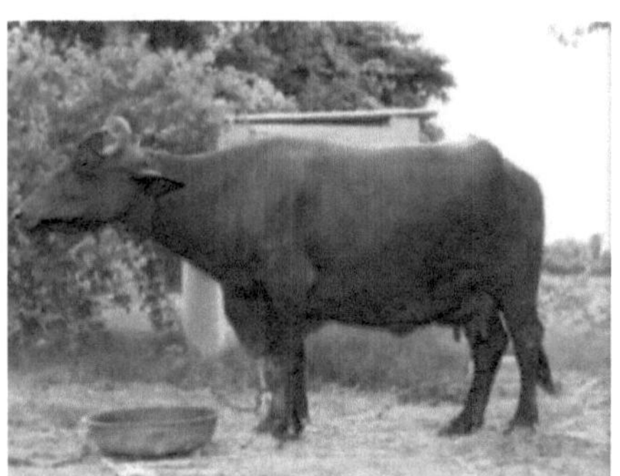

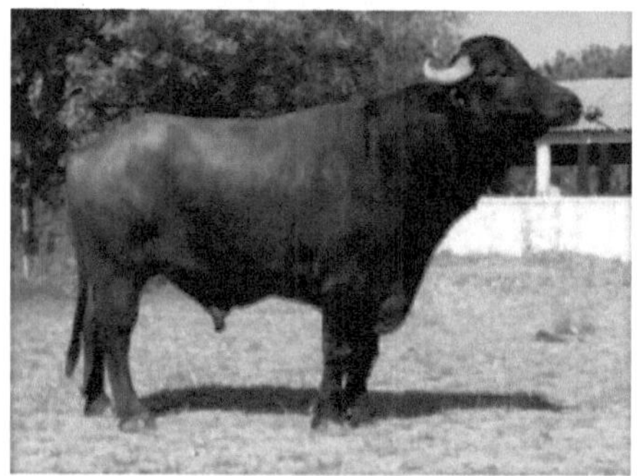

- Mehsana buffaloes are considered to be evolved by crossing Murrah and Surti breeds of buffaloes.
- The breed is named on the place of its origin that is Mehsana district of Gujarat and also known as "Mahesani" or "Mehsani".
- The breeding tract of the breed includes Mehsana, Sabarkantha, Banaskantha, Ahmedabad and Gandhinagar districts of Gujarat.
- The body is longer than Murrah buffalo with lighter limbs.
- Horns are generally sickle shaped and less curved than Murrah buffaloes and curve more upward than Surti buffaloes.
- Animals are mostly black in colour, a few animals are black brown or brown.
- **Eyes** are very prominent, black and bright bulging from their sockets with folds of skin on upper lids.
- The breed has good lactation persistency along with breeding regularity.
- Milk yield of the breed ranges between 598 to 3597 Kg per lactation with 5.2 to 9.5% fat. The average milk yield is 1988 Kg with 6.83 % fat.

For further details please see the following link

http://210.212.93.85/agris/breed.aspx

SURTI

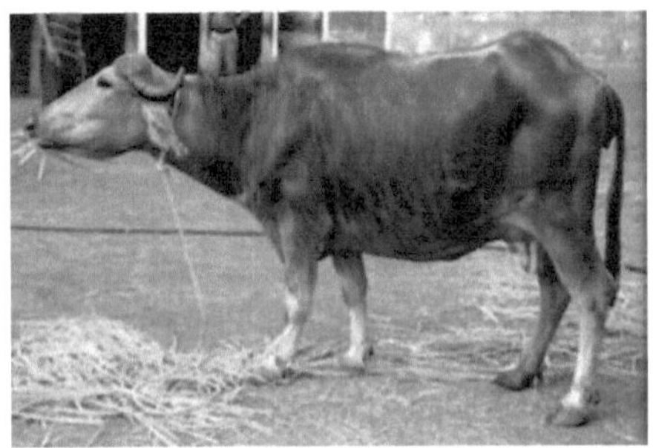

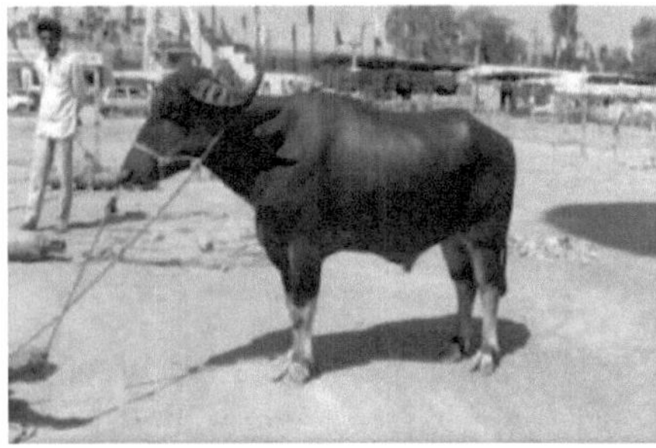

- Surti is also known as Charotari, Deccani, Gujarati, Nadiadi and Talabda.
- The breeding tract includes Vadodara, Bharuch, Kheda and Surat districts of Gujarat. The breed is named after its place of origin.
- Coat colour varies from rusty brown through silver- grey to black. Skin is black or brown in colour.
- Horns are flat, sickle shaped and are directed down ward and backward, and then turn upward at the tip to form a hook.
- Average milk per lactation & average fat % are 1667 kg with 7.02 % respectively.
- The Surti buffalo is lighter in body weight, as compared to heavy breeds, consume less feed, thrives well both on stovers and on limited or no green fodder, and produce milk with high fat and SNF content. It is popular with land less, small and marginal farmers.

For further details please see the following link

http://210.212.93.85/agris/breed.aspx

PANDHARPURI

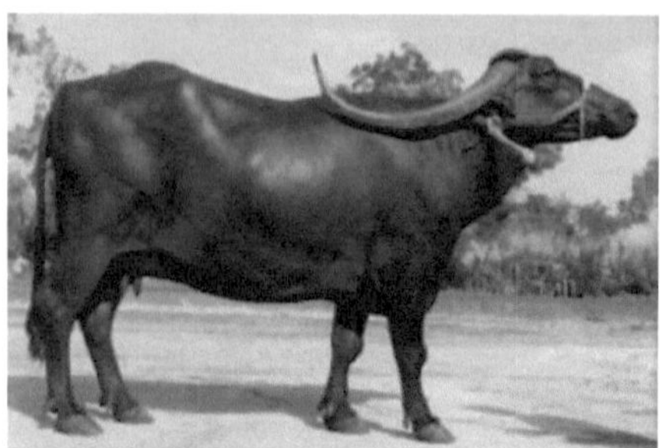
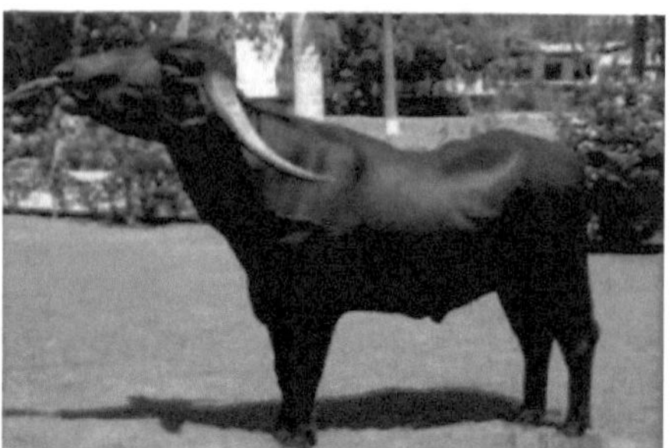

- Pandharpuri is native breed of Maharashtra. They are named after the name of the geographical area i.e. Pandharpur block in Solapur district of Maharashtra.
- The breeding tract includes Solapur, Sangli and Kolhapur districts of Maharashtra.
- The animals have multiple milk let down capability. Farmer takes animals to customer's door and milks as per requirement. Then the animals are taken to the next customer and are milked again.
- Pandharpuri buffaloes are usually black in colour but colour varies from light to deep black. White markings are found on forehead; legs and tail in few animals.
- Horns are very long and extend beyond shoulder blade, sometimes up to pin bones.
- The Nasal bone is very prominent, long and straight.
- The buffaloes produce on average 1790 Kg of milk per lactation with fat % of 8.

For further details please see the following links

- http://210.212.93.85/agris/breed.aspx
- http://www.buffalopedia.cirb.res.in/

20

Housing

An efficient management of animals will be incomplete without a well planned and adequate housing of animals. Improper planning of animal housing leads to additional labor charges. The housing should have proper sanitation, durability, arrangements for the production of clean milk under convenient and economic conditions.

a) General Housing Requirements

Dairy animals will be more efficient in the production of milk and in reproduction if they are protected from extreme heat, and particularly from direct sunshine. This can be achieved through provision of shade in tropical and subtropical climates. If dairy animals are confined, the area should be free of mud and manure in order to reduce hoof infection to a minimum. Concrete floors or pavements are ideal where the area per animal is limited. However, where ample space is available, an earth yard, properly sloped for good drainage is adequate.

Location of Dairy Buildings

The points which should be considered before the creation of dairy buildings animal houses are as follows:

1. Topography and drainage

The houses should be well raised / elevated for the surrounding ground to offer a **good slope for rainfall and more drainage of dairy wastes to avoid stagnation** and for the spread of diseases. A leveled area requires less site preparation and thus lesser cost of building. **Low lands and depressions should be avoided.**

2. Exposure to the sun and protection from wind

A dairy building should be located to a **maximum exposure to the sun in the north and minimum exposure in the south** and protect from prevailing strong wind currents whether hot or cold. **Buildings should be placed such that direct sunlight can reach the platforms, gutters and mangers in the cattle shed.** It is better to have, the long axis of the dairy barns set in the north-south direction to have maximum benefit of the sun.

3. Water supply

Abundant supply of fresh, clean and soft water should be available.

4. Surroundings

Narrow gates, high manger curbs, loose hinges, protruding nails, smooth finished floor in the areas where the cows move should be eliminated.

5. Labor

Honest, economic and regular supply of labor should be available.

6. Marketing

Dairy buildings should be in those areas where selling of dairy products can be done profitably and regularly. Owner should be in a position to satisfy the needs of the farm within no time and at reasonable price.

7. Facilities

Cattle yards should be situated in relation to feed storages, hay stacks, silo and manure pits as to effect the most efficient utilization of labor. Sufficient space per cow and well-arranged feeding mangers and resting contribute not only to greater milk yield of cows and make the work of the operator easier also minimizes feed expenses.

8. Orientation

In deciding which orientation to build, the following factors need be considered:

a. With the east-west orientation the feed and water troughs can be under the shade which will allow the animals to eat and drink in shade at any time of the day. The shaded area, however, should be increased to 3 to 4 m^2 per animal. By locating the feed and water in the shade, feed consumption will be encouraged, but also more manure will be dropped in the shaded area which in turn will lead to dirty animals.

b. With the north-south orientation, the sun will strike every part of the floor area under and on either side of the roof at some time during the day. This will help to keep the floored area dry. A shaded area of 2.5 to 3m^2 per animal is adequate if feed and water troughs are placed away from the shaded area.

c. If it is felt that paving is too costly, the north-south orientation is the best choice in order to keep the area as dry as possible.

d. In regions where temperatures average 30°C or more for up to five hours per day during some period of the year, the east-west orientation is most beneficial.

e. The gable roof is more wind resistant than a single pitch roof and allows for a centre vent. A woven mat of local materials can be installed between the rafters and the corrugated iron roof to reduce radiation from the steel and lower temperatures just under the roof by 10°C or more.

b) Systems of Housing

1. Loose housing system, and
2. Conventional dairy barn

The most widely prevalent practice in this country is to tie the cows with rope on a Kuccha floor except some organized dairy farms belonging to government, co-operatives or military where proper housing facilities exist. It is quite easy to understand that unless cattle are provided with good housing facilities, the animals will move too far in or out of the standing space, defeating all round and even causing trampling an wasting of feed by stepping into the mangers. The animals will be exposed to extreme weather conditions all leading to bad health and lower production.

Dairy cattle may be successfully housed a wide variety of condition, ranging from close confinement to little restrictions except at milking time.

1. Loose housing system

Loose housing may be defined as a system where animals are kept loose except milking and at the time of treatment. The system is most economical. Some features of loose housing system are as follows:

1. Cost of construction is significantly lower than conventional type.
2. It is possible to make further expansion without change
3. Facilitate easy detection of animal in heat.
4. Animals feel free and therefore, proves more profitable with even minimum grazing
5. Animals get optimum excise which is extremely important for better health production.
6. Over all better management can be rendered.

2. Conventional dairy barn

This system is comparatively costly and the cattle are protected from adverse climatic conditions. It further includes two systems of housing:

a. Head to head system.

b. Tail to tail system.

Both the systems are shown under next heading.

Advantages of head to head system

1. Dairy animals feel easier to get into their stalls.
2. Dairy animals make a better show for visitors.
3. Feeding of dairy animals is easier.
4. Sun rays shine in gutter where they are needed most.
5. It is better for narrow barns.

Advantages of tail to tail system:

1. Cleaning and milking of animals is easy.
2. Lesser danger of spread of diseases.
3. Any disease or change in hind quarters can be detected easily.
4. Dairy animals inhale fresh air from outside.
5. Inspection can be easier.

c) Housing of Dairy Cattle and Buffaloes in Animal Sheds:

Specifications of animal shed

- The entire shed should be surrounded by a boundary wall of 5 feet height from three side and manger etc., on one side.
- The feeding area should be provided with 2 to 2 ½ feet of manger space per cow.
- All along the manger, there shall be 10" wide water trough to provide clean, even, available drinking water. The water trough constructed can minimize the loss of fodders during feeding.
- Near the manger, under the roofed house 5" wide floor should be paved with bricks having a little slope. Beyond that, there should be open unpaved area (40'X35') surrounded by 5 feet wall with one gate.

- It is preferable that animals face north when they are eating fodder under the shade. During cold wind in winter the animals will automatically lie down to have the protection from the walls.
- Cow sheds can be arranged in a single row if the numbers of cows are small.
- In double row housing, the stable should be so arranged that the cows face out (tails to tail system) or face in (head to head system) as preferred.

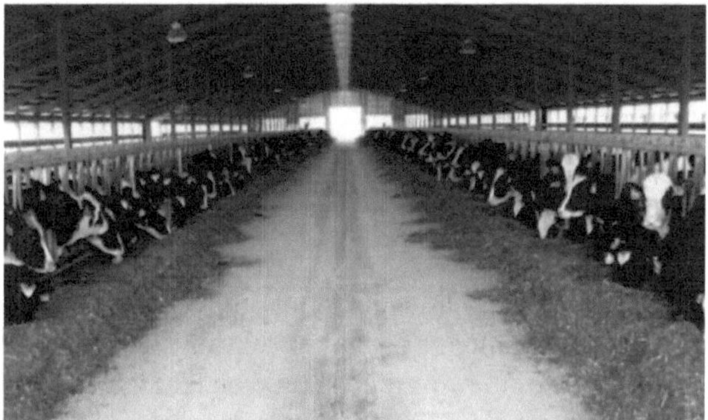

Head to head system of housing

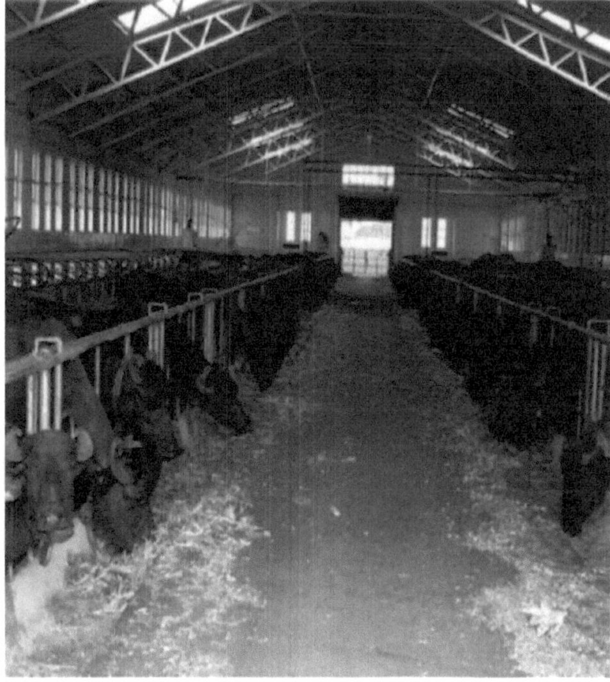

Head to head system of housing in buffaloes

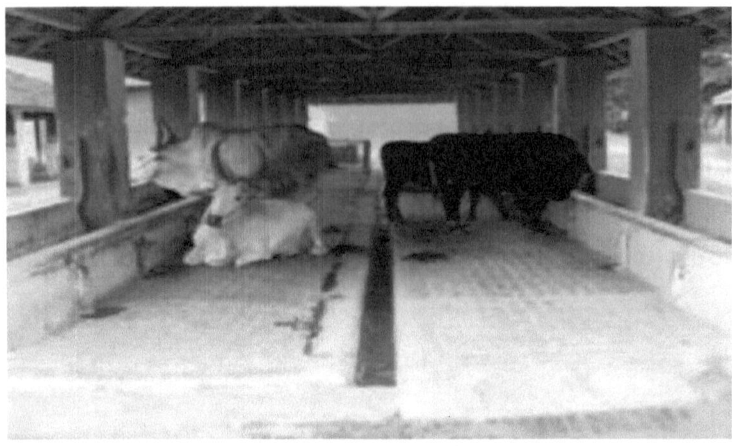

Tail to tail system of housing

Floor

The inside floor of the barn should be of some impervious material which can be easily kept clean and dry and is not slippery. Grooved cement concrete floor is still better. The surface of the cowshed should be laid with a gradient of 1" to 14" from manger to excreta channel. An overall floor space of 60 to 70 square feet per adult cow should be satisfactory.

Type of animal	Floor space per animal (sq. feet)		Manger length per animal (in inches)
	Covered area	Open area	
Cow	20-30	80-100	20-24
Buffalo	25-35	80-100	24-30
Young stock	15-20	50-60	15-20
Pregnant cows	100-120	180-200	24-30
Bull pen	120-140	200-250	24-30

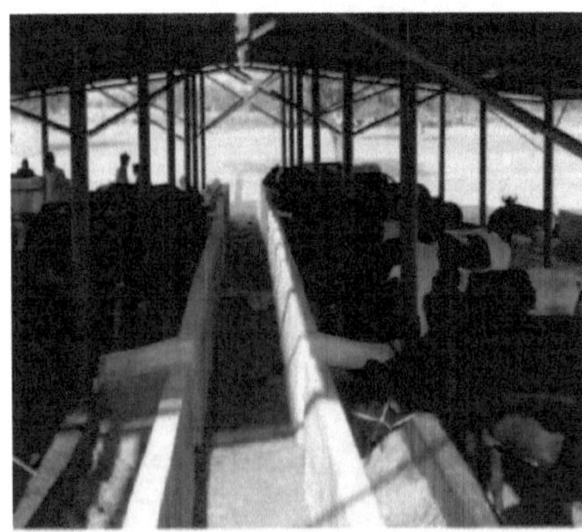

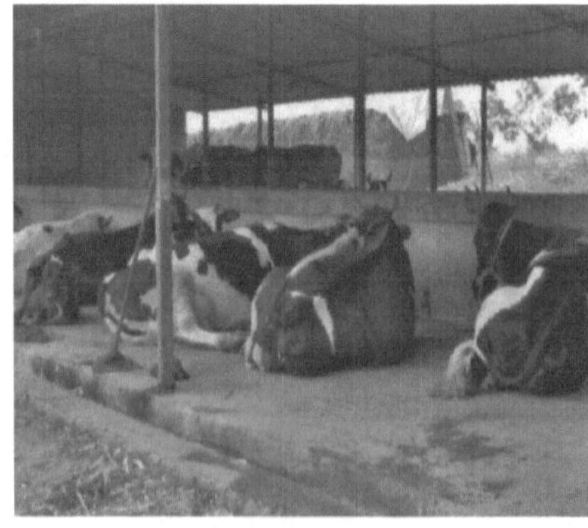

Wall

The inside of the walls should have a smooth hard finish of cement, which will not allow any lodgment of dust and moisture. Corners should be round.

Roof

Roof of the barn may be of asbestos sheet or tiles. However, iron sheets with aluminum painted tops to reflect sunrays and bottoms provided with wooden insulated ceilings can also achieve the objective. A height of 8 feet at the sides and 15 feet at the ridge will be sufficient to give the necessary air space to the cows. An adult cow requires at least about 800 cubic feet of air space under tropical conditions.

Manger

Cement concrete continuous manger with removable partitions is the best from the point of view of durability and cleanliness. A height of 16" for a high front manger and 6" to 9" for a low front manger is considered sufficient. Low front mangers are more comfortable for cattle but high front mangers prevent feed wastage. The height at the back of the manger should be kept at 30" to 36". An overall width of 24" to 30" is sufficient for a good manger.

Alleys

The central walk should have a width of 5'-6' exclusive of gutters when cows face out, and 4'-5' when they face in. The feed alley, in case of a face out system should be 4' wide, and the central walk should show a slope of 1" from the center towards the two gutters running parallel to each other, thus forming a crown at the center.

Manure Gutter

The manure gutter should be wide enough to hold all dung without getting blocked, and be easy to clean. Suitable dimensions are 2" width with a cross-fall of 1" away from standing. The gutter should have a gradient of 1" for every 10' length. This will permit a free flow of liquid excreta.

Door:

The doors of a single range cowshed should be 5' wide with a height of 7', and for double row shed the width should not be less than 8' to 9'. All doors of the barn should lie flat against the external wall when fully open.

Sheds for Young Stock

Calves should be kept in individual pens for the first month. The pens should be easy to keep clean, with shelter from direct sunlight, rain, snow and draught. Keeping the calves in separate pens makes it easier to check what they eat, that they are growing properly, and to detect illnesses. Also, naval suckling is avoided and diseases are less likely to spread.

The calves should have access to fresh and clean water at all times. Preferably, the buckets for milk and water should be outside the pen, in a steady holder within easy reach for the calf, but so the calves cannot splash liquid on the bedding. Humid bedding will facilitate growth of germs and parasites. The pen should contain a holder for hay and concentrate. These holders should be placed above the ground so that the calf cannot step or defecate in them.

- Calves should never be accommodated with adults in the cow shed.
- The calf house must have provision for daylight ventilation and proper drainage.
- Damp and ill-drained floors cause respiratory trouble in calves to which they are susceptible.
- For an efficient management and housing, the young stock should be divided into three groups, viz., young calves aged to one year bull calves, female calves.
- Each group should be sheltered in a separate calf house or calf shed.
- As far as possible the shed for the young calves should be quite close to the cow shed.

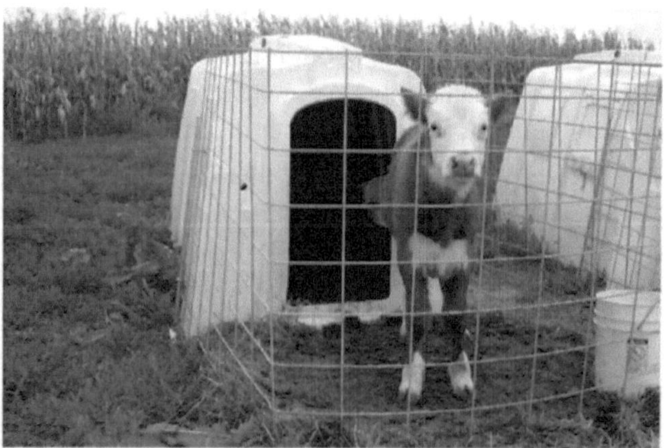

Modern individual calf pen

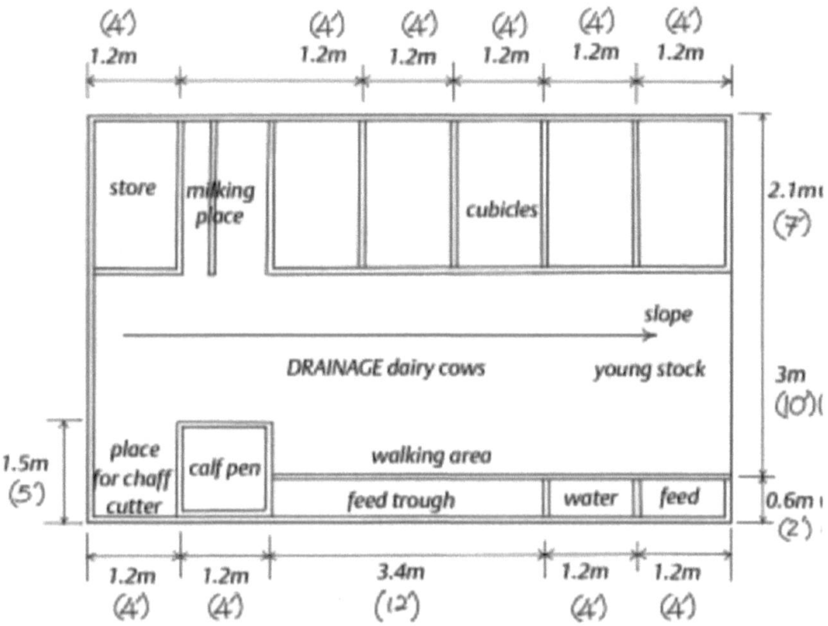

Layout of a stall fed unit for 5 dairy animals.

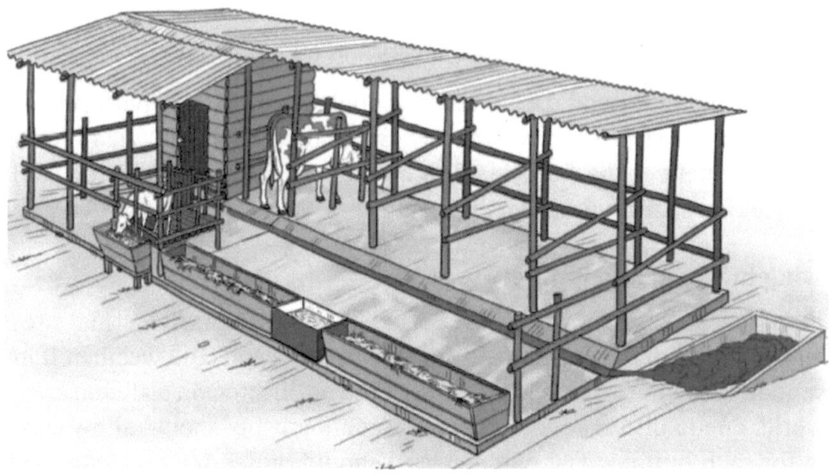

A complete sun shade structure for dairy animals

d) Special Housing Regimes

Improved housing and management of buffalo

- Production performances of Murrah buffalo in tied up housing and in loose housing were studied, and the result proved beyond doubt that loose housing was more profitable, with increased yields.

- In winter, curtains helped lactating buffalo to produce about 500 gm more milk daily than animals kept in an open shed.
- A higher conception rate of 80% was obtained in animals given showers in addition to wallowing facilities. This may also prevent early calf mortality.
- In areas where loose housing cannot be practiced buffalo should be tied up in a conventional half-walled shed through the daytime (after milking) from April to June.
- Over-herding of buffalo in the shed should be avoided, with a maximum 25 buffalo in a floor space of 25 ft x 50 ft.
- The animals should be let out into an open paddock or yard overnight, for exercise and to provide opportunity for natural breeding behaviour.
- They also need to be able to wallow for half an hour daily in clean water. Care should be taken to empty and disinfect the wallowing tanks at least once every weekday otherwise they can spread a variety of contagious diseases. With proper management buffalo farming is indeed profitable.
- By deciding at birth whether a calf should be a milk producer or not, proper care of the calves is easier and less costly. The farmer can then focuses on the future milk producers and cull the others.
- No matter how good the genetic potential, no animal will perform well if it is not cared for and fed properly. Bull calves from high yielding dams can be kept at the farm for future breeding. They can also be sold to breeding stations for progeny testing.

Housing in warm and temperate regions

As discussed, housing for water buffalo should protect against thermal stress – particularly from direct exposure to sun, heavy rains and cold weather. It must allow good ventilation. Housing may therefore be different in different areas of the world, due to differences in climate. But all housing should allow enough space for each buffalo. The outdoor yard should preferably be covered with grass or maybe concrete, in order to prevent it from becoming an unhygienic mud hole in rainy periods.

Buffalo may appear to be misplaced in a hot and humid environment as they are more or less dependent on water for their cooling. This is not entirely true. Buffalo protected from direct sunlight do very well even during hot and humid days, partly because of their ability to lose heat through the respiratory tract. But note that high milk production requires a high feed intake, and that leads to higher metabolic heat production. High yielding buffalo thus have a disadvantage over lower yielding animals, and need more cooling facilities. If buffalo are not provided with proper shelters, wallows or cool showers, their feed intake and growth rate declines, and there could even be loss of body weight. Water intake increases and in the case of lactating buffalo there could be a drop in milk production. There is also a marked reduction in fertility.

Guidelines to consider for good management

1. The feeding, watering and milking place should always give shade and protection from heavy rains, either by trees or by a roof.
2. Cool water either from a clean river or served in an earthen pit, helps the animals to maintain their temperature. Drinking bowls are used extensively for buffalo as an efficient way to provide clean, cool, fresh water at all times. Water troughs should always be placed in the shade.
3. A paddock with trees gives very cheap and effective protection from sun. However, the trees may need to be protected from the buffalo also.
4. In hot humid climates it is better not to have walls. Walls may lead to inadequate ventilation, favoring bacteria and mould growth which makes the stable unhygienic. To protect the interior from sunshine (or heavy rain), curtains made from straw, textile or other suitable material can be used.
5. If possible provide buffalo with a wallow. However, the wallow should be one with clean water and not far from the farm. Spending time walking in the sun to and from the wallow costs more than it saves.
6. Showering the buffalo with cool water for three minutes twice a day has proven to be an efficient way for them to get rid of excess heat.
7. In tied up systems it is advisable to provide partitions between buffalo. This helps to reduce the number of cases of teat trampling and other udder injuries. Partitions are also useful while milking buffalo with bucket milking machines or in a pipe-line milking system.

Thermal ameliorative measures to improve comfort levels of buffalo

The comfort or thermo neutral zone is described as the environmental temperature range in which no apparent demands are made upon physiological thermoregulatory mechanisms. This temperature range is from 2 to 21°C for Bos taurus and 10 to 27°C for *Bos indicus*. But buffalo are more sensitive than cattle to direct solar radiation and high ambient temperatures. There are several reasons for this.

1. The dark body color which absorbs heat well when the animals are exposed to sunlight.
2. The relatively fewer number of sweat glands per unit area of skin, which is unfavorable for high heat loss by sweating.
3. The thick epidermal layer of skin, which protects against heat loss by conduction and radiation.

Cattle have much more efficient thermoregulation mechanisms with their greater density of sweat glands which enable much more heat dissipation through sweating. In spite of their limitations buffalo adapt and thrive in hot and humid tropical and sub-tropical climates, principally due to the semi-aquatic behaviour by which a buffalo seeks water to immerse its body as a means of reducing the heat load. Buffalo are known to have a higher water turnover rate than both *Bos taurus* and *Bos indicus* cattle. They are also less efficient users of water per unit of dry matter intake, have higher urine outputs and a lower percentage of kidney re-absorption of water. Buffalo become more restless, nervous and aggressive during hot-dry and hot-humid climatic conditions. The percentage of restless, nervous and aggressive buffalo increases with increasing atmospheric temperature. During dry, hot and humid seasons almost all nervous and aggressive buffalo and more of the docile buffalo need oxytocin injections for milk letdown. Buffalo seem to tolerate cold better than is commonly supposed. However, cold winds and rapid drops in temperature appear to have caused illness, pneumonia and even death.

A study on the effect of certain summer management practices on lactating Murrah buffalo indicate that there is a definite increase in yield of about 20 to 25% by providing cooled drinking water and showering the animals during the afternoons. A distinct improvement in the summer breeding of buffalo following managerial changes in farm practices has been reported. A higher conception rate, of 80%, was obtained in animals given showers in addition to wallowing facilities. Showers may prevent early embryonic mortality. This study further established that there is no quiescence of reproduction rhythm during summer. Buffalo heifers whose age at puberty coincides with onset of summer can also be located in heat and can conceive during summer. Resting animals under a tree instead of the hot sun could also prevent pre-natal mortality.

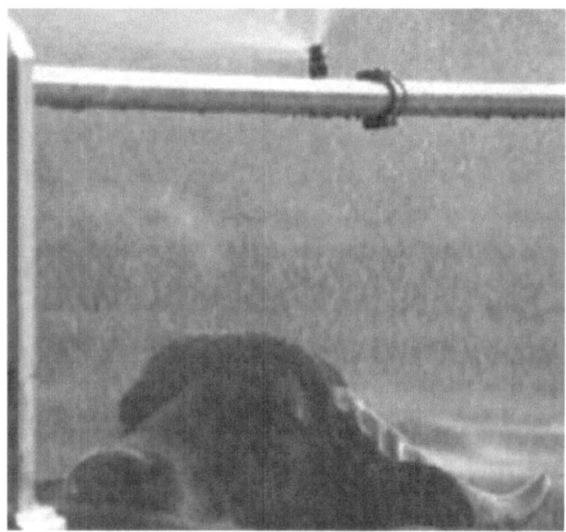

Sprinkler for buffalo in summer season

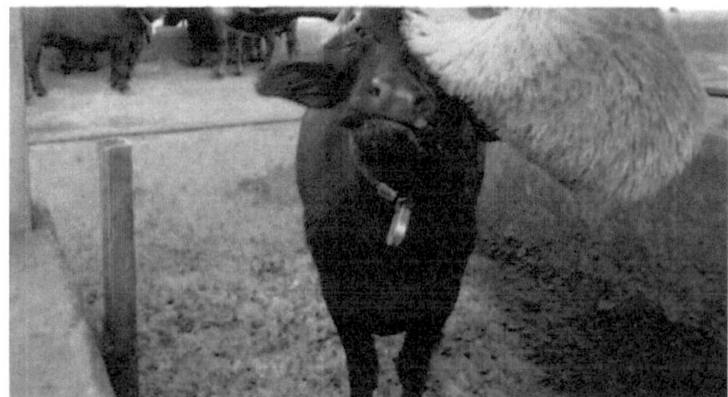

Buffalo using the swinging cow brush

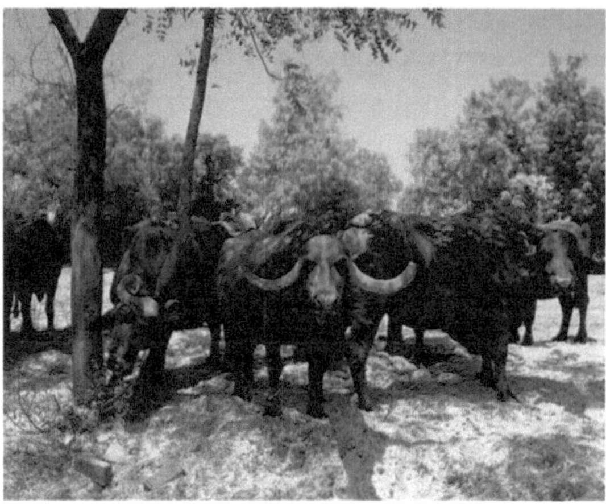

Buffaloes enjoying tree shade

Housing in cold regions

The shelter should protect the animals from rain, snow and strong wind. It may be a simple construction with a roof and three walls. This system will allow the buffalo to go outside to graze when the weather allows it. There should be a feeding area inside the shelter in case of several days with bad weather. A separate heated milking area is advisable. Dry and clean bedding is important in cold weather to maintain animal health.

Environment Controlled Housing (ECH)

Crossing of local cows with improved European breeds has been accepted by the farmers for getting more milk. The crossbreds obtained out of exotic inheritance needs to be managed in a different way to exploit their genetic potential. If this is not done, whatever the genetic quality of the cross bred cow-farmer may have, he will not get full return from the cow. This is because of the following:

1. The thermal stress in the warm tropical environment causes reduced growth rates, low milk yield and reduced reproductive performances. The animal's metabolism is altered to accommodate increased heat load. The heat stress is counteracted by the animal by increasing heat loss through evaporation and by decreasing heat production by lowering metabolic rate.
2. Heat loss is by radiation, conduction, convection and evaporation. When the ambient temperature is higher than the body temperature, the only means of heat loss is by evaporation. Ruminants depend upon respiratory heat loss, rather than sweating. This increases their respiratory rate. This causes reduced feed intake and rumination. When animal cannot dissipate entire heat, the body temperature rises. Rise in 1°C (or 1.80 F) in body temperature represents a storage of 410 kcal of heat - which is required to be dissipated.

The optimum thermal environment in which the animal enjoys optimum health and maximum performance is known as Thermo-neutral zone. This is between 13 to 18°C. The change in temperature by 10°C can bring about great discomfort and inefficiency in animal production.

The other managemental options to enhance animal production include protein to calorie ratio. Feeds differing heat increment needs to be manipulated during heat stress.

Let us see, what measures we can take to alleviate the heat stress in housing and other managemental practices.

Hot Weather Shelters

1. The roofs so designed reduce the radiant heat by 50% (Shining surface). Aluminum with white paint on the top is found to be the best.
2. Hay proves to be coolest of several materials used for sun roofs.
3. Shade provided by thorny tree is found to be slightly superior to shade provided by straw roofs for protecting calves from heat stress. (Acacia species, Ziziphus, Mauritiana, etc).
4. The best height of roof is suggested to be 10 - 12 feet. If these roofs are lower than 7 feet then they act as a shade from part of the cool sky. (The air near ground, in this case acts as a 'heat sink').
5. When evaporative coolers are used, for the shelters, they are found to increase humidity.
6. The sun-roof area for a dairy animal is suggested to be 50 to 60 sq./ft. per animal. It is observed that animals prefer shade-outside to shade inside a shelter.
7. Use of fans/coolers will be economical provided their use ensures 25% increase in milk production.
8. Showers and Fans: It was observed that higher crosses (75% blood level) spend more time (3 times) under showers when atmospheric temperature exceeds 35-36°C.

- Sprinkling water (on animal body) reduced their body temperature and respiratory rates, but did not increase the milk yield.
- Sprinkling water followed by shade was more effective than shade alone.
- Effect of sprinkling could be enhanced by fanning.
- Fanning the animals with sprinkling water every hour kept animal body temperature normal.
- In Air temperature, more than 39°C, it gives heating effect in fanning.

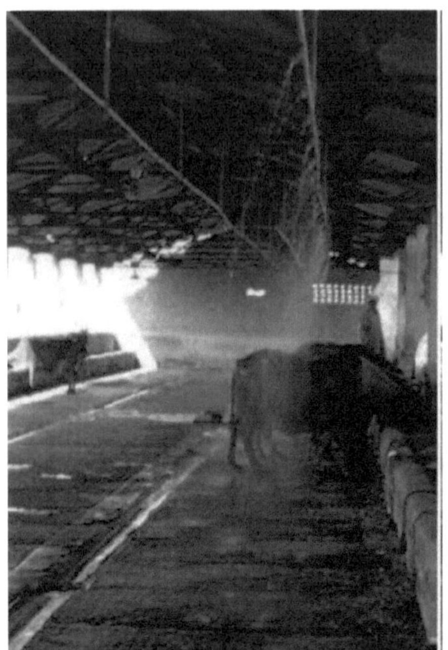
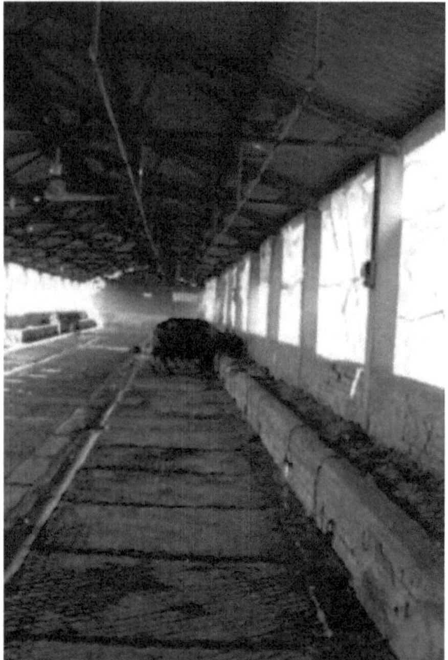

Showers and mist

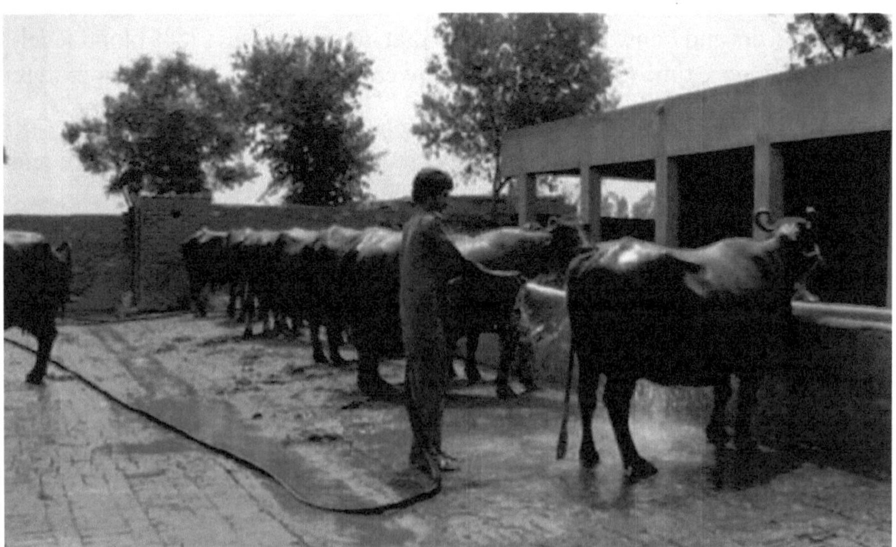

(A farmer giving shower to animals)

9. Other Methods:

- Providing cool drinking water +12° to + 18°C increases animal comfort, by cooling the body by conduction.
- Providing a wide hood around the head of animal with a cool air of temperature 10° or 16°C for breathing (when atmospheric temperature is more than 29°C) was found to be useful. However, under field conditions this method cannot be suggested to the farmers.
- A traditional system in which farmer allows his animal to roam about, in the so called grazing land for scavenging its feed should be stopped. Crossbreds fail to show any advantage over local cow, when sent out for grazing. Therefore, crossbreds should be kept under stall feeding.
- Thatching of roofs helps in cooling the byre. The layer of a thatch should be at least 6 to 8 inches.
- Clipping the animal body coat helps body cooling. Clipping of body coat helps easy dissipation of heat. (Otherwise hair act as insulator and does not allow air-current to come in contact with the skin). Clipping twice a year will be beneficial.
- When there is shortage of water, sponging of animal body with cool water is beneficial, when done, an hour before milking.
- Feeding of roughages during cool hours of the day - correct ratio of protein and cncrgy, feeding of potassium salt (as it is more needed in hot climate) and vitamin 'A' powder (One gram/day/animal - two to three times a week) for improving heat tolerance of the animal is also suggested.

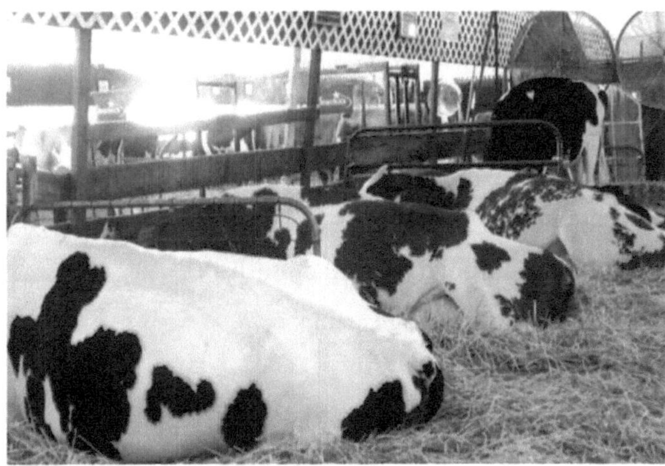

Good bedding and ventilation

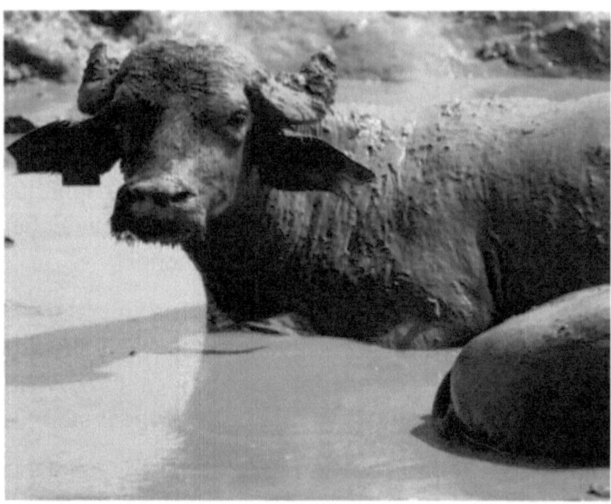

Buffaloes wallowing in mud pool during hot summer day

e) Housing for Medium to Large Scale Herds

For the farmer with up to 30 dairy animals (cattle or buffaloes) a yard with paved shade and feed area would be suitable. The yard and feeding area may alternatively be combined with an open sided barn designed for deep bedding or equipped with free stalls and where the herd consists of high yielding cows the milking shed may be equipped with a bucket milking machine. Some farmers with up to 30 cows may even consider using an open sided tie-stall shed.

In general a medium or large scale dairy unit may include the following facilities:

1. Resting area for cows:
   a. Paved shade, or
   b. Deep bedding in an open sided barn, or
   c. Free-stalls in an open sided barn
2. Exercise yard (paved or unpaved)
3. Paved feed area:
   a. Fence line feed trough (shaded or unshaded), or
   b. Self-feeding from a silage clamp
4. Milking Centre:
   a. Milking shed or parlor,
   b. Collecting yard (part of the exercise yard),

   c. Dairy including milk store
   d. Motor room
5. Calving pen(s)
6. Calf accommodation
7. Young stock accommodation (yard with paved shade and feed area)
8. Bulk feed store (hay and silage)
9. Concentrate feed store
10. Veterinary facilities:
    a. Diversion pen with Artificial Insemination stalls
    b. Isolation pen
11. Waste stores:
    a. Slurry storage, or
    b. Separate storage of solids and effluents
12. Office and staff facilities

Each of the parts of the dairy unit may be planned in many different ways to suit the production system and the chosen method of feeding. Some requirements and work routines to consider when the layout is planned are as follows:

a. Movement of cattle for feeding, milking and perhaps to pasture.
b. Movement of bulk feed from store to feeding area and concentrates from store to milking shed or parlor.
c. Transfer of milk from milking shed or parlor to dairy and then off the farm. Clean and dirty activities, such as milk handling and waste disposal, should be separated as far as possible.
d. The diversion pen with Artificial Insemination stalls and any bull pen should be close to the milking centre as any symptoms of heat or illness are commonly discovered during milking and cows are easily separated from the rest of the herd while leaving the milking.
e. Easy and periodical cleaning of accommodation, yards, milking facilities and dairy, and transfer of the waste to storage and then to the fields.
f. The movements of the herdsman. Minimum travel to move cows in or out of milking area.
g. Provision for future expansion of the various parts of the unit.

21

Nutrition (Feed and Fodders)

Introduction

The dairy farmers mostly keep cows (indigenous and crossbred) along with few buffaloes for milk production. However, the genetic potential of the dairy animals is exploited fully, when they are fed with well balanced ration. Further, as feed cost is around 75% of the total cost of production, the success of the dairy farming depends not only on the quality of the ration, but also on the economy of the ration. Therefore, knowledge on the feeds and feeding of dairy animals is highly essential.

What is Feed?

Feed may be defined as supplementation of nutrients for development, maintenance and operation of day to day activities by animals.

Types of feed

The important feed components are carbohydrates, proteins, fats, minerals, vitamins and water. These ingredients are supplied through roughages and concentrates. Before embarking on a dairy farming enterprise it is important to find out the type of feeds available affordably in your area. Types of feeds can be divided into:

1. Forages (Roughages): these include Napier grass, hay, grass, maize (Stover and residues) plants, and banana pseudo stems. Fodder legumes like leucerne (Leucaena leucocephala), calliandra (Calliandra calothyrsus), sesbania (Sesbania sesban) and gliricidia (Gliricidia sepium). Different types of forages have different nutritional value to the animal. It is therefore necessary to mix or change between forages over time.

2. Concentrates: these include wheat bran, maize germ, dairy meal, and pollard or maize bran. These types of feeds cannot be produced on small or medium scale farms, as they require large capital investments. However, in almost all areas where dairy farming is suitable there are industries that specialize in producing and selling these types of feeds. Concentrates are usually used in small quantities, unlike forages.

3. Other byproducts: e.g. cotton seed cake, fishmeal, molasses, brewer's waste and poultry waste. These are usually by products of other industrial or farm enterprises, but are rich in nutrients that increase productivity of dairy animals.
4. Feed additives: e.g. minerals and vitamins, livestock salts, buffers, enzymes, probiotics yeast and urea. These also have to be purchased and are an essential component of costs in a dairy enterprise.

Examples of nutrient content of common feedstuffs used for feeding dairy animals

Feed name (live weight kg)	Energy (ME in Mcal)	TDN (kg)	Total crude protein (g)	Calcium (g)	Phosphorous (g)
Alfalfa hay	2.36	0.63	200	15.4	2.2
Napier grass	2.0	0.55	87	6	4.1
Rape fresh	3.16	0.81	164	-	-
Oats	2.73	0.6	140	-	-
Sorghum fresh	2.36	0.63	88	4.3	3.6
Sorghum silage	2.14	0.58	62	3.4	1.7
Maize silage	2.67	0.7	81	2.3	2.2
Wheat straw	1.51	0.44	0	1.8	1.2
Rape seed	2.93	0.76	390	7.2	11.4
Cotton seed cake	2.71	0.71	448	1.9	1.2
Wheat bran	2.67	0.7	171	11.8	3.2
Molasses	2.67	0.7	103	11	1.5
Urea	0	0	281	0	0

Common feed ingredients

Cereals:

1. Maize:

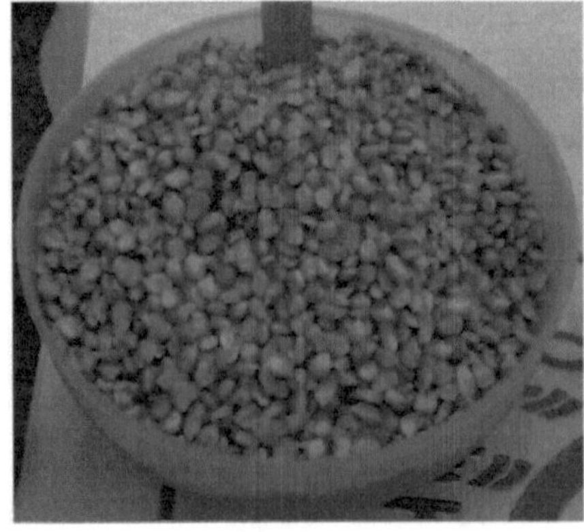

Grain form

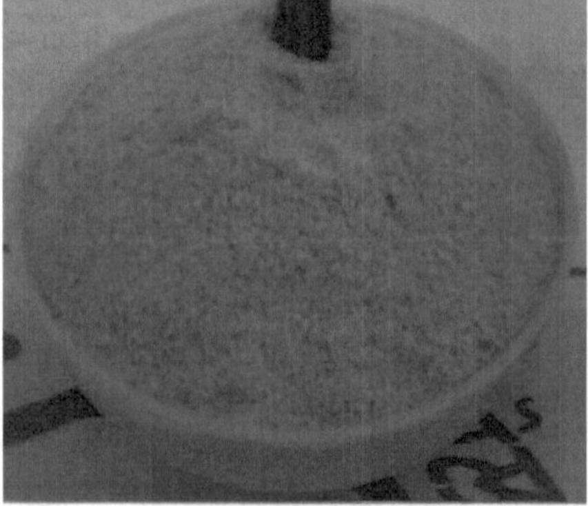

Ground form

(Crude Protein-10%; Ether extract-2.5%)

2. Rice kani: (Crude Protein-10%; Ether extract-1.5-2.0%)

3. Rice polish:

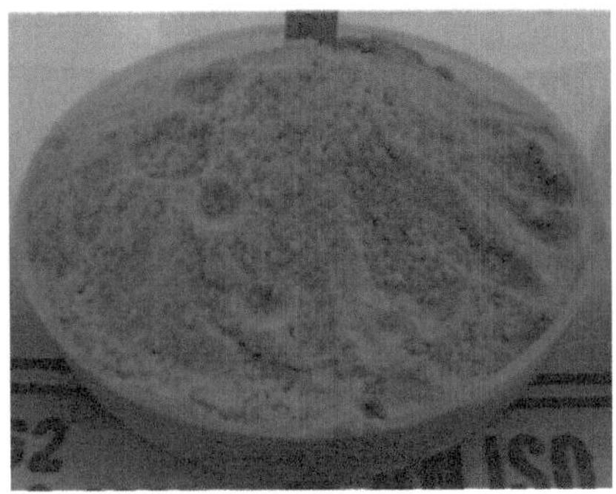

Ground form
(Crude Protein-12-14%; Ether Extract-14-16%)

4. De-oiled Rice Polish:

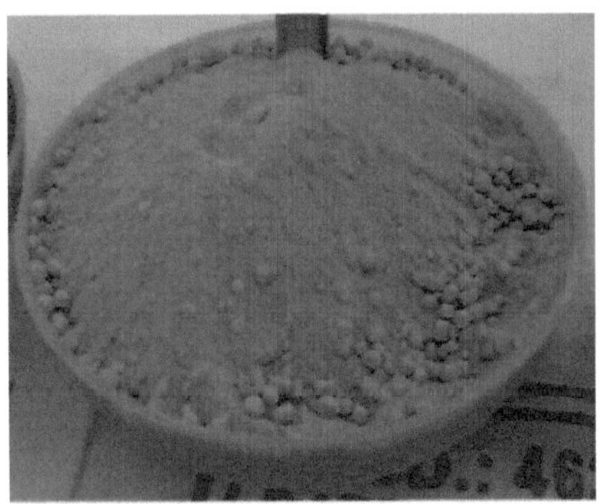

Ground form
(Crude Protein-14-18%; Ether Extract-0.5-1.0%)

5. Brewers's Dried Grains:

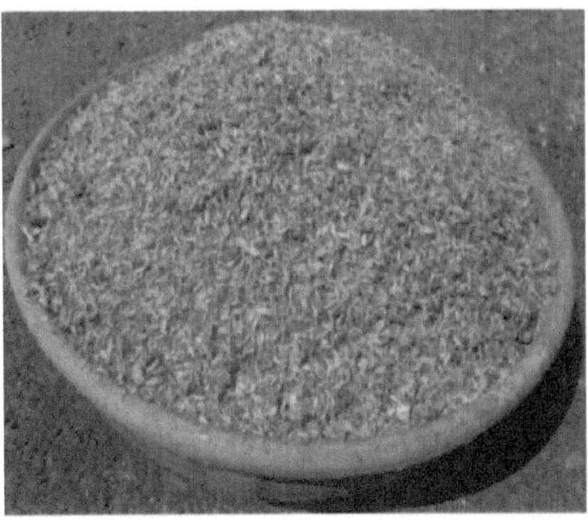

(Crude Protein-25%; Ether Extract-5%)

6. Soybean Meal:

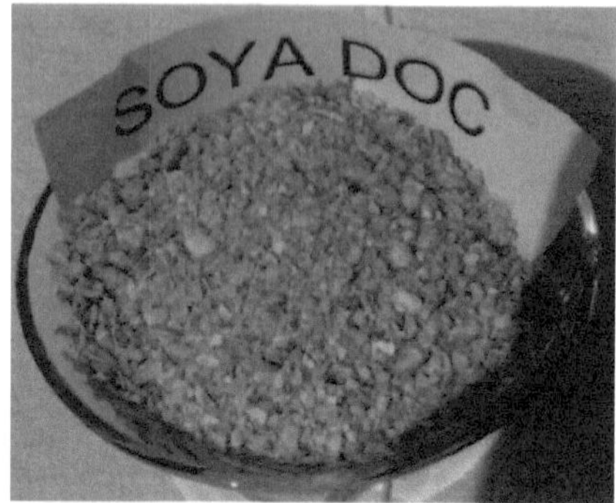

(Crude Protein-48-50%; Ether Extract-0.5-1.0%)

7. Groundnut Cake:

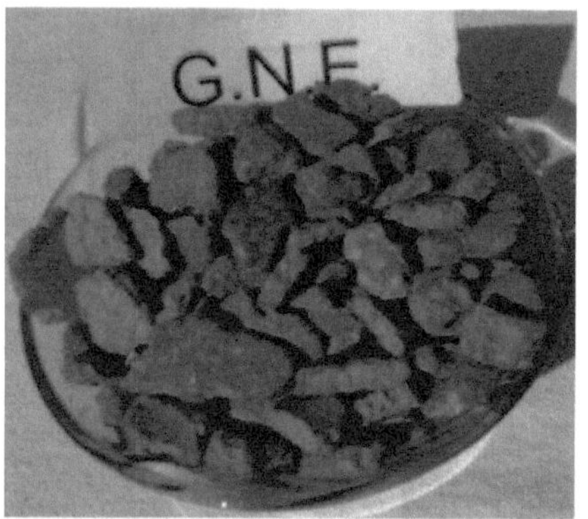

(Crude Protein-45%; Ether Extract-0.5-1.0%)

8. Mustard Seed Cake:

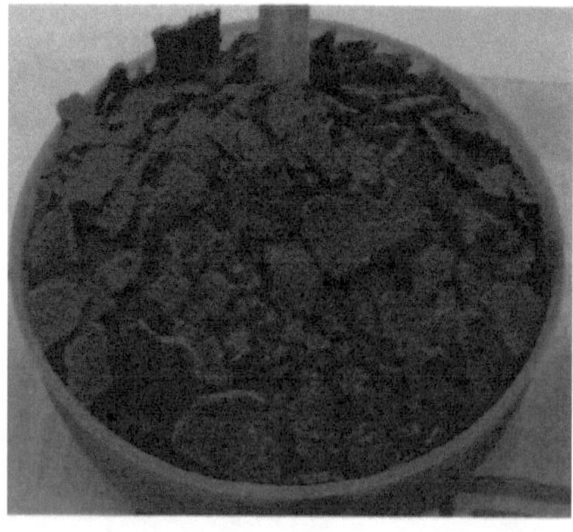

(Crude Protein-35%; Ether Extract-7%)

9. Cottonseed Cake: (Crude Protein-25%; Ether Extract-7%)

10. Mineral Mixture:

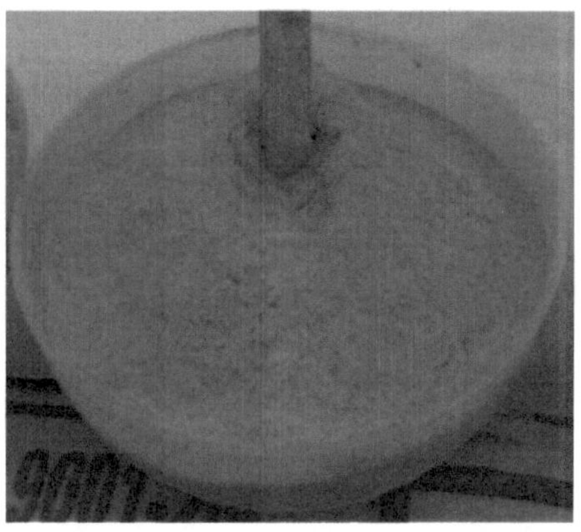

(Calcium-20%; Phosphorus-16%)

11. Common Salt:

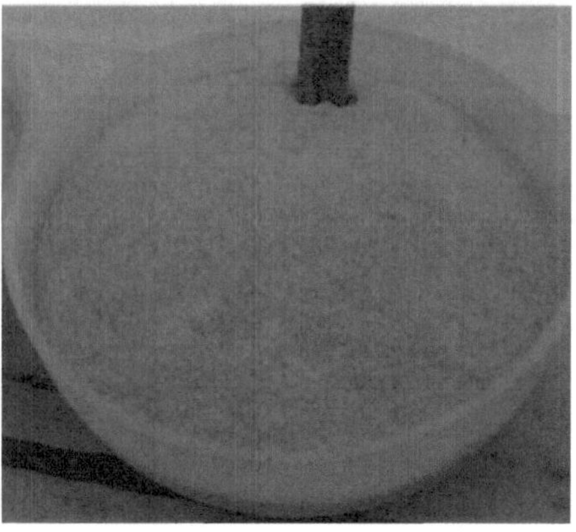

Green Fodder:

1. Cowpea Green Fodder:

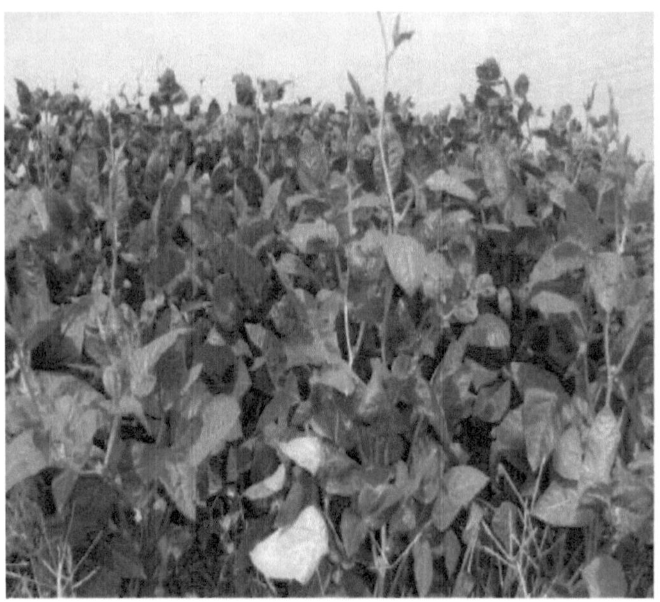

(Crude Protein-15-20%)

2. Maize Green Fodder:

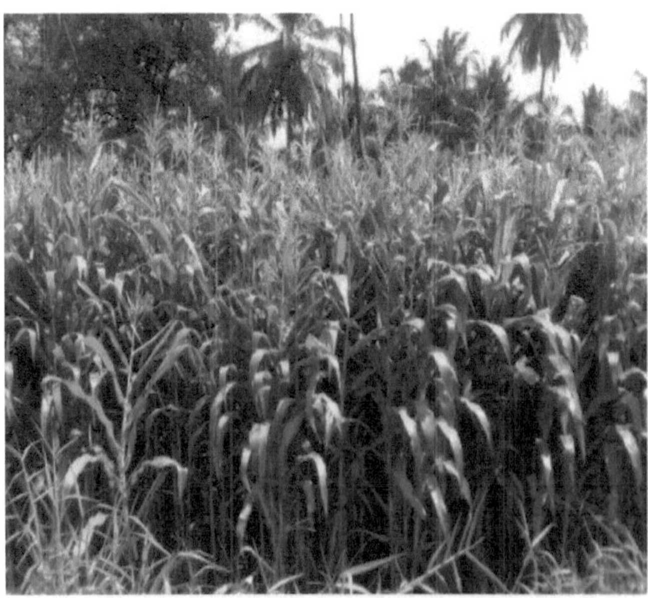

(Crude Protein-8-10%)

3. Napier Bajra Hybrid (CO-3) Green Fodder:

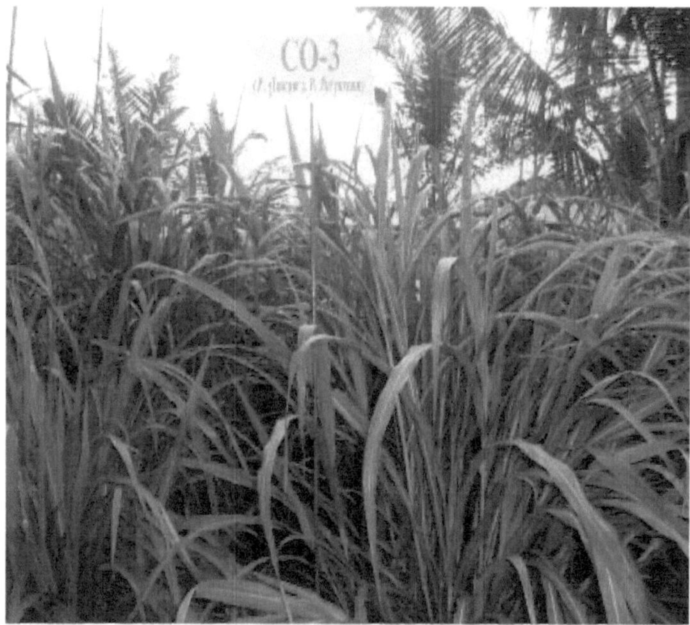

(Crude Protein-8-10%)

4. Napier Bajra Hybrid (CO-4) Green Fodder:

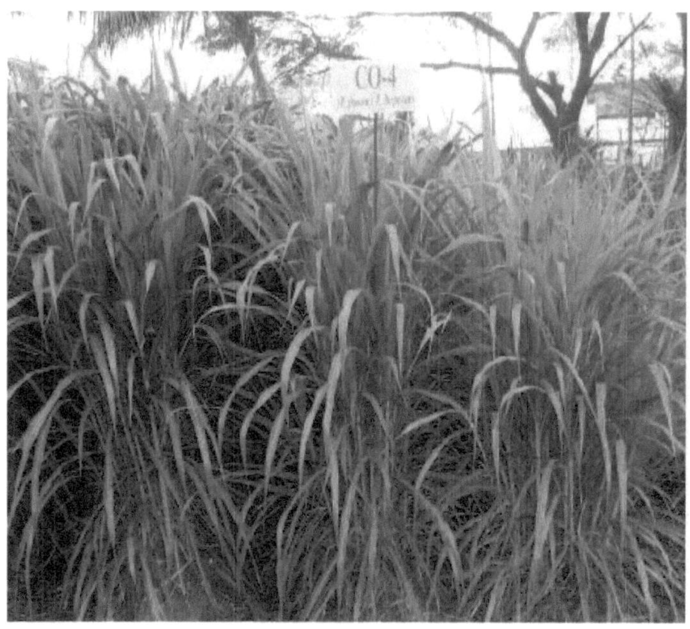

(Crude Protein-8-10%)

5. Green Karad Grass:

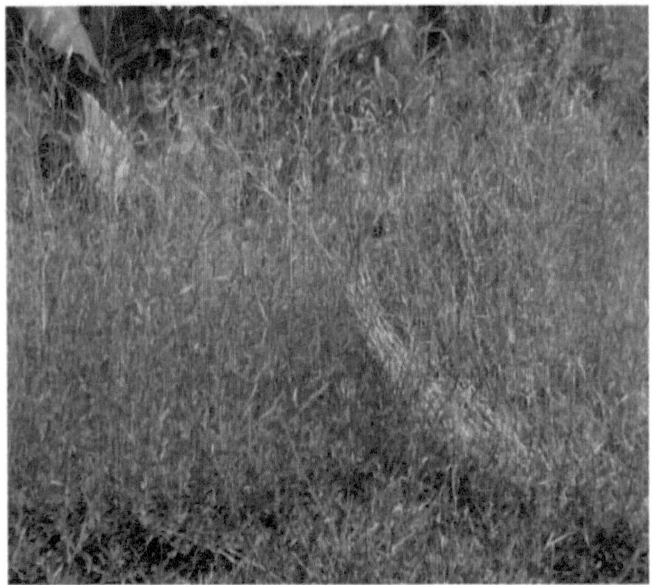

(Crude Protein-2.5-3.0%)

Dry Fodder:

1. Paddy Straw:

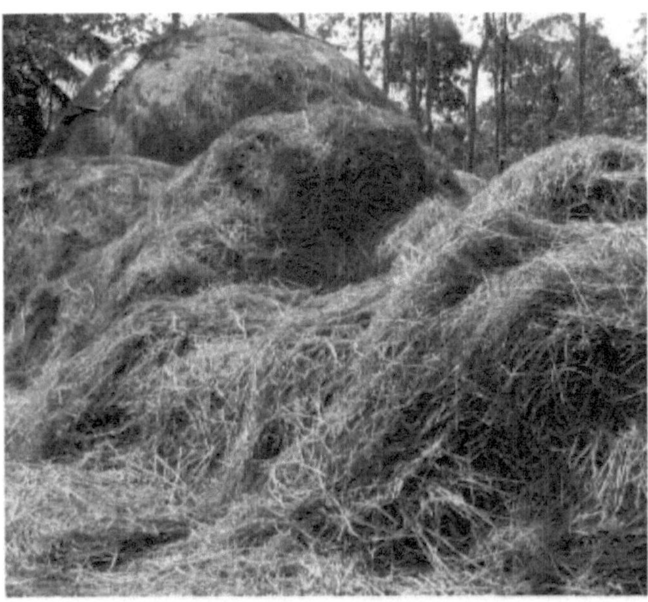

(Crude Protein-2.5-3.0%)

2. Dry Karad Grass:

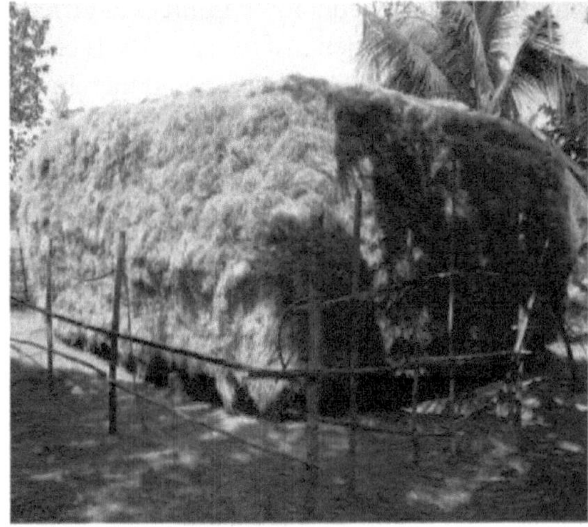

(Crude Protein-5-6%)

3. Jowar Straw (Kadaba Kutti):

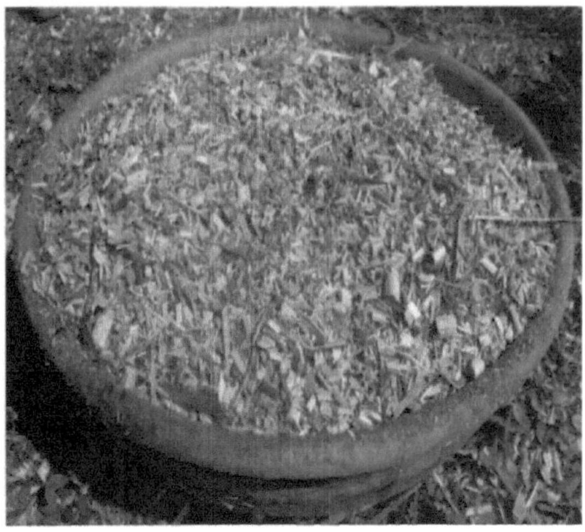

(Crude Protein-3.5-4.5%)

Guideline for preparation of 100kg feed:

1. Crushed maize: 42kg
2. Oats/wheat/rice bran: 35kg
3. Oil cakes: 20kg
4. Mineral mixture: 2kg
5. Salt: 1kg

General nutrient requirements:

In order to utilize animal, feed and economic resources as efficiently as possible, one must know the nutrient requirements of the animals. If an animal is wrongly fed this may lead to diseases, loss of production and thereby economic losses. By knowing what a specific animal needs, proper advice concerning purchase, cultivation and feeding systems can be given.

Requirements for buffalo are more or less the same as for cattle, so nutrient requirement tables for dairy cattle may be used as a guide. A farmer must observe the animals and change the feeding system, with guidance from an extension officer, if the feed seems unsuitable.

Energy:

Sources of energy are predominantly carbohydrates like fibre and starch, and fat to a lesser extent. For buffalo, fibre in the form of roughage is the most

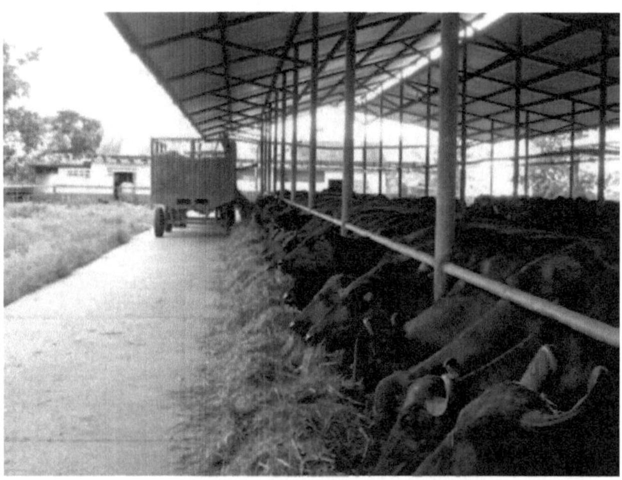

Forages being fed to buffaloes in large farm by help of distribution trolley

important and cheapest energy source. When calculating feed ratios for buffalo the term metabolizable energy (ME) is used.

Energy is measured in calories (cal) and joules (J) (1 cal equals 4.18 J). It is most common to use the term Megacalories (Mcal) or Megajoules (MJ) which means a million cal or J. Another measurement is Total Digestible Nutrients (TDN). The unit for TDN is kg or gram.

The energy ratio in the feed may be increased by adding fat in protected form, thus transferring its digestion from the rumen to the intestinal tract. Feeding of protected fat has been proven to increase nutrient utilization. Feeding of unprotected fat in similar amounts has been shown to adversely affect nutrient utilization.

Protein

Protein is required for growth, tissue repair and milk production. Good sources of protein are leguminous forage, grain and oilseed cakes. Protein requirements are measured in Crude Protein (CP) in kg or gram (CP = nitrogen x 6.25).

Minerals and vitamins

Minerals are essential for many body functions. The macro-minerals calcium (Ca) and phosphorus (P) are especially important in milk production. They are also vital for the skeleton and the function of nerve impulses. Phosphorus is the mineral included in the body's energy metabolism, ATP. When considering Ca and P requirements for the animal it is equally important to consider the ratio in which they are given. The Ca:P ratio should be 2:1 since there is an antagonist relationship between the two minerals concerning uptake from the small intestine.

Vitamins are essential for total body function. Most vitamins are synthesized by the animal or its rumen microbes. Such vitamins, B, C and K (and to some extent D) do not need to be fed. Vitamin B is synthesized by ruminal microbes, vitamin K by intestinal microbes and vitamin C in the tissues. Vitamin D is formed when the precursor, found on the skin on animals and on grass, is exposed to UV rays, so in tropical countries vitamin D deficiency is rare. Vitamins A and E are not synthesized in the animal but must be supplied. Vitamin A is found in silage, fresh grass, dark green leaves, peas and carrots. Cereals are a source of vitamin E. Mineral and/or vitamin mixture should always be supplied in order to fully meet the requirements.

Animals which do not receive a readymade concentrate mixture with a mineral and vitamin supplement, must be fed a supplement in the form of "lick stones" to which the animals have free access, or fed a powder individually once or twice a day. Vitamins may be included in the mineral feed, but vitamins are sensitive and may be destroyed if exposed to sunlight. Care must therefore be taken to store vitamin supplements correctly.

Water

Water is essential for most body functions, such as body temperature control, milk production and maintaining blood plasma volume. Thermal regulation of the animal is the most water consuming process. The animal receives water in three different ways:

- Drinking water
- Water in feed
- Metabolic water = water made from feed degradation.

Drinking water is the most important water source and should be of good hygienic quality. The water available in feed is highly dependent on the dry matter in feed. Straw, hay and cereals include little water, whereas silage and fresh grass may contain as much as 70% or more.

The water requirements of buffalo depend on:

- Diet (dry matter)
- Environment (humidity, temperature)
- Physiological function (growth, pregnancy, lactation).

Generally, buffalo require more water than cattle under the same circumstances and should have access to clean cool water ad-libitum. Restricted water intake leads to a decrease in dry matter intake and thus negatively affects milk production and growth.

Salinity of water is seldom a problem in dairy buffalo feeding. **A salt content of up to five grams per litre of water can be used for buffalo.** However, temporary diarrhea may be caused by water approaching the higher levels.

b. Balanced Ration

- During formulation of dairy cow rations, the daily requirements for all the above nutrients must be taken into consideration.

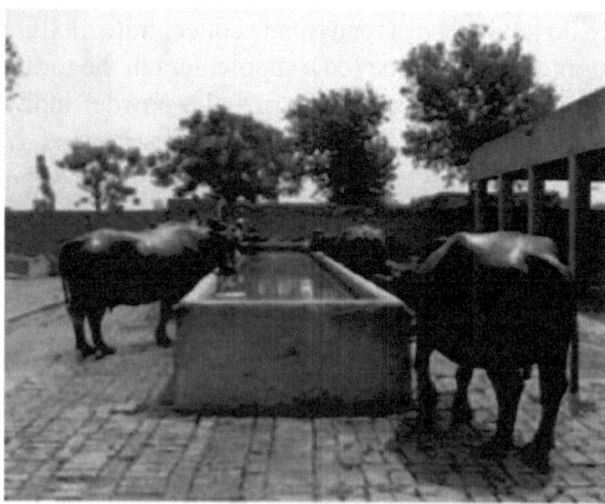

Watering buffaloes in watering alley

- The available feed resources should then be mixed to meet the cow's nutrient requirements, which are dependent on bodyweight, milk yield, reproductive (pregnancy) requirements and growth.
- A balanced ration will consist of combined feed ingredients which will be consumed in amounts needed to supply the daily nutrient requirements of the cow, both in correct proportion and amount.
- A ration will be balanced when all the required nutrients are present in feed eaten by the cow during a 24 hour period.
- When a ration is not balanced, the cow eats some nutrients in excess or in insufficient amounts.
- Some excesses and deficiencies, if not checked, can lead to death (e.g. calcium deficiency resulting in milk fever). However, some imbalances are difficult to identify because they result in some degree of loss thus not permitting the cow to exploit its genetic potential.
- A properly balanced ration will therefore be a mixture of all the ingredients.

Feeding Regimen

Bureau of Indian Standard (BIS) Specifications for Compounded Cattle Feed

Nutrients (%)	Type-I	Type-II	Calf Starter	Calf Grower
Moisture (Max)	11	11	10	10
Crude Protein (Min)	22	20	23-26	22-25
Ether Extract (Min)	3.0	2.5	4.0	4.0
Crude Fiber (Max)	07	12	07	10
Acid Insoluble Ash (Max)	3.0	4.0	2.5	3.5
Salt as NaCl (Max)	2.0	2.0	-	
Calcium (Min)	0.5	0.5	-	
Available Phosphorus	0.5	0.5	-	
Vit A (IU/kg)	5000	5000	-	

Composition of Calf Starter

Calf starter is a balanced concentrate mixture, which is fed to the calves from 10th day of age to supplement the nutrients, when they are raised on limited milk intake.

Composition of calf starter

Ingredients	Parts (kg/100 kg)
Maize/ wheat shorts/ barley/ oats	50
Groundnut cake/ soybean meal	30
Skimmed milk powder	07
Wheat bran/ rice bran	10
Mineral mixture	02
Common salt	01
Vitamin A and D supplement (g/q)	10
Available Phosphorus	0.5

Composition of Concentrate Mixture

It is a mixture of different concentrate feed ingredients like cereal grains (maize, rice kani etc), cereal grain byproducts (rice polish, brewers' dried grains etc), oil cakes (soybean meal, ground nut cake, cotton seed cake etc), mineral mixture and common salt in different ratios as per the requirement.

Examples of Concentrate Mixture

Feed Ingredients	Parts by Weight (kg)				
	Ex-1	Ex-2	Ex-3	Ex-4	Ex-5
Maize grain (ground)	35	35	35	35	35
Soybean meal	15	20	—	10	10
Groundnut cake	15	—	24	—	15
Cotton seed cake	—	12	24	27	14
Rice polish	32	30	14	—	23
Brewers' dried grains	—	—	—	25	—
Mineral mixture	02	02	02	02	02
Common salt	01	01	01	01	01

The concentrate mixture may be either in Mash Form or Pellet Form.

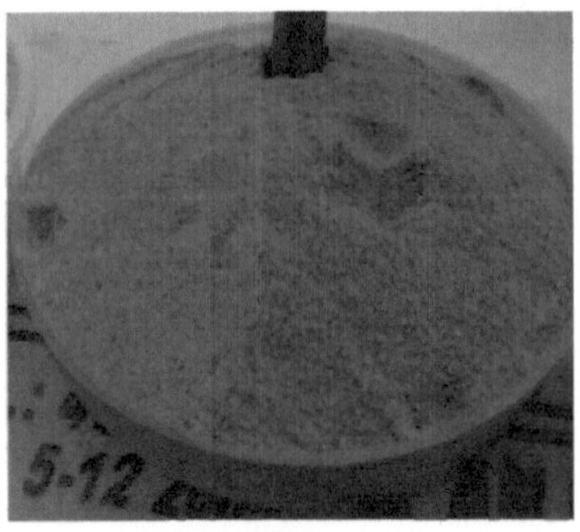

Mash Form

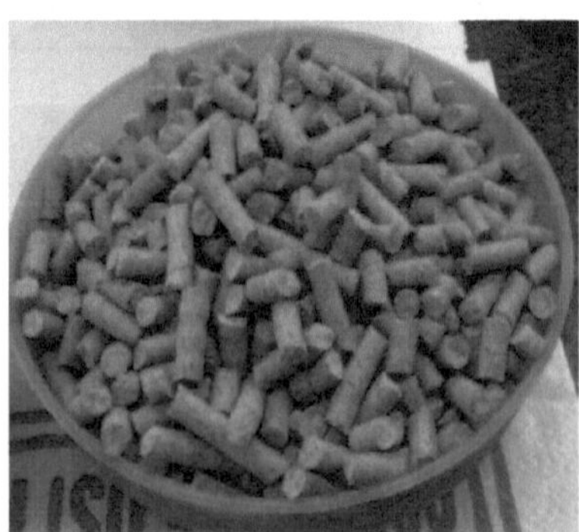

Pellet Form

Feeding Schedule for Calves, Heifers, Pregnant and Lactating Cows:

Feeding schedule for calves (per day):

Age	Whole milk (liters)	Calf starter (kg)	Legume (Cow pea) green fodder (kg)
1-3 days	3.0 (colostrums)	-	-
4-15 days	3.0	-	-
16-30 days	3.5	Ad lib.	Ad lib.
1-2 months	2.5	0.25	Ad lib.
2-3 months	2.0	0.50	2-3
3-4 months	1.0	0.75	5-7

Feeding schedule for heifers (per day):

Age	Diet (kg)	
	Maize/ CO-3/ CO-4 Fodder	Concentrate Mixture
4-6 months	6-7	1.5
6-12 months	12-15	1.5
12-18 months	20-25	1.0
18-30 months	25-30	1.0
Pregnant (last quarter)	30-35	2.0

Feeding schedule for pregnant animals 8-10 weeks before calving:

Feeds	Quantity (kg/ day)
Maize/ CO-3/ CO-4 fodder	30-35
Paddy straw/ Maize stover/ Kadaba Kutti/ Dry karad grass	5
Concentrate mixture	2-3

Feeding schedule for lactating animals:

Rations for lactating animals (for cows producing up to 7 kg milk and buffaloes producing up to 5 kg milk per day):

Feeds	Quantity (kg/ day)
Maize/ CO-3/ CO-4 green fodder	10-20
Paddy straw/ Maize stover/ Kadaba Kutti/ Dry karad grass	7-8
Concentrate mixture	3-4

Rations for lactating animals (for cows producing more than 7 kg milk and buffaloes producing more than 5 kg milk per day):

- If the dairy animal i.e. cows producing more than 7 kg milk and buffaloes producing more than 5 kg milk per day, then provide extra concentrate mixture @ 400g per kg increase in cow milk and 500 g per kg increase in buffalo milk.

- If the dairy animal is pregnant, then besides the maintenance and production requirement, one kg concentrate mixture as pregnancy allowance should be offered extra only in the last three months of the pregnancy.

Feeding of high producing animals

The high yielding dairy animals need very special feeding strategies. Low quality roughages like straw or stovers should not be offered to high producing animas. The concentrate mixture of high yielders must contain energy and protein rich ingredients like soybean meal, roasted soybeans, by pass nutrients etc. Buffers like sodium bicarbonate, magnesium oxide and vitamin mixture should be added in the diet for better utilization of the feedstuffs. The composition of concentrate mixture for high yielders is presented in Table below.

Concentrate mixture for high yielding animals:

Ingredients	Kg
Maize	40
Mustard cake	20
Soybean meal	10
Roasted soybean	05
Rice bran	15
Wheat bran/ Deoiled rice bran	07
Mineral and vitamin mixture	02
Common salt	01

Ranking of Top Feeds

On the basis of composition, in-sacco kinetic parameters for nutrients, in vitro gas production data and the estimated DOM, ME and intake potential, the ranking of the top feeds is as follows:

1. **Very good:** *Leucaena leucocephala, M. azedarach, Zizyphus jujube*
2. **Good:** *Carissa spinarum, Z. nummularia, Hippophae rhamnoides*
3. **Average:** *Ficus raxburghii, Robinia pseudoacacia*

Poor: *Quereus incana*

Examples of feeding regimes for a lactating dairy animal weighing 550 kg:

Milk yield (7% fat)	4% FCM	Kg dry matter of roughage	Kg dry matter of concentrate
4kg	5.8kg	3.5 alfalfa hay + 3.2 maize silage + 4 wheat straw or	2 wheat bran
5kg	7.40kg	2 alfalfa hay + 4 maize silage + 4 fresh sorghum	
7 kg	10.15 kg	5.3 alfalfa hay + 5.5 maize silage or 4.5 alfalfa hay + 5 maize silage + 2 wheat straw or 3.5 alfalfa hay + 5.5 maize silage and	2 wheat bran
9 kg	13.05 kg	5.6 alfalfa hay + 5.5 maize silage + 3 wheat straw or4.5 alfalfa hay + 5.5 maize silage and	2.5 wheat bran
10 kg	14.50 kg	6 alfalfa hay + 7 maize silage or 9 alfalfa hay + 3 maize silage and	1 cotton-seed-cake
12 kg	17.40 kg	7 alfalfa hay + 5 maize silage + 2 wheat straw and	1.5 wheat bran
15 kg	21.75 kg	7.5 alfalfa hay + 6 maize silage and	2.2 wheat bran + 0.5 molasses + 0.3 urea

Feeding of Dairy Cattle

Practical feeding

During the formulation of rations for lactating dairy cows, the quality of the ration should be commensurate with the requirements of the cow. The requirement is directly related to the milk yield, which is in turn dependent on the stage of lactation. As such, cows in early lactation will require more nutrients compared to those in late lactation. Since it is not practically possible to formulate a separate ration for each cow, the cows should be fed in groups (strings) with common nutrient requirements. Cows in the same stage of lactation will have almost similar requirements and can therefore the rations can be formulated according to the phase (stage) of lactation.

Phase 1: Early Lactation Phase (1-70 days)

- During this phase, milk production increases more rapidly than feed intake resulting in higher energy demand than intake leading to a negative energy balance.
- The health and nutrition of the cow during this phase is critical and affects the entire lactation performance.

- Excessive weight loss may be detrimental to cow's health and reproductive performance (cow may not come on heat at the optimum time) leading to long calving intervals.
- Concentrates should be added to the basal diet to increase the energy and protein content as forage alone will not be sufficient.
- Cows that are poorly fed during this early phase do not attain peak yield and milk production drops from 1st week.
- If excessive concentrates are added too rapidly (non-accustomed cows) to the ration, they can lead to digestive disturbances (rumen acidosis, loss of appetite, reduced milk production, low milk fat content). It is therefore recommended that concentrates should be limited to 50-60% of diet dry matter, the rest being forage to ensure rumination (proper function of the rumen).
- If high amounts of concentrate are fed during this time buffers (chemicals that reduce the acid in the rumen and available commercially) can be helpful.
- At this stage, high protein content is important since the body cannot mobilize all the needed protein and bacteria protein (synthesized in the rumen by bacteria) can only partially meet requirements.
- A ration with protein content of 18%CP is recommended for high yielding cows. If the cow is underfed during this stage, milk production cannot recover even when balanced rations are fed at later stages.

Phase 2: Mid Lactation Phase (70-150 days)

- During this phase the dry matter intake is adequate to support milk production and either maintain or slightly increase body weight.
- Feeding should be to maintain production peak as long as possible.
- Decline of 8-10%/month in milk production are common after peaking.
- The forage quality should still be high and a CP content of 15-18%.
- Concentrates high in digestible fiber (rather than starch) e.g. wheat or maize bran can be used as energy source.

Phase 3: Late Lactation Phase (151-305 days)

- During this phase feed intake and milk production decline.
- The body weight increase is due to replenishment of body reserves and, towards the end of lactation, due to increased growth of fetus.

- It has been shown that it is more efficient to replenish body weight during late lactation than during the dry period.
- The animals can be fed on lower quality roughage and limited amounts of concentrate compared to the other two phases.

Phase 4: Dry Period (305-365 days)

- During this phase the cow continues to gain weight primarily due to weight of fetus.
- Proper feeding of cow during this stage will help realize the cow's potential during next lactation and minimize health problems at calving time (milk fever and ketosis).
- At the time of drying, cows should be fed a ration to cater for maintenance and pregnancy but two weeks before calving, the cow should be fed on concentrates in preparation for next lactation.
- This extra concentrate (steaming) enables the cow to store some reserves to be used in early lactation and to adapt rumen microbial population to digest concentrates in early lactation to minimize digestive disturbances.
- During this phase the cow can be fed good quality forage or poor quality supplemented with concentrate to provide 12% CP.
- The cows should not be fed high amounts of concentrate to avoid over conditioning. If the diet is rich in energy, intake should be limited.
- Bulky roughages can be fed to help increase rumen size to accommodate more feed at parturition.
- The amount of calcium and phosphorous fed should be restricted during the dry period to 0.4% and 0.25% to minimize incidences of milk fever.

Important tips on feeding of dairy cows

- The green fodder must be chopped before feeding to the dairy cows for better utilization.
- If possible, soak the concentrate mixture in water for 6-8 hours and then feed to the animals.
- The required concentrate mixture, green fodder and straw may be offered either separately or mixing together as total mixed ration (TMR).
- The total ration to be offered daily should be divided and offered twice (morning and afternoon) for better utilization.

- Do not feed calcium rich feed ingredients or mineral mixture to the dairy cows 15 days before parturition, as high calcium intake during this period increases the chances of milk fever.
- Provide clean fresh water free of choice to the dairy cows. For easy accessibility, a cemented water tank should be constructed near to the cow shed and the tank should be painted with lime at frequent intervals to make the water clean.

Feeding of Dairy Buffaloes

General on feeding and feedstuffs

Buffalo are, like cattle, ruminants. This means that they utilize micro-organisms in the rumen to digest the feed. Feed eaten by ruminants is of vegetable origin. The ruminant is an expert in converting cellulose and other fibrous materials into high quality milk and meat. Their digestive capacity is greater than the non-ruminant. Ruminants **"chew the cud"**, that is they regurgitate partly digested food to the mouth to chew it again, thus helping to breakdown this plant material.

Buffalo have slower rumen movement than cattle, which leads to a slower rate of ingesta outflow. The pH of the rumen content is similar to that of cattle, and it is affected in the same manner. Normal pH is between six and seven, depending on feed and time of feeding.

Feed components can be divided into protein, energy (carbohydrates), fat, minerals and water.

The breakdown and utilization of the different feed components are reviewed below.

The waste end products of the microbial attack are methane and carbon dioxide that are eructated. Volatile fatty acids (VFA) of which acetic, propionic and butyric acids are the predominant ones, are together with ammonia, absorbed through the rumen wall and transported via the blood.

The main diet for buffalo is roughage such as grass, legumes and straw. The roughage can be fed either fresh as pasture or in a cut-and-carry system, or conserved as hay or silage. Roughage is often complemented with grains, concentrate and agro-industrial by-products such as oilseed cakes, sugar cane tops etc.

- Roughage should form the base of the feed ration and contribute to meeting at least the total maintenance requirements.
- Grains and concentrate should be fed only to meet additional requirements such as growth, pregnancy and milk production.

- Too much non-fibrous feed will alter the rumen environment. In the long run this could lead to serious problems in feed digestion causing loss of appetite, weight loss and a drop in milk yield. This is especially important for animals under stress, for instance from high growth rate or high milk yield.
- The roughage should be of good quality – of both nutritional quality and hygienic quality. This cannot be emphasized enough.

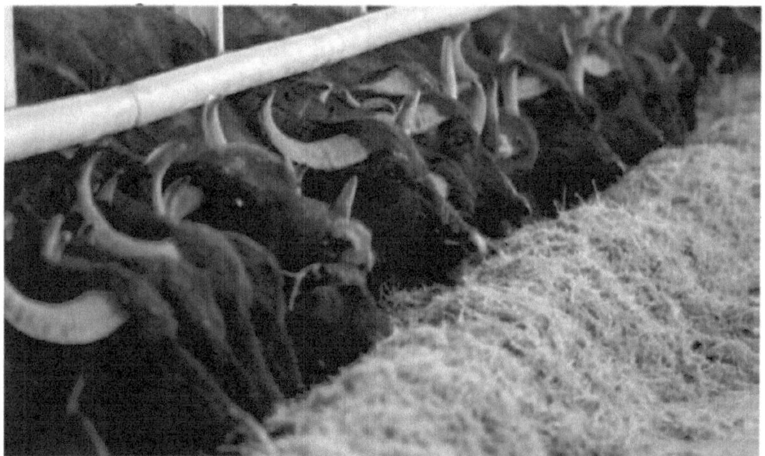

Roughages being fed to the buffaloes

Practical feeding of buffalo calf

- Calves should be fed on colostrum (first milk from a cow that has calved down) as soon after birth as possible (within 30 minutes and certainly within 4 hours) so as to protect the new calf against diseases.
- Commercial colostrum supplements can also be given when colostrum is not available e.g. if cow dies during calving or quality is poor e.g. if cow is too sick and is being treated with drugs that can affect the newborn calf if they are taken in through the colostrum. These supplements contain bovine immunoglobulin and are prepared from cheese whey or colostrums from immunized cows. Milk or milk replacer should be fed by open pail method and calves are fed twice daily. For example, a 50 kg calf can be fed 2 kg of milk in the morning and 2 kg of milk in the afternoon.
- Weaning of calves from milk should be between 4 and 8 weeks after birth. Abrupt weaning is good as it usually stimulates dry feed consumption.

- Calf mortality can be very high in some countries. In India it is often 30 to 40% before three months of age. This is caused by malpractice such as negligence, limited milk feeding, injuries and diseases. By increasing the amount of feed to the calf's requirements and by following sound calf management practices as outlined here, mortality can be decreased.
- Colostrum is the most important and most suitable feed for the newborn calf. It contains all the nutrients needed along with the vital antibodies. It is crucial for the survival of the calf that it receives colostrum during the first 12 hours of its life, the earlier the better. The calves should be given colostrum as long as the mother provides it, e.g. three to four days. Any surplus colostrum can be frozen and then thawed and carefully heated to 39°C before feeding. If no freezing facilities are available colostrum can stay fresh for a couple of days if it is cooled in a hygienic container. Colostrum can be fermented with living lactic acid culture. Fermented colostrum can be kept for at least a week and up to two weeks if cooling facilities are available.
- Colostrum should be fed to the calf several times a day, preferably more than twice a day, at equal intervals.
- The calf should be trained to drink from a bucket. The easiest way to do this is to dip clean fingers into the milk and then allow the calf to lick and suck the fingers. The hand is then gradually drawn into the milk in the bucket while the calf is still suckling. Once the calf has learnt to drink it is easy to feed. The calf may need assistance for five days. There are special nipples that can be put in the bucket. Once the calf suckles those, it will need less assistance from the trainer (the practice is known as pail feeding).
- After the colostrum period, whole milk should be provided to the calf until 15 days of age at a level of 1/8th to 1/10th of the calf's body weight. Milk replacer can be fed along with the whole milk provided that it has a certain composition of nutrients. It is not advisable to completely substitute whole milk with milk replacer. Milk and/or replacer should be offered to the calf on at least two occasions per day. The milk and/or replacer should be served at body temperature (38-39°C).
- At two weeks of age, the calf should be introduced to good quality green feed and concentrates, as a calf starter (see table). This stimulates the rumen to grow and function properly.

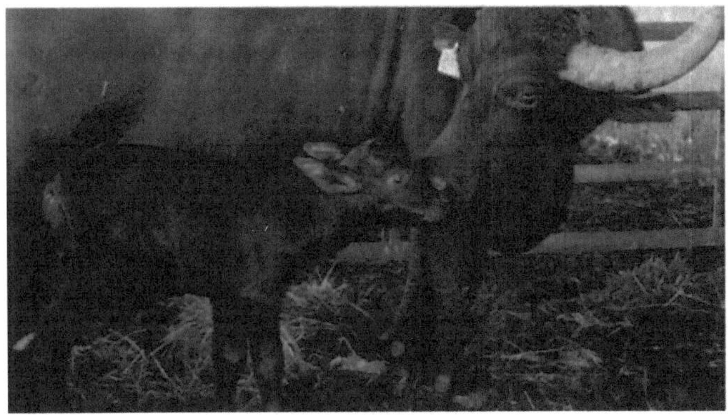

Buffalo calf with dam

Calf starter mixture:

Feed source	Amount
Crushed barley	50%
Groundnut cake	30%
Wheat bran	8%
Skim milk powder	10%
Mineral mixture	2%
To increase palatability, add per 100kg of starter:	
Molasses	5-10kg
Salt	500g

- Buffalo calves fed with stovers of maize, bajra and oat cannot meet their nutrient requirements and are often in negative energy and protein balance. However, feeding the calves treated stovers with a urea-molasses-salt complex both enhances the palatability of the stovers as well as the digestibility and nutrient value.
- Buffalo male calves weighing 150 to 200 kg have been proven to increase their intake of treated stovers compared to untreated ones, thus increasing weight gain and improving nitrogen balance and health.

Practical feeding of the buffalo heifer

- The heifer is a future milk producer and has to be given a fair chance to produce well. She must have an average daily gain of at least 500 grams per day in order to reach the optimum size for calving within a reasonable time (500 kg at 32 to 40 months).
- Heifers should be fed seasonal green feed of about 4 to 7 kg dry matter (DM) together with some straw and concentrate or grain per day.

- If the green feed is leguminous the ration of green feed and concentrate or grain can be reduced and the amount of straw increased. However it is important to feed the heifers a small amount of grain or concentrate, not less than 0.5 kg per day, to help both them and their rumen to become accustomed to this type of feed prior to partus.
- If available, ammonia treated straw could be given along with low quality green feed and concentrate.
- Silage could be given to heifers, but it is often a very valuable feed saved for milk producing animals. However, a few months before partus the heifer should slowly be introduced to the feed she will have as a milk-producing buffalo.
- Maximum voluntary intake for the heifer is obtained at approximately 1 to 1.5 kg DM of straw together with 3 kg DM of green feed and 1 kg concentrate.
- Straw fed to appetite is not enough to keep or increase the body weight of growing buffalo. Straw fed to growing stock should preferably be ammoniated and further supplemented with green feed or hay and some kind of concentrate to give the best result.

Practical feeding of the lactating buffalo

- Lactating buffalo should be given the best feed the farm can offer. Producing milk is one of the most energy demanding biological processes. Weight loss is common in high producing animals during the first month of lactation because they cannot consume a sufficient amount of energy.
- A popular term is that the animals are milking off the fat. It is therefore important that the buffalo is in good health status at partus.
- In Table c, examples of various feeding regimes for lactating buffalo are given. A well balanced ratio of protein, energy, vitamins and minerals in a palatable and tasty feed is the best way of increasing milk production and live weight, as well as improving health and fertility.
- Traditional feeding patterns for buffalo all over the world are subject to seasonal forage and crop production, which affects the level of milk production.
- Forage is insufficient during the dry season and abundant during the rainy season. Shortages are overcome by conserving forages as hay or silage.

Formulating balanced feed ration for lactating buffaloes

- Formulating feed rations for milk producing buffalo starts with theoretical calculating of the requirements.
- As there are no standardized international tables for dairy buffalo requirements, the calculations in Table a, are based on dairy cattle nutrient requirement tables (NRC, 1988).
- It is important to know the buffalo live weight. This is most accurately done by weighing the animals three times in one week and calculating the average.
- Once the weight is known, requirements for maintenance can be extracted. Milk yield should also be known, as well as fat percentage.
- Recommendations are to use at least three days of milk records to calculate the average yield and fat percentage. For simplicity, the yield is then calculated as four percent fat corrected milk. Total requirements are gained by summing the requirements for maintenance and for milk production.
- The requirement for milk production is based upon the calculation of fat corrected milk (FCM) using the formula:

  4% FCM, kg = 0.4 x (milk yield, kg) + 15 x (milk yield, kg x fat%/100)

Table a: Nutrient requirements of buffalo

Requirements for live weight (kg)	Energy (ME in Mcal)	TDN (kg)	Total crude protein (g)	Calcium (g)	Phosphorous (g)
450	13	3.4	341	18	13
500	14.2	3.7	364	20	14
550	15.3	4.0	386	22	16
600	16.3	4.2	406	24	17
Requirements for milk yield per kg 4% fat corrected milk:					
	1.24	0.32	90	2.73	1.68

For a buffalo weighing 550 kg and yielding 7 kg of milk with 7.2% fat per day, the amount of 4% fat corrected milk comes to 0.4 x 7+15 x (7 x 0.072) = 10.36 kg per day.

- If the animal seems to be too fat at the time of weighing, the maintenance requirements may be reduced by ten percent. Similarly, if the animal is too skinny, ten percent may be added to the maintenance requirements. The feeding regime of the buffalo can then be decided.
- Primarily, crops grown on the farm should be included in the diet. For optimal economic feeding regimes the feed should be analyzed at a

laboratory for dry matter content, energy and crude protein, and for calcium and phosphorus.

- It is important to note that silage should not form the sole source of roughage because it has a high amount of easily fermentable carbohydrate and a physical structure which does not really stimulate rumen contraction. As a rule of thumb, the amount of silage in a diet should not exceed 30% of the total dry matter intake if concentrate is also given. If the diet is solely made from roughage the silage ration may be increased to 60%. On the other hand, alfalfa hay contains much too much protein and therefore it is important to give a mixture of silage, hay and perhaps straw.
- Including urea in the diet may be a cheap and good way to "help up" a low protein diet. One must remember, however, that a source of highly soluble carbohydrates such as molasses must be included in a urea diet. The maximum level of urea should correspond to less than 25% of the crude protein. An alternative is to feed readymade urea-molasses blocks.
- Controlling the animals' intake of feed is a good practice. Low yielders tend to eat more than they require and at the same time it is difficult for the high yielders to eat enough. It is therefore vital that the feed is analyzed and the milk yield known, in order to provide the correct nutrient requirement for each animal.

Practical feeding of the dry buffalo

- Feeding the dry buffalo is concerned with preparing for partum and high milk production.
- In the last two months of gestation the buffalo has increased requirements for nutrients for foetal growth.
- Experiments with Murrah buffalo has shown that the best economical way of feeding dry buffalo two months before calving is at 125 percent of the recommended level for cattle (NRC, 1988).
- By giving the dry buffalo a little more than she needs, her chance of building up body reserves and being in good physical condition is improved.

Techniques for Enhancing Nutritive Value of Poor Quality Feeds of Dairy Animals

1. **Treatment of crop residues:** The roughages are eaten by animals less voluntarily because of their slow passage through alimentary canal. Only limited use can be made of straws in animal nutrition if fed without any treatment. Animals spend more energy in chewing and digesting such

roughages than they gain from them. Often the digestibility of poor roughage is limited not due to the lignification only but also due to the low N content. Physical (particle size reduction), biological (pre-feeding fermentation, addition of fibrolytic enzymes), and chemical treatment have been extensively explored to improve the utilization of crop residues in animal diets. Among various chemicals (acids and alkalis) employed for the treatment of cereal straws, ammonia and alkali have shown good results.

2. **Urea treatment of straws:** Urea is used to treat straws for enhancing their protein content from zero to upto 3%. 4kg urea is dissolved in 50 liter water and is sprinkled on 100kg straw.

3. **Urea molasses mineral blocks (UMMB):** Although the cellulosic feedstuffs are the primary basal feed for ruminants, seasonal shortages do occur during weather extremes and drought and flood situations, which adversely affect the buffalo productivity. A combination of urea, molasses and minerals in the form of solid blocks has been extensively prepared and fed to animals. These blocks, as a source of fermentable carbohydrates and nitrogen, are preferred over ammoniation of crop residues because they are easy to ship and safe to handle by farmers. The supplementation of urea molasses block (UMB) to animals fed straw based diets has increased the growth and supported moderate milk production.

4. **Ensiling legumes and grasses:** Ensiling multi-cut high yielding legumes (Lucerne, Berseem) and grasses (corn, sorghum, barley, oat, millet, mott (*Pennisetum purpureum*) and jambo fodders) offer a good promise to bridge the escalating gap between supply and demand of fodder for buffaloes. However, because of continuous use of fresh green fodders over the years through the "cut and carry system", dairy farmers in south Asia believe in a strong myth that feeding silage could animal productivity. Berseem and lucerne are highly nutritious, high yielding and abundantly available multi-cut legumes in India.

5. **Complete feed blocks:** These blocks consist of all the major nutrients which are necessary for dairy animals for producing milk and general body maintenance. These blocks are present in a compressed form and require very less space for storage and its keeping quality is optimum. These blocks are mainly used by dairy farmers which are city-based and have less spacious farms. These can also be used as a major source of nutrients during natural calamities and disasters.

Feed Conservation

Pasture and fodder production is rain fed and thus seasonal resulting in times of plenty and times of scarcity. The aim of conservation is to harvest the maximum amount of dry matter from a given area and at an optimum stage for utilization by animals and allow for re-growth of the forage. The two main ways of conserving fodder are making hay or making silage.

1. Hay

Hay is fodder conserved by drying to reduce the water content so that it can be stored without rotting or becoming mouldy (reducing moisture content stops microbial growth). The moisture content should be reduced to about 15%. The grasses that are very suitable for hay making include Rhodes grass, Lucerne and vetch.

Steps in haymaking

1. Harvesting and curing

- Harvest the fodder for haymaking when flowering is 50%. At this stage protein and digestibility are at maximum, after which they decline with age.
- The fodder should be harvested after 2 to 3 days of dry weather so that drying will be possible.
- Where possible, drying should be done under shade so that the dried fodder retains its green color, which is an indicator of quality.
- Turn the fodder using farm fork to ensure even drying.
- Check the dryness by trying to break the stem.
- If it bends too much without breaking, there is still much water.
- Legumes and grasses can be mixed to make better-quality hay, e.g. Rhodes grass + lucerne.

2. Baling hay

Baling the hay allows more material to be stored in a given space. A good estimate of the amount stored makes feed budgeting easier. Baling can be manual or mechanized, manual baling being more economical for small-scale dairy farmers. Manual hay baling is done using a baling box with dimensions 85 cm long x 55 cm wide x 45 cm deep, open on both sides. If the hay is well pressed, the box will produce an average bale of 20 kg.

3. Storage

Hay should always be stored away from direct sun and rainfall, e.g. in hay barns. Rodents like rats should be controlled as they can damage the hay.

Characteristics of good-quality hay: Quality of the hay should be evident on physical examination. Good-quality hay should;

a. be leafy and greenish in color.

b. have no foreign material mixed with it.

c. have no smell.

2. Silage

Silage is high-moisture fodder preserved through fermentation in the absence of air. These are fodders that would deteriorate in quality if allowed to dry. Silage can be made from grasses, fodder sorghum, green oats, green maize or Napier grass. An ideal crop for silage making should;

a. contain an adequate level of fermentable sugars in the form of water-soluble carbohydrates.

b. have dry matter content in the fresh crop above 20%.

c. possess a physical structure that will allow it to compact readily in the silo after harvesting.

Crops not fulfilling these requirements may require pre-treatment such as:

a. Field wilting, to reduce moisture.

b. Fine chopping, generally 20–25 mm preferred to allow compaction.

c. use of additives, to increase soluble carbohydrates

Harvesting stages

Napier grass should be harvested at about 1 meter when protein content is about 10%. Maize and sorghum should be harvested at dough stage that is when the grain is milky. The grains will provide water-soluble sugars and molasses is not necessary when ensiling. When ensiling napier grass, molasses should be added to increase the sugar content. To improve silage quality, poultry waste and legumes like lucerne and desmodium may be mixed with the material being ensiled to increase the level of crude protein.

Types of silos

A silo is an airtight place or receptacle for preserving green feed for future feeding on the farm. Silos can be either underground or above ground, the qualification being that the silo must allow compaction and be air tight. Five types are described here: tube, pit, above-ground, trench and tower.

- Silage can be made in large plastic sacks or tubes. The plastic must have no holes to ensure no air enters. This is popularly referred to as ***tube silage.*** Silage can also be made in *pits* that are dug vertically into the ground and then filled and compacted with the silage material.
- An *above-ground silo* is made on slightly slanted ground. The material is compacted and covered with a polythene sheet and a layer of soil is added at the top. When finished, it should be dome-shaped so that it does not allow water to settle at the top but rather collect at the sides and drain away down the slope.
- The *trench silo* is an adaptation of the pit silo, which has long been in use. It is much cheaper to construct than a pit silo. Construction is done on sloping land. A trench is dug and then filled with silage material. This method is ideal for large-scale farms where the tractor is used. Drainage from rain is also controlled to avoid spoiling the silage.
- ***Tower silos*** are cylindrical and made above-ground. They are 10 m or more in height and 3 m or more in diameter. Tower silos containing silage are usually unloaded from the top of the pile. An advantage of tower silos is that the silage tends to pack well due to its own weight, except for the top few feet.

Qualities of good silage

- Well-prepared silage is bright or light yellow-green, has a smell similar to vinegar and has a firm texture.
- Bad silage tends to smell similar to rancid butter or ammonia.
- Natural microorganisms turn the sugars in the plant material or any added as molasses into weak acids, which then act as a preservative. The result is a sweet smelling, moist feed that cattle like to eat once they get used to it.

Storage and feeding

- Tube silage should be stored under shade, for example in a store.
- Rodents like rats that could tear the tube need to be controlled.
- When feeding, open the tube and scoop a layer and remember to re-tie without trapping air inside.

- When feeding from the pit, scoop in layers and cover after removing the day's ration, making sure the pit is air tight.
- Drainage from the top should be guided to avoid rainwater draining into the pit.
- When feeding from the above-ground method, open from the lower side of the slant, remove the amount you need for the day and re-cover it without trapping air inside.
- To avoid off-flavors in milk, feed silage to milking cows after milking, not before, or feed at least 2 hours before milking.

Losses

- Nutrient losses may occur during silage making. In the field during cutting, losses due to respiration during wilting will be about 2% per day. If it rains, leaching may cause some loss.
- Overheating due to poor sealing gives a brown product, which may smell like tobacco and result in severe damage to nutrients e.g. proteins.
- Effluent losses of 2–10% that occur from moisture seepage contain soluble and highly digestible nutrients; seepage should be avoided by wilting the herbage.

Silage additives

- During silage preparation, different types of additives can be added to improve the quality. These include fermentation stimulants. Most inoculants contain Lactobacillus plantarum.
- *Fermentation inhibitors* include acids such as propionic, formic and **sulphuric.** Inorganic acids are more effective but are strongly corrosive thus not recommended.
- Of the organic acids, formic is more effective than propionic, lactic or acetic.
- Substrate or nutrient sources (grains, molasses, urea or ammonia) are used when there are insufficient soluble carbohydrates in the material to be ensiled (e.g. legumes, Napier grass, crop residues). They are also used to increase the nutritive value of the silage.
- Molasses can be added at about 9 kg/ton of silage.

Note: Use of additives is not a prerequisite for making good silage, but it is good for problem crops.

Foddder

Fodder Crops

Seasonal cultivation of green fodder in North India

July-October	Napier Sorghum Bajra/Jowar Cowpea
November-April	Napier + Lucerne Berseem + Mustard Lucerne + Oat
May-June	Napier + Lucerne Sudan grass Lucerne Early Maize

Scarcity Fodders

India is a facing a shortage of feeds and forages for feeding the livestock population. Moreover this situation aggravates due to natural calamities like droughts and floods. Although the feed reserves in the form of hay and silage can bridge these gaps but owing to the large livestock population of the country, the need arises to search for an alternate resource in feed sector which comes through non-conventional feeding of various by-products emerging from different industries. Although these by-products consist of different toxins and these toxins are to be neutralized before they are being fed to the livestock. These resources form a category of feedstuffs called as scarcity feeds or lean period feeds and are enlisted as:

1. Agro-industrial by-products

a. Mango seed kernel

b. Mahua cake

c. Babul

d. Tamarind seed

e. Rain tree

f. Sun hemp

g. Date stones

h. Maize gluten feed

i. Virginia tobacco seed cake

Agronomical Practices for Production of Leguminous Fodder in Different Seasons:

S.No	Name of the crop	Time of sowing	Ploughing	Seeding	Manuring and irrigation	Yield and nutritive value	Crop rotations
1.	Cow pea	June-July	After harvesting Rabi crop	Broadcast @ 25-30 kg/ hectare	40-50 quintals/ hectare.	200-300 quintal/ hectare. 30-45% DM3-4% DCP17-18% TDN	1. Cow pea-sorghum -wheat. 2. Cow pea-maize-oat.
2.	Guar	End of march to July	One ploughing and 2 harrowings	25-30 kg/ha	Green manure	250-400 quintal/ha 13-15% CP	Guar-sorghum-wheat
3.	Berseem	September-October	After harvesting kharif crop, 2 harrowings required	20-25 kg/ha	Kisan khad 150kg/ha. Superphospahte 500kg/ha	5-6 cuttings can be obtained.500-600 Q/ha16-21% CP	-
4.	Lucerne	October-November	Disc plough with 2-3 harrowings	15-18 kg/ha	500kg/ha kisan khad and 100 kg superphosphate	1000-1200 Q/ha	Maize-lucerne Paddy-lucerne
5.	Senji	September-October	One ploughing and 2 harrowings	20-25 kg/ha	250kg superphos phate per hectare.	250-300Q/ha Productive ration	-

Agronomical Practices for Production of Non-Leguminous Fodder in Different Seasons:

S.No	Name of the crop	Time of sowing	Ploughing	Seeding	Manuring and irrigation	Yield and nutritive value	Crop rotations
1.	Maize	March-September	Disc plough with 2-3 harrowings	30-40kg/ha	Kisan khad 350 kg/ha.	350-450 Q/ha 8-10% CP	-
2.	Sorghum	April-August	Land is ploughed once	55-60 kg/ha	100kg nitrogen/ha in the form of urea.	250-450 quintal/ha 4-5% CP	Cow pea-sorghum-wheat. Cow pea-sorghum-oat
3.	M.P. Chari	February-March	2 ploughings and a harrowing	20-25 kg/ha	100kg nitrogen/ha in the form of urea.	700-800 Q/ha. 6-8% CP	M.P. Chari-Berseem. M.P. Chari-Lucerne
4.	Mak-Chari	March-September	Disc plough with 2-3 harrowings	35-40 kg/ha	350kg/ha kisan khad	350-500 Q/ha	-
5.	Pearl millet	March-August	One ploughing and 2 harrowings	30-40 kg/ha	100 kg/ha nitrogen in the form of urea.	250-400Q/ha 4-5% CP	-
6.	Oats	September	One ploughing and 2 harrowings	75-80 kg/ha	250 Quintals of farm yard manure	400-500 Q/ha. 7-9% CP	Cow pea-Oat Sorghum +Guar-Oat

Perennial Fodders

S.No	Name of the crop	Time of sowing	Ploughing	Seeding	Manuring and irrigation	Yield and nutritive value	Utility
1.	Pusa giant napier grass	February-August	Stem and root cutting	-	Kisan khad 250 kg/ha.	Grass assume a height of 12 feet. 4% CP	Hay making
2.	Buffal (Anjan) grass	Monsoon months	Land is ploughed once	4-5 kg/ha	100kg nitrogen/ha in the form of urea.	450-500 quintal/ha 4-5% CP	Hay and silage making
3.	Blue panic	Dry spells	-	-	100kg nitrogen/ha in the form of urea.	400-500 Q/ha. 8% CP	Silage making
4.	Jerga grass	Monsoon months	Root stumping	-	-	500-600 Q/ha 7% CP	Silage making
5.	Doob grass	Spring season	Creeping growth through roots	-	-	300-350 Q/ha 10-12% CP	Silage making
6.	Para grass	Summer season	Root and stem cuttings	-	-	400-500 Q/ha.	Hay making
7.	Guinea grass	Summer season	-	-	-	120-150 ton/ha	Hay making
8.	Sewan	Summer season	Root and stem cuttings	-	100kg superphosp hate and 300 kg ammonia per hectare	10 ton/ha	-

j. Silk cotton seed
k. Rubber seed cake
l. Tapioca waste
m. Neem seed cake

2. Sugar industry waste

a. Molasses
b. Bagasse
c. Sugarcane tops

3. Inferior quality roughages

a. Wheat straw: can be fed after urea molasses treatment.
b. Sunflower straw
c. Spent straw: can be fed to animals after mushroom cultivation
d. Sorghum ear husk
e. Cotton seed hull
f. Mustard straw: after treating with urea
g. Paddy straw

4. Root crops

Root crops like turnips, carrots, and fodder beet can be best used for feeding during winter season when other succulent fodders are not available. They have low crude fibre and are easily acceptable by the animals.

5. Grasses and weeds

Water hyacinth can be used as a feed. Various weeds van be neutralized by ensiling and can be fed to the animals during lean periods.

Schedule for green fodder production throughout the year

Fodder Trees

During recent years, with the promotion of social forestry programme, cultivation of fodder trees to support dairy cattle feeding is becoming a possibility. These tree species can be established in rows on field bunds, under agro-forestry **system.** Trees and bushes can also be developed into plantations on marginal lands where agricultural productivity is extremely poor. Cultivation of fodder trees has several advantages over seasonal fodder crops, in terms of wide adaptability to harsh agro-climatic conditions, ability to utilize limited quantity of water and sustain fodder production for a long period. This would also bring down the cost of production.

Type of Fodder Trees

Depending on the management of trees and the type of feed produced, the fodder trees can be categorized into the following groups. However, these groups signify only the method of management and a particular species can be put into any category depending on the situation. The categories are:

1. Trees for fodder hedges.
2. Trees for lopping side branches.
3. Trees for fruits and pods.

1. Trees for Fodder hedges

- Trees *like Leucaena, Albizia amara, Gliricidia, Pithecellobium dulce,* Hedge lucern, (*Desmanthus vergatus*), *Sesbania sesban* (shevri) and *Calliandra calothyrsus* can be established closely in rows and managed in hedges by cutting the main trunk at a convenient height.
- As these species re-grow vigorously after harvesting the shoots, the forage can be harvested regularly at an interval of 30- 50 days, depending on the soil fertility, moisture availability and climatic conditions.
- Under a high density plantation with a population from 50,000 to 1,00,000 plants per hectare, it is possible to harvest dry matter up to 20 tonnes per hectare per year, even on marginal soils with assured irrigation.
- *Leucaena* plantation can be maintained over a period of 15 - 20 years without any significant reduction in forage yield. While *Calliandra* and *Gliricidia* can be maintained for a period of 9- 10 years, Sesbania and hedge lucern can be managed as fodder hedge for 2 to 3 years.
- As all these species belong to the family of legumes, they have the capacity to fix atmospheric nitrogen and enrich the soil.
- The nutritive value of these fodder crops is high because of high protein content and higher digestibility.
- Regular supply of fodder throughout the year is another significant benefit of growing fodder trees.

2. Fodder trees for Lopping Side Branches

Many tree species are browsed by livestock. The foliage of these tree species can definitely be utilized for feeding the animals. However, it may not be very economical for growing these trees as fodder crops because of low fodder yield as well as poor tree regeneration capacity. Some of these species are ideal for poles, timber and other specialized use like oilseeds, medicines, etc. and in the process of shaping the trees, side branches can be lopped from time to time without causing any serious economical loss. Some of these tree species, which have the potential of providing fodder through side branches are:

- *Ailathus excels* (Maharukh)
- *Albizia amara* (Amara)
- *Albizia lebbeck* (Shins)
- *Albizia falcataria* (Albizia)
- *Albizia procera* (White Shins)
- *Albizia saman* (Rain tree)
- *Azadirachta indica* (Neem)
- *Bauhina perpuria* (Kanchan)
- *Dalbergia sissoo* (Shisham)
- *Erythrina indica* (Pangara, or Coral tree)
- *Ficus* Species (Peepal, Banyan, Umber)
- *Hardwickia binata* (Anjan)
- *Leucaena leucocephala* (Subabul)
- *Pithecellobium dulce* (Madras thorn)
- *Prosopis cineraria* (Khejdr)
- *Mella azedarach* (Bakain)
- *Sesbania sesban* (Shevari)
- *Sesbania grandiflora* (Agastha)
- *Safvadora percica* (Pilu)
- *Terminalla arjuna* (Arjun)
- *Ziziphus mauritiana* (Ber)
- *Ziziphus numularia* (Jagli ber) and many other species.

Under this system, the supply of fodder is erratic and inadequate. Nevertheless, they help farmers by providing fodder in an emergency, when other fodder and feeds are in short supply. It is advisable to keep foliage of these trees in reserve and use on days when farmers do not find adequate fodder for their livestock. Some of these species are not capable of producing vigorous shoots if lopped frequently and the growth of such trees remains stunted. Foliage of certain species such as Ailanthus, Neem and Melia are bitter in taste and cattle generally do not prefer them except during the period of fodder scarcity.

3. Trees Producing Edible Pods

Pods and fruits of several tree species are highly palatable and can become an excellent substitute for concentrate. Some of the tree species which produce edible pods are: *Prosopis juliflora, Acacia nilotica, Albizia saman, Pitheceiobium dulce* and *Parkia speciosa.*

- It has been estimated that a hectare of well maintained *Prosopis juliflora* plantation can yield 2 - 5 tonnes of pods every year. Information about the yield of pods of other species is not readily available.
- Species like *Leucaena leucocephala* produce 1 - 2 tonnes of seeds every year per hectare and the seeds can be crushed and used to feed the animals as a substitute for concentrate.
- Matured pods of *Sesbania prandiflora, Sesbania sesban* and almost all other legumes are highly nutritious and can be fed to cattle. The tender pods of *Sesbanias* are also used as vegetable in many parts of India.
- Seeds of tamarind (*Tamarindus indica*) and jackfruit are very rich in starch and can be used for feeding cattle. There are several trees which produce oilseeds of economic importance.
- Oils of *Madhuca indica* (Mahua) and *Madhuca latifolia* are edible and popularly used in tribal areas throughout the country. The cake is a source of animal protein.
- Cakes of neem, palas (*Butea monosperm*) and *Pongamia* are also fed in a limited way to livestock, particularly during the period of scarcity.
- Mahua flowers are fleshy, sweet and edible. The corolla drops down naturally after the fruit set and the villagers collect and consume the flowers directly or after drying.

22

Management

Management of Calf

Management before birth

- As calf management begins before birth, a few days before the calf is born, the pregnant cow is transferred to a maternity paddock, which should be near the homestead (for closer observation), well watered and free from physical objects.
- The signs of imminent parturition (calving) include filling of udder with milk and is turgid, vulva swollen with a string of mucus hanging from vagina.
- Insemination records can also be used to estimate the expected calving date.

Management at calving

- After the calf is born, ensure that calf is breathing. Should breathing not commence, the calf should be assisted (remove mucus from nostrils and if breathing does not start hold calf by hind legs upside down and swing several times).
- The umbilical cord should be disinfected using disinfectant (iodine or copper sulphate solution).
- If the calf is unable to suckle, it should be assisted and be allowed to suckle colostrum from the dam *at will* during the first week. Any excess colostrum should be milked and stored or fed fresh to other calves.
- During the second week of life and thereafter, the calf should be separated from dam and fed by hand.

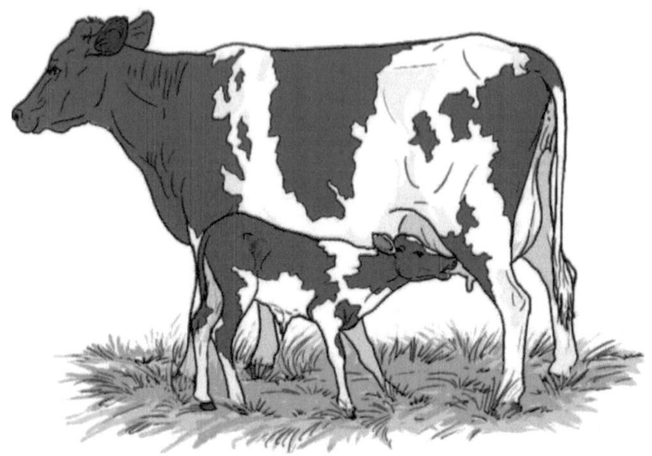

Calf Suckling

Care and management of calf

We must give good feeding and management for the calves so that they develop well and useful for replacement stock. The feeding and care of the calf begins before its birth. The dam should be dried 6-8 weeks before expected calving and should be fed well. Underfed animals will give weak and small calves.

A) Early Management

1. Immediately after birth remove any mucous or phlegm from those nose and mouth.
2. Normally the cow licks the calf immediately the birth. This helps to dry off the calf and helps in stimulating breathing and circulation. When the cows do not lick or in cold climate, rub and dry the calf with a dry cloth or gunny bag. Provide artificial respiration by compression and relaxing the chest with hands.
3. The Naval should be tied about 2-5cm away from the body and cut 1cm below the ligature and apply Tr. Iodine or boric acid or any antibiotic.
4. Remove the wet bedding from the pen and keep the stall very clean and dry in condition.
5. The weight of the calf should be recorded.
6. Wash the cow's udder and teats preferably with chlorine solution and dry.
7. Allow the calf to suckle the first milk of the mother i.e. Colostrum.
8. The calf will be standing and attempts to nurse within one hour. Otherwise help weak calves to stand.

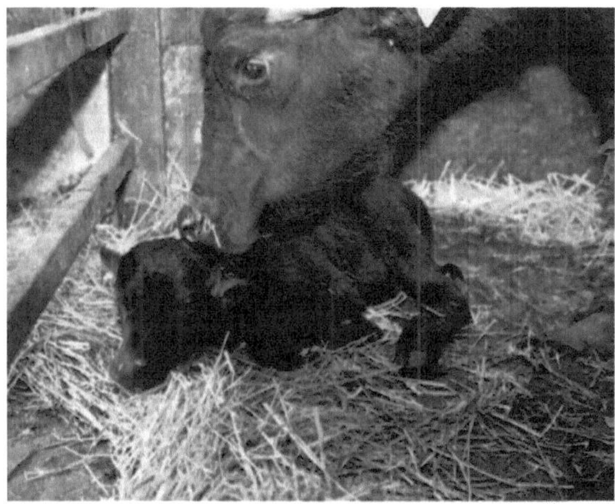

Buffalo licking her new born & transferring the desirable microflora

B) Feeding of Calves

1. Feed colostrum i.e. the first milk of the cow for the first 3 days. The colostrum is thick and viscous. It contains higher proportions of Vit. A and proteins. The proteins are immunoglobulins which gives protection against many diseases. Colostrum contains antitrypsin which avoids digestion of immunoglobulins in the stomach and is absorbed as it is.
2. Whole milk should be given after 3 days it is better to teach to drink the milk from the pail or bucket. Feed twice a day which should be warmed to body temperature. For weak calves feed thrice a day.
3. The limit of liquid milk feeding is 10 % of its body weight with a maximum of 5-6 liters per day and continues liquid milk feeding for 6-10 weeks. Over feeding causes 'Calf Scours'.
4. The milk replacers can be given to replace whole milk.
5. Give calf starter after one month of age.
6. Provide good quality green fodder and hay from 4th month afterwards.
7. Feeding of antibiotics to calves improves appetite, increases growth rate and prevents calf scours. E.g. Aureomycin, Terramycin etc.

Other Management Practices

1. Identity the calf by tattooing in the ear at birth, and branding after one year.
2. Dehorn the calf within 7-10 days after birth with red hot Iron or caustic potash stick or electrical method.

3. Deworm the calf regularly to remove worms using deworming drugs. Deworm at 30 days interval.
4. Fresh water should be given from 2nd week onwards.
5. House the calves in individual calf pens for 3 months afterwards in groups. After six months males and females calves should be housed separately.
6. Weigh the calves at weekly interval upto 6 months arid at monthly interval afterwards to know the growth rate.
7. Mortality in calves is more in first month due to pneumonia, diarrhea (calf scours) and worms. House them under warm condition, clean condition to avoid above condition.
8. Extra teats beyond 4 should be removed at 1-2 months of age.
9. 8-9 weeks of age, males should be castrated.
10. Keep the body clean and dry to avoid fungal infection.
11. Mineral-blocks should be provided, so that the calves lick and no chances for mineral deficiency occur.
12. Wean the calf from the mother and feed through pail feeding system.

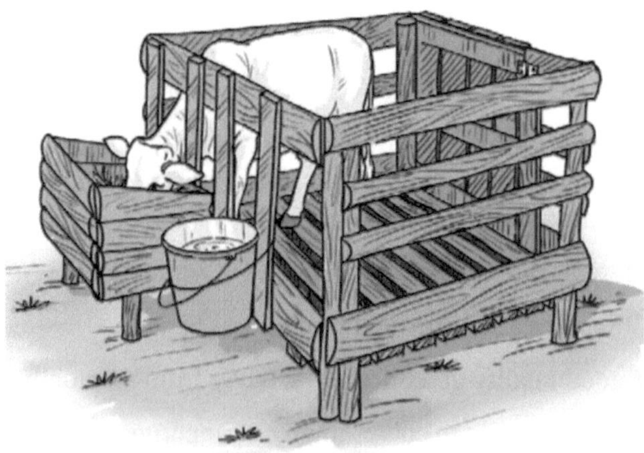

Feeding the calf

Calf health

Most of the common health problems experienced by calves are due to poor management. Diligent feeding management and housing is therefore essential to ensure calf health is maintained. Some of the common problems associated with management practices are diarrhoea and pneumonia.

Common Diseases

1. Scours (diarrhoea): Scours could be caused by nutritional disorders, viruses or bacteria. Digestive upsets leading to scours are a major cause of death in young calves. The problem can however be minimised through:

a. Ensuring calves receive adequate colostrum within 6 hours of birth and therefore acquire some natural immunity.

b. Feeding the correct amount of milk.

c. Early recognition, isolation and treatment of scouring calves.

d. Maintenance of hygiene and cleanliness of feeding utensils and the environment.

e. Not rearing calves continually in pens, dirt yards or small paddocks that become heavily contaminated. Paddock rotation will help prevent disease.

f. Separation of sick animals to avoid cross infection.

g. Close observation of calves at feeding to identify scouring animals as soon as possible for remedial treatment will prevent dehydration and secondary disease leading to chronic ill-thrift and mortality.

To minimize scours, the following should be avoided:

a. **Overcrowding**: Provide about 20 – 24 square feet of building floor space for calves raised in confined, elevated stalls.

b. **Inadequate ventilation**: Provide fresh air circulation in the calf pen but avoid direct drafts on the calf.

c. **Wet, damp calves:** Provide adequate bedding and good ventilation, and avoid spraying calves with water when cleaning the pen to prevent calves becoming chilled.

d. **Overfeeding**: Irregular amounts and too much of the wrong concentration or wrong kind of liquid diets are common causes of calf scours.

e. **No first-milk colostrums**: Don't assume the newborn calf has nursed. Many newborn calves don't receive enough colostrum to be protected from calfhood diseases. Feed colostrum, preferably by hand, as soon as possible after birth.

f. **Dirty utensils**: Clean the feeding utensils thoroughly after each feeding. Store upside down to drain all water out. Small amounts of excess wash water that remains in utensils are perfect areas for bacteria to multiply rapidly.

Most scour incidents can be treated simply by:

- Feeding water with salts.
- Avoiding milk for 1-2 feeds. Give fresh water, concentrates and forage.
- Antibiotics should not be used to treat scours resulting from over feeding or digestive upsets. Blood scours (mostly caused by coccidia) require veterinary treatment and management changes to improve hygiene.

2. Pneumonia

One cause of pneumonia in young calves is fluids going to the lungs via the windpipe (trachea). The first feeding of colostrum can cause problems if the feeding rate is faster than swallowing rate. If colostrum is bottle fed it is important to use a nipple that matches the calf's ability to swallow. Greedy calves swallow large quantities of milk from the bucket, some of which may end up in the windpipe leading to pneumonia.

3. Navel-ill

Clinical signs: Umbilical region inflamed, Joints swell.

Management: Dress umbilicus with antiseptic at birth, Maintain good hygiene at parturition.

Management of Heifer

Better care and management of heifer will give high quality replacement stock to the dairy farm.

During the early stage relatively more protein than energy is needed. Most heifers grow well if excellent hay is given. The amount of growth depends upon the quality of forage fed. Feed the heifer sufficiently to produce normal growth.

- The heifers should be provided with a dry shelter free from drafts. A loose housing system with a shelter open to one side is sufficient.
- Breeding undersized animals is never profitable. Small heifers are more likely to have difficulty in calving.
- Place the heifer in a separate shed about 6-8 weeks before she is due to calve.
- Feed 2 - 3 kg of concentrate daily and all other green.
- Animals lagging behind below the required standards should be removed from the herd.
- For the heifer the calving is first time and it may have difficulty in calving. So take extra care during calving.

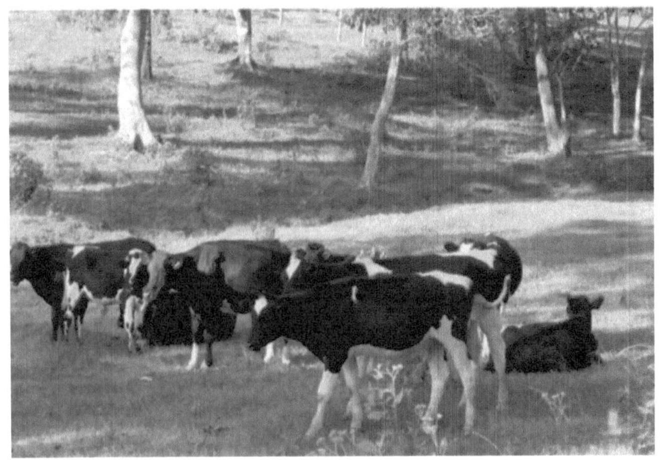

Healthy heifers

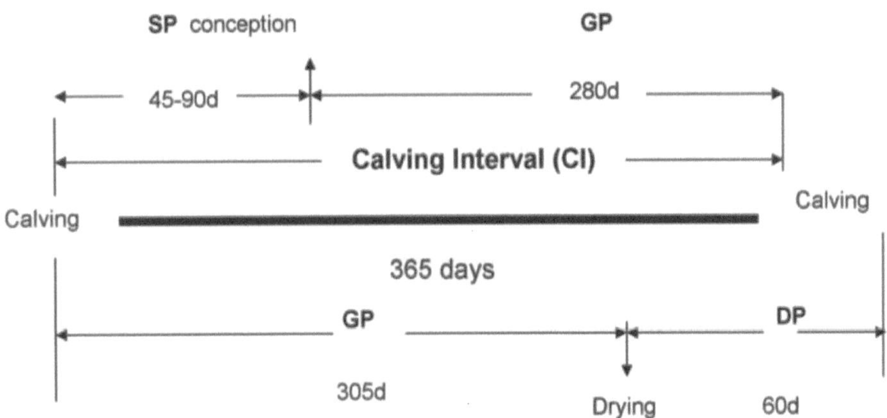

SP+GP = CI and LP+DP = CI

Different periods of dairy cow cycle
(SP: service period; GP: gestation period; LP: lactation period; DP: dry period)

Management of Lactating Animals

To get high milk during any lactation, the milch animal should be properly fed along a proper care and management practices.

- Provide green succulent forage together with leguminous hay or straw to the extent of animal can consume, so that all its maintenance requirements are met with through forage only. Extra concentrate at the rate of 1 kg for every 2 to 2.5 liters of milk should be provided. Salt and mineral supplements should be given to maintain the lactation.

- Never frighten or excite the animals.
- Concentrate mix is fed before or during milking, where as roughages after milking. This practice will avoid dust in the shed.
- Water should be provided adlibitum.
- Regularity in milking is essential. Increase of milk in the udder will reduce further secretion of milk. Milking thrice is better than twice since 10 - 15 % more milk can be produced.
- Milking should be done with whole hand. Avoid knuckling.
- Cows should be trained to let down milk without calf suckling. This will help to wean the calves early.
- Loose housing with shelter during hot part of the day should be provided.
- The animals will get maximum exercise in loose housing system.
- Grooming of the cows and washing of the buffaloes before milking help in clean milk production.
- Daily brushing will remove loose hair and dirt from the coat.
- Grooming will also keep the animal hide pliable.
- Wallowing of buffaloes or water spraying on their bodies will keep the buffaloes comfortable especially in summer.
- Provide at least 60 days dry period between calving. If the dry period is not sufficient, the milk yield is subsequent lactation will be reduced.
- Vaccinate the cows- against important diseases.
- Every animal should be numbered and particulars pertaining to milk, fat %, feed taken, breeding, drying and calving dates should be recorded.
- Check for mastitis regularly.

Cow as a milk factory

A dairy cow can be compared with a factory. The raw materials that go into milk manufacturing are the feeds consumed by the cow. To get more milk, feed the cow on good quality feed in large quantities. The size of the factory can be compared to the size of the cow where a large factory will hold more raw materials, so will a large cow have a larger rumen.

Animal Feeding

Good Practice

- Timely provision of feed to meet livestock nutritional requirements.
- Always give the animals clean and healthy feed.
- Input must be adequate in both nutritional and economic terms. Feed cows according to the stage of lactation.
- Make sure adequate water available after milking.
- Cows need clean potable water and free access to it.

Bad Practice

- Insufficient quantity of feed supplied.
- Use of poor quality feed stuffs, Inadequate to meet the animal's requirement, feeding unbalanced rations leads to wastage and poor performance.
- Feeding fodder that has been recently sprayed with pesticide.
- Using dirty water for drinking.

Environment

Good Practice

- Cleaning away waste every day.
- Separating medicine and chemical containers from other organic waste.
- Use the manure for land improvement.
- Keep the area clean and safe for animals.

Bad Practice

- Wet unventilated dirty environment.
- Burning rubbish in the vicinity of the cows.
- Excessive use of chemicals, fertilizers and pesticides, contaminates the soil and ground water.

Management of Dry Animals

The dairy animals should be rendered dry before parturition for four principle reasons:

1. To rest organs of milk secretion.
2. To permit nutrients in feed to be used solely for development of fetus.
3. To make animal replenish its body.
4. To permit to build up a reserve of body flesh before parturition.

It has been seen that the cows denied of dry period yields less milk in their successive lactations

The following points should be considered for drying off dairy animals:

1. Before 80 days of parturition, incomplete milking of the animal should be done i.e. all the milk should not be extracted out. This should be done at the beginning of the dry period.
2. Before 60 days of parturition, intermittent milking should be done i.e. the animal should be milked only once a day.
3. Before 40 days of parturition, there should be complete cessation of milking. It is seen that complete cessation of milking can be done safely in cows producing as much as 10 litres of milk per day.
4. The animal should be kept on adlibitum roughages and 12% CP should be supplemented in diet.
5. The level of calcium and phosphorous should be checked.
6. Feeding of extra concentrates is helpful for animal.

Management of Breeding Bulls

- The maintenance of breeding bulls in good condition and suitable for breeding is highly essential requirement for the success of breeding programmes. A rising condition is better for reproduction than a falling one. Fat males may produce semen of inferior quality or they may be slow or fail at service. Breeding bull should receive plenty of exercise; will usually produce large ejaculation containing more sperms of higher activity.
- A breeding bull should be housed separately known as "Bull Shed" with sufficient area of floor and proper covering. It is sound practice to provide cool conditions and adequate drinking water.

- A balanced ration should be fed containing adequate energy, proteins, minerals, and vitamins. Green fodder must be available both before and during breeding season.
- Most of the bulls are ferocious and so control them properly using nose rings, etc.
- It is of great importance that males should be, fed regularly and not too much at one time, and too little at another.
- For bulls two mating a day has been found to be profitable.
- Moderate exercise should be provided to keep the breeding bull in active and non fatty conditions.
- Regular grooming of the breeding bull is practiced.
- In buffalo bulls regular shaving may be practiced.

23

Reproduction

Breeding of Heifers

- Regardless of age, puberty is reached when a heifer weighs approximately 40% of her mature body weight.
- Breeding however, is recommended when a heifer has reached 60% of her expected mature body weight. This is normally achieved when the heifer is 14 to 16 months old.
- Smaller breeds may be bred one or two months earlier than large breeds because they mature faster.
- Heifers in good condition and gaining weight at breeding time generally show more definite signs of estrus and have improved conception rates over heifers in poor condition and/or losing weight.
- Over-conditioned or fat heifers have been reported to require more services per conception than heifers of normal size and weight.

Heat Detection

Behavioral signs and physical changes

This is an extremely important exercise as a missed heat translates into a wasted 21 days while efficient heat detection makes it possible to serve the animal at the right time. The average heat interval is 21 days with a range of 18 to 24 days. Duration of heat is 24 to 36 hours in exotic and crossbred cows. Several methods are used to detect heat. The most commonly used by farmers are behavioral signs and physical changes.

1. Early Heat: watch the animal closely.

- Increased nervousness/restlessness.
- Mounting other cows.
- Swollen vulva.
- Licking other cows.
- Sniffing other cows and being sniffed.
- Reduced feed intake.

2. Standing Heat: take the animal for service.

- Standing to be mounted.
- Clear mucus discharge.
- Sharp decline in milk production.
- Tail bent away from the vulva.
- The animal may stop eating.

3. After heat: keep records.

- Dried mucus on the tail.
- Roughened tail head.
- The animal refuses to be mounted.
- Streaks of saliva or signs of leaking on her flanks.

Symptoms of heat

The various symptoms of heat are

1. The animal will be excited condition.
2. The animal will be in restlessness and nervousness.
3. The animal will bellow frequently.
4. The animal will reduce the intake of feed.
5. Peculiar movement of lumbo-sacral region will be observed.
6. The animals which are in heat will lick other animals and smell other animals.
7. The animals will try to mount other animals.
8. The animals will standstill when other animal try to mount. This period is known as standing heat. This extends 14-16 hours.
9. Frequent micturition (urination) will be observed.
10. Clear mucous discharge will be seen from the vulva, sometimes it will be string like mucous will be seen stick to the near the pasts of vulva.
11. Swelling of the vulva will be seen.
12. Congestion and hyperarmia of membrane.
13. The tail will be in raised position.
14. Milk production will be slightly decreased.
15. On Palpation uterus will be turgid and the cervix will be opened.

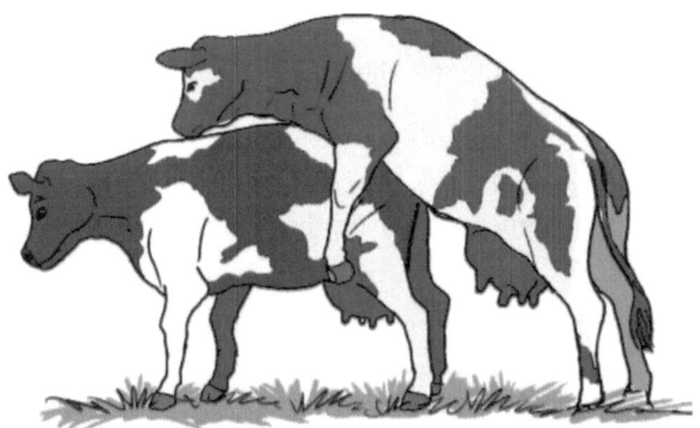

(a) Standing to be mounted: The positive sign of heat is standing to be mounted. The cow in heat stands to be mounted and does not move away.

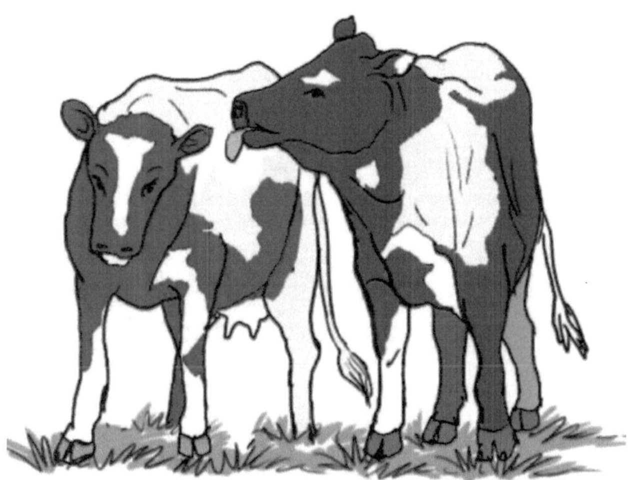

(b) Licking: Both cows may be in heat.

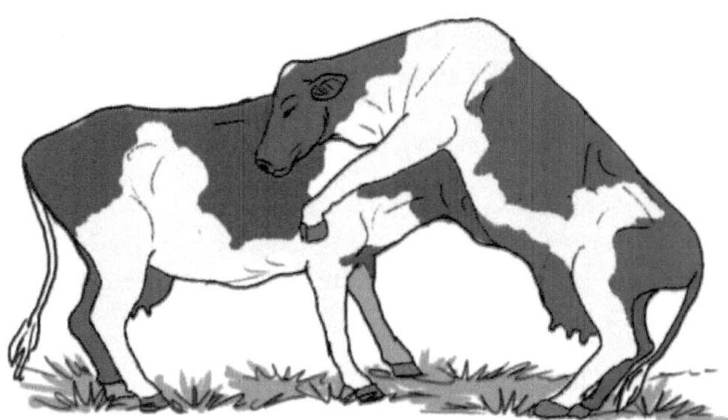

(c) Mounting head to head: The cow mounting is in heat.
Fig. (a) to (c): Behavioral signs of heat in cows.

Mating

Once heat has been detected, cows should be mated.

When to serve

Present the cow for insemination at the right time to increase the chances of conception. Below is a guide as to the best time to present the cow for insemination:

AM – PM Rule		
Standing heat observed:	Before 9 am	Late evening the same day
Present for insemination:	Late afternoon or evening	Early next morning.

Breeding Methods

Breeding can be achieved through natural service or artificial insemination, and irrespective of the method, the aim should be to achieve increased chances of conception.

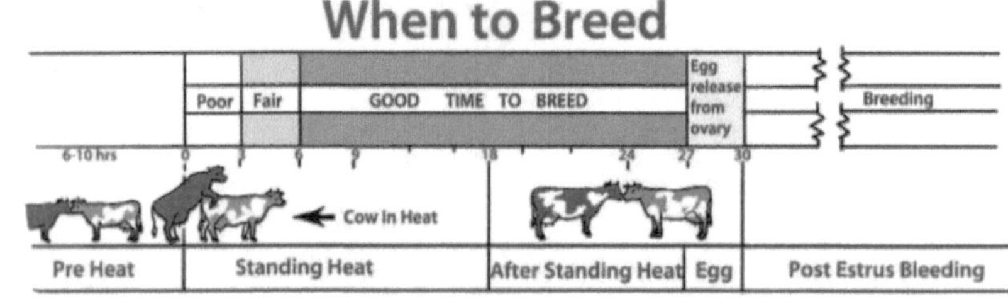

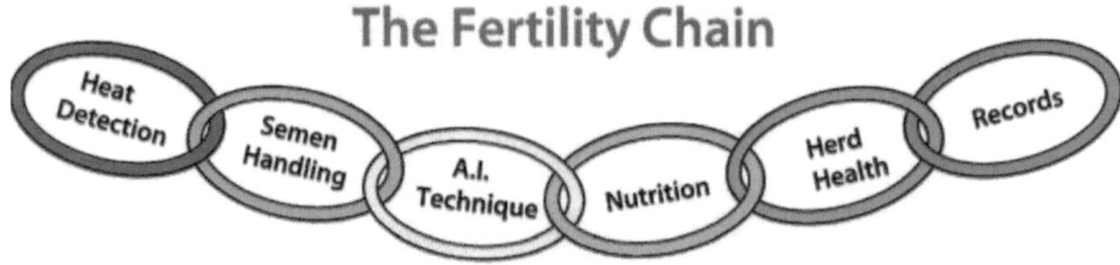

Natural service

This is where the cow is taken to a bull and left for some time for the bull to serve.

The advantages of this method are

1. The cow has an opportunity to be served more than once; this increase the chance of conception.

2. The semen is fresh and of good quality since there is no handling.
3. Where the farmer does not own a bull, cost of service is lower compared to A.I.

Natural service has the following disadvantages

1. Rearing a bull is not economical especially to a small holder farmer.
2. There is risk of spreading breeding diseases.
3. There is risk of inbreeding if the bull is not changed frequently.
4. There is no opportunity to select the type of bull the farmer wants.

Some tips for natural breeding

1. Take the cow to the bull as soon as it is detected to be in heat and leave it for at least twelve hours.
2. Young inexperienced heifers should be mated with old experienced bulls.
3. Young inexperienced bulls should be given to old experienced cows.
4. The bull should be kept fit and in good health particularly the legs and feet.

Natural mating can be done in two ways

1. **Free/pasture mating**: This method of mating is practiced by farmers who own bulls which run full time with the cows. One bull can serve 20-25 cows.

   It has the advantage that no heat detection is required and disadvantage of lack of accurate records and possibility of transmission of reproductive diseases e.g. brucellosis.

2. **Hand mating:** The bull is enclosed in its pen and the cows are brought in when they show signs of heat. Most small-scale farmers will practice this method since bulls are owned by few farmers and others bring their cows for service at an agreed fee. The advantage is keeping accurate records while the disadvantage is the farmer has to detect heat.

Artificial Insemination

Artificial Insemination popularly referred to as AI is one of the breeding methods that has contributed to the development of the dairy sector in the last sixty years in India and also worldwide. The process of artificial insemination starts with a healthy bull, that is disease free and producing ample quantities of high quality semen. The fertility of the cow is also important, the competency of the inseminator and a clean environment. Farmers are encouraged to use semen from proven bulls which is obtained from AI centers and registered service providers.

Advantages of Artificial Insemination

1. Prevention of venereal diseases.
2. Indefinite preservation of genetic materials of low cost enabling wide testing and selection of bulls.
3. Enhances genetic progress as best bulls are used widely nationally and internationally.
4. Small scale farmers through AI can access good bulls cheaply.
5. One is able to select the bull of interest.
6. When handled properly, there is no chance of spread of breeding diseases.
7. It is easy to control inbreeding.
8. A.I. is the best method of improving the genetic make-up of local breeds because it enables semen from the very best bulls to be widely available.
9. It is **cost effective** since the farmer does not have to rear a bull.

Disadvantages of AI

1. It requires very accurate heat detection and proper timing of insemination for greater chances of conception.
2. The inseminator must be trained on the technique.
3. It requires high investment in equipment.

Pregnancy Diagnosis

The success of pregnancy diagnosis shows the profitability of the dairy unit. It can be done as early as 1 ½ months after service by a skilled veterinarian. However in case of cattle it is performed at 2 months after service and in buffalo after 3 months after service in field conditions.

PD can be done by following methods:

1. Manual method or per rectal examination: it should be carried out only by a skilled and experienced veterinarian. The per rectal palpation of the genitalia is done manually by a vet and hence the diagnosis is made.
2. Ultrasonography: in this case, the use of ultrasound is done for PD. It is more reliable than per rectal palpation. Still this should be only carried out by a veterinarian or by a skilled veterinary technician.

Reproductive Management in Dairy Cows

- Reduced fertility is one of the commonest reasons for vets being called onto dairy farms. In many cases cows presented to vets have obvious problems such as "whites" or ovarian cysts.
- However, not every cow failing to hold to service has an obvious problem. A significant number (around 10 to 15%) of cows require four or more inseminations to get pregnant despite apparently cycling normally.
- Most of these are indeed "normal" since, assuming no cows are culled after earlier services, then even in a herd with every cow becoming pregnant at a rate of 50% (a good rate for our dairy farms these days) there will be 12.5% of cows presented for a 4th service.
- However, in some cases there is an underlying problem reducing the chance of the cow getting pregnant. These may be either cow factors that require ultrasound examination or even other more sophisticated tests e.g. oviduct patency, or the result of a wide range of external factors, such as poor management.
- An obvious example is inefficient estrous detection. On farm, without extensive testing, it is very difficult to distinguish between all these factors, as their only sign is a cow that is apparently normal but hasn't got pregnant. Such cows get lumped together as having 'repeat breeding syndrome'.

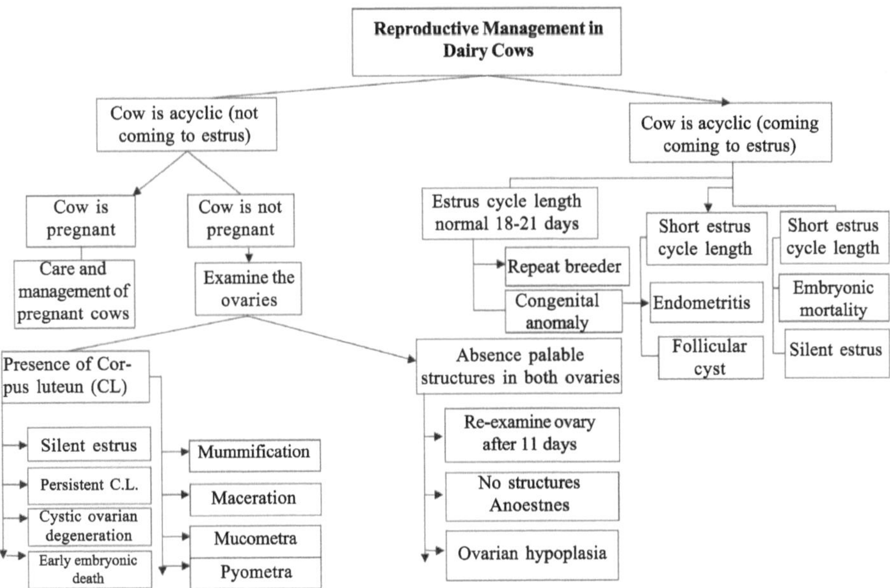

Care and management of pregnant cow

- Pregnant animals should be watched carefully, particularly during the last stages of pregnancy to avoid abortion due to fights or other physical trauma.
- During early stages of pregnancy, there is no need of special feeding for heifers. The system of feeding and management recommended for heifers before breeding may continue. During last three months of pregnancy when foetal growth is very rapid, a special pregnancy allowance of about 1-2 Kg of concentrate should be offered.
- Special care should be taken regarding mineral and vitamin deficiencies because they can have a serious adverse effect on the newborn calf. Feeding trace mineralized salt plus recommended amounts of calcium and phosphorus is usually sufficient to avoid these problems. Care must be taken that calcium and phosphorus should not be taken in excessive amounts.
- During the last few weeks of pregnancy there is a tendency of prolapse of vagina which may be caused by constipation, mineral deficiency and debility. Balanced and laxative rations should be fed to maintain the normal tone of the reproductive tract.
- Sometime udder oedema occurs before calving. This can be avoided by moderate exercise for a half an hour, two to three times per day. Massaging the udder for a few minutes is also helpful. Use of diuretics and prepartum milking may be helpful in severe cases.
- Isolate the pregnant animal 8-10 days before the expected date of calving and keep it in a clean well bedded, dry and disinfected maternity pen. The animal should be watched closely as calving time approaches at least every two to three hours.
- A good calving environment reduces the exposure of cows and newborn calves to infectious disease. A clean and comfortable area that provides cows with good footing minimizes the potential for injuries. Calving areas should be landscaped to allow for adequate drainage. Shade structures are recommended.
- Calves are usually born without assistance. Any abnormality in their presentation requires immediate attention by a competent person to correct the position of the calf so that it can be delivered. Strict sanitation must be observed during assistance.
- After removal of calf, milk animal it will help in removal of placenta. Placenta is normally expelled within 2 to 6 hours after calving. If placenta

fails to be expelled with 12 hours it is considered retained placenta. In case of retained placenta veterinarian should be called for its removal.

- After normal birth, the dam is alert and willing to eat and drink within one or two hours of calving. Warm water and some wheat bran should be offered to dam after calving. It is necessary to encourage the dairy animals to rise and to move to the manger for feeding after calving, especially on the day of calving and the first 2 days after calving.
- The animal should be closely watched for health problems after calving. In addition to observing feed intake and milk production, rectal temperature and ketone levels should be monitored daily. Animals having health problems should be identified and treated accordingly, whereas healthy animals can join the general population 3 to 4 days postpartum.

Approaches in achieving better reproductive efficiency in cattle

Steaming up

During the last two months of pregnancy, the feeding regime can affect milk production during the first lactation. The exact amount of concentrates to feed before calving will depend on forage quality, size, and condition of the heifer. A rule of thumb the heifer should be fed concentrate at 1 percent of body weight starting about 6 weeks before calving with a ration balanced in protein, minerals, and vitamins.

Feeding concentrates allows the rumen bacteria to get used to digesting high levels of concentrate, which is very important during early lactation. If practical, concentrates should be fed in a milking parlor as this accustoms the heifer to the milking parlor.

Well managed heifers will have a minimum of problems at calving, but ease of calving can be affected by plane of nutrition in two ways:

- an effect on calf size, and
- an effect on fatness of the dam.

Fat heifers have higher rates of difficult calving because of small pelvic openings and usually a larger-than-normal sized calf at birth. Underfed or poorly grown heifers also will require more assistance at calving and have a higher death rate at calving than normal sized heifers.

Improvement of reproductive efficiency in the animals can be obtained by directing attention to management systems and utilizing controlled breeding techniques:

The application of oestrus induction techniques permits the possibility of inducing fertile oestrus in non cycling heifers, in order to increase fertility in the low breeding season and reduce the intercalving period. Different treatments are utilized to induce oestrus, such as prostaglandin, gonadorelin, progestagen, however improved results have been obtained using PRID plus PMSG and prostaglandin.

- To identify animals in heat, in order to apply AI, the presence of a teaser bull can be helpful.
- New approaches are being developed to provide automated systems of detection of oestrus using electronic technology such as pedometry and radiotelemetry.
- To apply a fixed time AI, thereby overcoming the problem of oestrus detection, different hormonal treatment schedules have been proposed.
- Protocols using fixed time insemination and only prostaglandin treatment have not provided good results. The use of GnRH, in association with that of prostaglandin, improves the efficiency of fixed time insemination because it synchronizes the ovulation in a short period of time but this treatment is efficient when animals are cyclic.
- The use of PRID associated with PMSG and prostaglandin can be successfully employed in the low breeding season thereby proving to be the preferred treatment when oestrus synchronization and AI are programmed out of the breeding season.

Reproductive Management in Buffaloes

Buffalo are said to be seasonal breeders. However, this is not entirely true as buffalo are polyestral animals and may breed all year round. The buffalo's reputation as a difficult breeder is because of its inherent susceptibility to environmental stress, which causes anoestrus and sub-oestrus. These conditions are responsible for prolonged inter-calving periods, resulting in great economic losses for the buffalo dairy industry. Susceptibility to heat stress also affects feed intake and in turn the nutritional balance and this also inhibits reproductive efficiency.

Reproductive management of buffalo bull

- **Bulls reach sexual maturity at two to three years of age.**
- Semen is produced all year round but it is highly affected by heat stress and low quality feed.

- The buffalo bull seems to be most fertile in spring, when the volume of ejaculate and sperm concentration is highest.
- Sperm vitality is also much higher in spring than at other times of the year. Corresponding values are lowest in summer time.
- Heat stress may have a negative effect on libido.

Reproductive management of she-buffaloes

- Wild or feral female buffalo reach sexual maturity at two to three years of age. Domesticated buffalo that are cared for and fed properly may reach puberty earlier. Puberty is highly affected by management factors.
- Size is more important than age, and a Murrah heifer should weigh around 325 kg at insemination or mating and 450 to 500 kg at her first calving.
- The age of puberty in buffalo is 36 to 42 months in India. It is comparatively late compared to other countries like Italy, where the age at first calving is between 28 to 32 months on average.
- Delayed puberty in both male and female buffalo is common in India. This is due to neglect of calves during their growing period. Buffalo have the potential to gain 400 to 800 gm daily after about four to six months of age, and can attain the 300 to 450 kg body weight suitable for breeding at about 24 months of age.
- In a majority of dairy buffalo calving occurs at four to six years of age. This is mainly due to an inadequate supply of feed and nutrients during the growing phase.

The reproductive cycle of a buffalo

The oestrus cycle varies between 21 and 29 days depending on breed. The total duration of oestrus is usually 24 hours but varies from 12 to 72 hours. The most reliable sign of oestrus is frequent urination. The signs of oestrus are much less pronounced in buffalo than in cattle. Many buffalo show oestrus only at night time, and then it is difficult to detect. A lactating animal may have a slight decrease in milk yield when in heat, although it is seldom as pronounced as in cattle. The buffalo may be more restless and be difficult to milk.

- **Age at puberty:** 36 to 42 months
- **Length of oestrus cycle:** 21 days
- **Duration of heat:** 12 to 24 hrs
- **Time of ovulation:** 10 to 14 hrs after end of oestrus

- **Period of maximum fertility:** last 8 hrs of oestrus
- **Gestation period:** 310 days
- **Period of involution of uterus:** 25 to 35 days.

Reasons for poor reproductive performance in buffaloes

1. Climate affects both production and reproduction in all farm animals. However as buffaloes are very susceptible to extreme conditions of heat and cold they show a tendency towards better performance during the cool months. In India 70 to 80% of buffalo conceive between July and February. In India it is reported that a lower number of services are needed during the July to February breeding season than in the March to June season. Buffalo are sexually activated by decreased daylight.

2. As mentioned earlier buffalo have poor thermal tolerance on account of an under developed thermo regulatory system and are unable to get rid of excess body temperature. If their housing is not designed to take care of this special species-specific requirement for adequate shade and ventilation, it will affect production and reproduction.

3. Nutrition plays a major role in the reproductive performance of buffalo, as with other farm animals. However there is a strong possibility that the consequences of poor nutrition are often interpreted as seasonality of breeding in buffalo. Under feeding, over feeding or unbalanced feeding, as well as deficiencies in minerals, vitamins or trace elements will cause reduced fertility in buffalo just as in other farm animals. A poor body condition score at calving affects fertility, characterized by prolonged post-partum intervals, reduced conception rates, and more services per conception. A very low protein diet can cause cessation of oestrus.

4. One of the reasons buffalo suffer from long post-partum anoestrus is because their natural behavior of rolling in dirty water pools, and unhygienic shed conditions, cause buffalo to suffer from a high incidence of endometritis. The loose broad uterine ligaments and rolling in water cause torsion of uterus cases in buffalo. Buffalo also suffer from uterine prolapse and retention of the afterbirth. All these lead to uterine infections, delayed involution of the uterus and endometritis in buffalo resulting in the need for repeat breeding.

Approaches for improving reproductive efficiency

1. Providing the right kind of housing for buffalo to suit their natural behavioural requirements is important for their optimum performance. Free stall as well as tied systems work well for buffalo. However it is important that the housing provides sufficient shelter from both heat and extreme cold. During summer they have to be protected from extreme heat while in winter they have to be protected from extreme cold as well.

2. Showers or foggers with fans or wallowing tanks should be made available to buffalo during the hottest part of the day. Thermal ameliorative measures such as sprinkling and cooling are known to increase comfort levels and feed intake in buffalo.

3. Balanced feeding with mineral supplements, plenty of green fodder, and concentrate as per each animal's specific need, is necessary to bring buffalo into normal reproductive cycles.

4. Regular testing of all buffalo and bulls for infectious reproductive diseases like brucellosis and regular culling of infected animals are crucial for good reproductive health in the herd. Attending cases of difficult birth and retained placenta in time and maintaining good hygiene during parturition are also crucial to prevent reproductive disorders such as endometritis.

5. Wall charts, breeding wheels, herd monitors and individual buffalo records are important oestrus detection aids. The key to successful use of these inexpensive management aids is to accurately record every heat, beginning with the first heat after calving, and to make daily use of the information to identify those buffalo that are due to return to oestrus.

Breeding buffalo

1. Calving interval: Calving interval in buffalo is highly dependent on management, climate and nutrition. It is therefore shorter in some regions and longer in others. In order to shorten the calving interval the female should be serviced again as soon as possible after calving, after providing a sufficient period of rest. Weaning of calves at birth has been shown to decrease the service period in comparison to unweaned buffalo. A shorter service period will lead to a shorter calving interval – a calving interval of less than 410 days is recommended.

2. Natural mating: Except for a very small percentage of the world's buffalo, most are bred through natural mating. In most cases at the village level and in the home tracts of buffalo there is no information on the buffalo bull or on the dam's milk yield, and this information is seldom considered

while breeding. This has been one of the major reasons for the diversity in both the productive and reproductive traits of buffalo. However as this method persists on the farms it is crucial to avoid the spread of venereal diseases which cause infertility and sterility in both sexes.

Utility of breeding buffalo bull

- Having a breeding bull with the dams all the time enhances the chances of fertile mating. This bull seldom misses a female in heat.
- However, to be able to calculate the time of calving it is advisable to keep some sort of record of expected heat.
- The observant farmer will soon learn how his buffalo behave when in heat and when to expect conception and calving. The females can be teased with a bull twice a day around expected oestrus.
- A breeding bull can be put into service from three years of age. One bull, if managed correctly, can serve 20 to 25 females.
- On a smaller farm, the bull should be exchanged more often to avoid interbreeding.
- If the bull shows signs of loss of interest in the females or is otherwise ill, he should be taken out of service immediately.
- In order to perform best, bulls must be fed high quality feed and be protected from heat and cold stress in the same way as the rest of the herd.
- Bulls should not be used for service more than twice a week.

3. **Artificial insemination (AI):** With the help of AI improved genes are transmitted to a large number of offspring, and the interval between generations is reduced. Buffalo generally have more difficulty conceiving by artificial insemination than cattle do. Reports from the National Dairy Research Institute, Karnal, India, show that the conception rate for first insemination is around 40% and the conception rate for third insemination is around 77%. In the state of Gujarat in India, the National Dairy Development Board has a breed improvement programme called Dairy Herd Improvement Programme Actions (DIPA). The genetic gain of buffalo is being improved through selective mating of both sire and dam, to breed sires with the desired genetic traits. A progeny testing programme is being followed, producing 100 completed first lactation records of progeny per bull. Twenty bulls are put to test every year, with 2 000 doses of frozen semen from each bull being distributed to the selected villages, and 5 000 doses being stored until the test results are available.

Some Common Reproductive Disorders

1. Anovulation

Ovum not released from ovary. The animal has normal cycle, normal reproductive tract but fails to conceive.

Causes

- Inadequate level or absence of Luteinizing Hormone.
- Ovaro-bursal adhesion. It may be diagnosed by palpation of matured Graffian Follicle on the ovary more than 48hrs after the end of estrum.

Treatment

- L.H preparations (HCG- Human Chorion Gonadrotropin)- 3000 IU. I/V. when the animal is in heat.
- Inj. Buserelin - 5 ml I/m.
- Improved feeding.

2. Delayed Ovulation

Ovulation takes place 48-72 hours after the onset of oestrus but the spermatozoa would be dead by then.

Cause

- Due to low level of LH.

Treatment

- As for anovulation.

3. Early embryonic death

Embryonic mortality is generally defined as loss of the conceptus which occurs during the first 42 days of pregnancy, which is the period from conception to completion of differentiation when organ systems develop.

- Approximately 30 percent of all embryos and foetuses will not survive to birth.
- About 80 percent of this loss occurs before day 17, 10-15 percent between day 17 and 42 and 5 percent after day 42.
- These losses to be much higher in "repeat breeders" those cows and heifers inseminated three or more times.
- This has a significant economic impact on dairy herd profitability.

- Because of the complex interactions among the various processes involved in establishment and maintenance of pregnancy, no single factor can be identified as the primary cause of embryonic death.

Causes

- It is well documented that short term exposure to **heat stress** several days before and after insemination results in low conception rate or embryonic death. This is due to elevated temperature of the uterine environment. This has been a serious problem affecting reproductive performance this spring and summer.
- Chromosomal abnormalities are known to be a cause of embryo mortality. Unfortunately, this problem cannot be controlled through management.
- Nutritional factors have been shown to contribute to low conception rates resulting from embryonic mortality.
- Abnormal hormonal situation such as reduced progesterone secretion or ovulation of a defective oocyte has not been determined.
- Several reports showed that feeding excess crude protein, excess degradable intake protein or low levels of fermentable carbohydrate and the various combinations of these nutrients can cause low conception rates. Such situations can produce excessive levels of ammonia in the blood and uterus of cows. Some researchers believe this could be toxic to the gametes and the developing embryo.
- Infectious agents can cause uterine infection or directly affect the embryo causing death. The major organisms adversely affecting reproduction are: Corynebacterium pyogenes, Campylobacter fetus (Vibriosis), Haemophilius somnus, Leptospirosis, Neospora and the viruses bovine virus diarrhoea (BVD), infectious bovine rhinotracheitis (IBR) and to a lesser extent Ureaplasma and Mycoplasma.
- **Subclinical mastitis and other systemic infections** can substantially increase the incidence of early embryo loss. Furthermore, nutritional deficiencies or an environmental challenge can alter uterine immune function.
- Hormonal patterns or imbalances associated with embryonic mortality have been identified.

4. Endometritis

- Endometritis is an infection of the uterine endometrium.
- Cattle endometritis is a common condition that is known by the layman as 'whites'.
- It occurs three weeks or more after calving and should not be confused with the more severe condition of metritis which occurs immediately post-partum.
- The main consequence of endometritis is poor fertility. Therefore it has a major economic impact by increasing calving interval, services per conception and cull rates and by decreasing milk yield.
- It is reported to have an incidence of between 10-15 percent in dairy herds however it is very variable from herd to herd), with the total cost of Rs. 1600/- per case.

Cause

- The main bacteria involved in endometritis is *Actinobacillus pyogenes*, however, numerous gram-negative anaerobes may also be involved.
- The presence of these opportunistic bacteria can delay return to service and cyclical activity, prevent fertilisation and cause early embryonic death by producing a hostile uterine environment. It is also reported that it increases incidence of ovarian cysts.

Signalment: Endometritis can occur in any cow post-partum however incidence is increased by the following predisposing factors:

- Retained foetal membranes
- Dystocia
- Caesarian section or assisted calving
- Induced parturition
- Still Birth
- Twins
- Unhygienic calving environment - includes seasonal effect as indoor calving has higher endometritis rates.
- Ovarian inactivity
- Parity

- Concurrent disease and nutrition - fatty liver disease and hypocalcaemia are reported to increase endometritis rates.

Clinical Signs

- Mucopurulent vaginal discharge should be evident on vaginal exam 21 days or more post-calving. Discharge is relatively odourless (dependant on severity) and whites in colour, hence the name 'whites'.
- The discharge should not be confused with lochial discharge or vaginitis.
- Rectal palpation should reveal a poorly-involuted, oedematous uterus.
- On an individual or herd level there may be a history of subfertility.

Diagnosis

- Diagnosis should be based on the calving history and clinical signs following vaginal and rectal exam.
- Vets may use a scoring system to categorise the colour and odour of the vaginal discharge which indicates how severe the infection is and whether treatment is necessary.
- Measurements of the uterine and cervical diameter may be included in the scoring system. Definitive diagnosis can only be achieved by endometrial biopsy, however this is rarely indicated.

Treatment

- **Antibiotics:** Generally, a broad spectrum antibiotic, active against *Actinobacillus pyogenes* and gram-negative anaerobes should be used. Ideal antibiotics are cephalosporins and oxytetracycline as they match the majority of criteria listed above. Some resistance to oxytetracyclines is reported and additionally some formulations cause irritation to the endometrium, therefore intrauterine cephalosporin should be considered the most effective antibiotic treatment. Sulphonamides, aminoglycosides, nitrofurazones and penecillins have decreased activity as a result of the uterine environment and bacteria present. Metranidazole and chloramphenicol should not be used as they are banned from use in food-producing animals.
- **Hormones:** Prostaglandins, PGF2a or analogues can be administered parenterally. They should be considered the treatment of choice if a corpus luteum is present. There is no milk withdrawal period for prostaglandins, making them ideal for use in dairy cattle. These are mainly used in chronic cases.

- **Antiseptics:** Chlorhexidine and metacresol sulphonic acid (Lotagen), povidone iodine antiseptic administered intrauterine are reported to be a effective alternative to antibiotic treatment, however few studies have been carried out to confirm this and detrimental effects on fertility are reported.

5. Pyometra

Pyometra is characterised by a progressive accumulation of pus in the uterus and by the persistence of functional luteal tissue in the ovary.

Causes

- In most cases, pyometra occurs as a sequel to chronic endometritis when, as noted above, the infection is not eliminated because the cervix remains fairly tightly closed the purulent exudate accumulates within the uterine lumen, although occasionally there is a slight purulent discharge. Occasional cases of pyometra occur in the presence of a luteal cyst.
- The second main cause of pyometra is the death of the fetus, invasion of the uterus by A. Pyogenes and retention of the corpus luteum of pregnancy. This is a relatively infrequent cause of the condition.
- Venereal infection with organisms such as *Trichomonas fetus*, which cause embryonic death, also causes pyometra.

Signs & Symptoms

- Cows which suffer from pyometra show few or no signs of ill health; the main reason for them being examined is the absence of cyclical activity, or, perhaps, the presence of an intermittent vaginal discharge.
- The uterine horns are enlarged and distended, quite often to an unequal degree, owing to incomplete involution of the previously gravid horn or to recent conceptual death.

Differentiation of pyometra from a normal pregnancy can sometimes be difficult, but there are a number of distinguishing points

- The uterine wall is thicker than at pregnancy.
- The uterus has a more 'doughy' and less vibrant feel.
- It is not possible to 'slip' the allantochorion.

- In most cases of pyometra, no uterine caruncles can be palpated. However, when the infection occurred in a non-involuted uterus, involution of the caruncles is delayed and they may remain palpable for quite a long time.
- Transrectal ultrasonography will demonstrate the absence of a fetus and the presence of a 'speckled' echotexture of the uterine contents compared with the black anechoic appearance of normal fetal fluids.

6. Repeat Breeding

To identify repeat breeder cows you need two things: good records and good heat detection. Given what has been said above and that on many farms the efficiency of oestrous detection is less than 60% (i.e. for every 10 cows potentially cycling only 6 are served) it can be seen that this is quite a need.

However if done well they allow the farmer or herdsperson to pick up cows that are cycling normally but not getting pregnant or most importantly those not fitting a normal pattern. Using this information these possible problem animals can be identified quickly, subjected to veterinary examination and a treatment protocol applied. This reduces the potential days open and so saves money.

Other aids, such as beacons, tail paint pedometers and milk progesterones can also improve heat detection but there is still no really cost effective substitute for the astute observer apart from the bull. Even the latter can be overwhelmed if there are too many cows in season at one time.

Causes

• Early Embryonic death

In this case the retention of Corpus Luteum of pregnancy, which has been terminated early, occurs. This is usually encountered during 90-120 days of gestation where the embryo is too small to be detected when aborted or it may be reabsorbed. This may be a characteristic feature in served cows coming into heat after a period longer than the normal oestrus cycle.

Treatment

- Improved nutrition.
- Suspect for Trichomoniasis and Vibriosis and treat them.
- Inj. Buserelin, 11 days after insemination is known to improve embryo survival.

7. Prolapse

Prolapse of the vagina usually involve a prolapse of the floor, lateral walls and a portion of roof of the vagina throuogh the vulva with the cervix and uterus moving caudal. Vagino-cervical prolapsed is seen in all animals but cattle are more prone to it.

Cause: there are many causes but mostlt observed during last 2 to 3 months of gestation in case of cattle. The relaxation of pelvic ligaments during late pregnancy causes prolapse.

Once the prolapse of the vagina or the cervix occurs, the mucus membranes become very edematous, inflamed and necrotic.

Treatment

1. Raise the hind quarters of the animal in early stages of prolapsed.
2. Progesterone therapy can be given.
3. Vulvar truss can be applied.
4. Surgical manipulation is required for advanced prolapse.

8. Retention of placenta

In normal parturition, the placenta falls off within 3 to 8 hours following calving, but if is retained more than 12 hours, the condition is pathological and require attention.

Cause: failure of villi of the fetal cotyledon to detach themselves from maternal crypts of the caruncle.

Treatment

1. Manual removal, it should only be done by a skilled veterinarian.
2. Use of hormones like oxytocin.
3. Use of antimicrobials like aureomycin.
4. Intra-uterine medications can be practiced.

9. Anoestrus

Anoestrus is the failure of a cow to cycle and display oestrus (heat). Anoestrus is normal before puberty, during pregnancy and for a short period after calving (postpartum anoestrus, PPA). All cows undergo varying degrees of PPA. On average, 20% of seasonal-calving cows are anoestrus at the start of mating, with extreme cases of over 50% of the herd also being reported.

Causes

- Factors responsible for anoestrus are environmental stress, endocrine (endogenous opioid peptide, lower insulin concentration, imbalance in hormones such as LH, FSH, prolactin, melatonin and thyroid), nutritional (negative energy balance, micro and macronutrient deficiency), managemental factors such as lactational stress, suckling etc. A lower level of body weight, total serum protein, blood haemoglobin, blood glucose, blood insulin, inorganic phosphorus, calcium, manganese, iodine, cobalt, copper, iron, cholesterol and vitamin A deficiency also causes anoestrus.

Diagnosis

Anoestrus may be diagnosed by per-rectal palpation of reproductive organs and frequent activity of reproductive cycles of buffaloes using ultrasonography.

Negative energy balance; a cause of anoestrus

NEB happens when energy intake is lower than output in milk production and maintenance. It is seen as a loss of body condition as body fat is mobilised to meet the energy demands of lactation.

Some degree of NEB is inevitable in nearly all dairy cows in the month after calving. Resumption of cyclic activity after calving is influenced by:

- nutrition
- body condition
- suckling
- lactation
- breed
- age
- uterine pathology
- debilitating disease

Fewer than 10% of cows fail to ovulate in most well-managed dairy herds by day 40 post partum. It is well established that poor nutritional status and Negative Energy Balance are responsible for the majority of anoestrus cases in both dairy and beef cattle.

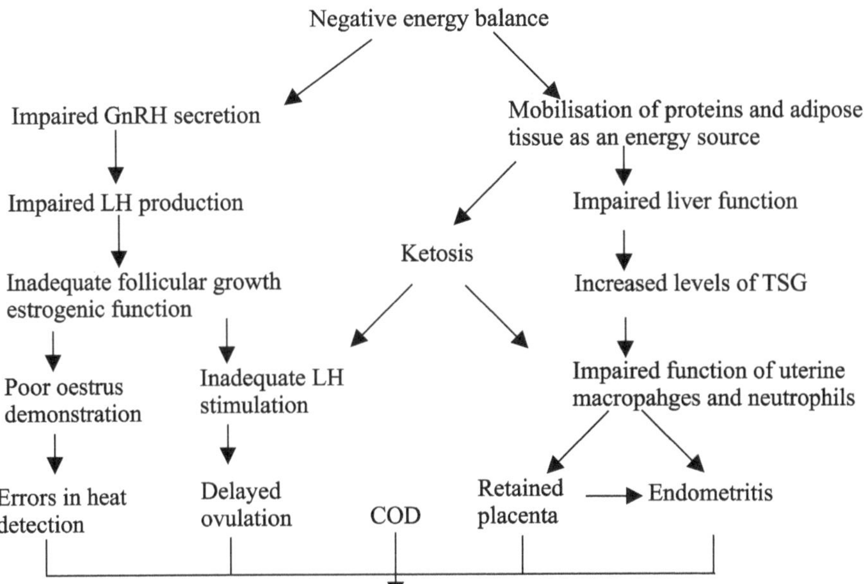

Treatment of anovulatory/anoestrus conditions in cattle

Treatment is based on:

1. **Improvement in energy status**: optimal nutrition during the transition period and during early lactation.
2. **Hormonal treatments**: combined with increased energy supplementation or reduced suckling stimulus may also help to stimulate oestrus.

10. Silent heats (unobserved and subestrus)

- Incidence of subestrus in cattle and buffaloes has a wide variation in the frequency (15-73%).
- The intensity of heat signs in buffaloes is generally lower and also homosexual activity is not pronounced as in cows.
- The intensity of expression of estrus is generally affected by housing, floor surface, yield, lameness and number of herd mates in estrus simultaneously.
- Summer anestrous is an important condition is buffaloes contributing to infertility in buffaloes.
- Heat stress has a pronounced effect on the estrus behaviour of the female animals as heat stress reduces the length and intensity of estrus. Changes caused by heat stress reduce the likelihood of estrus detection.

11. Dystocia

Difficult birth or difficulty in parturition is termed as dystocia.

Causes: Hereditary, nutritional and managemental, infectious, traumatic,etc.

- Small sized primipara often lead to dystocia.
- Ventral hernia also leads to dystocia.
- Early mating yields dystocia.
- Torsion.

Treatment

- Rolling the dam to relieve torsion.
- Traction can be applied.
- Use of relaxin during parturition.
- Surgical manipulations can be performed.

Artificial Insemination (AI); Strategy for High Breeding Efficiency in Dairy Animals

- In dairy cattle, there is immense potential for intensive selection amongst males (bulls) and their wider use through artificial insemination (Al) on females.
- Al is the single most important tool which has revolutionized the field of cattle breeding throughout the world.
- In natural service, a good bull could be mated with 50 -100 females per year. On the contrary, the Al with frozen semen technology has been possible use of an Al bull on about 10,000 females per year almost 100 times more utilization over the natural service.
- Al offers challenging opportunities for wider dissemination of desired inheritance per unit of time in the next generations of animals.
- The future course of large scale dairy cattle breeding in the developing countries depends on how best we adapt and adopt the Al technology to our advantage.
- The initial taboos are now disappearing, the farmer's acceptance is on the increase, but much remains to be done to avoid disappointments of the cow-owners and to achieve desired breeding goals.

- In lieu of adequate productivity by indigenous stocks, numerous countries attempted to increase output per animal by importation of improved exotic breeds of upgrading their local stock with males or semen of bulls of exotic dairy breeds.
- The importation of large number of breeds has proved prohibitively expensive and met with reasonable success only when maintained under good management and feeding regimes.
- The improved pure-bred exotic dairy cattle have failed to function with reasonable efficiency where feed supplies have been inadequate and health control measures unsatisfactory.

Methods to Improve Fertility in Dairy Animals

For improving fertility of the herd so many tools were in practice since last fifty years, and many will be added in times to come - these tools are:

1. Use of artificial insemination technique.
2. Use of frozen semen.
3. Use of high quality, progeny tested bull's semen.
4. Improving different managemental practices like -
    - Maintenance of good health record/breeding records.
    - Offering balanced and nutritious fodders and feed.
    - Breeding at proper time.
    - Use of heat detection methods.
    - Doorstep services of A.I.

Now days in most of the western developed countries where dairy development has reached to its peak, many new technologies are in vogue, these are -

1. Oesturs synchronization.
2. Embryo transfer.
3. Early pregnancy diagnosis tests.

Culling of Unproductive Dairy Animals

Dairymen should develop a checklist of culling reasons to use in their decision making process. The following list of 10 questions is one that could be used for each cow before deciding her future in the herd.

1. Is her yearly production 20 per cent or more below the herd's rolling average?
2. Is she a chronic mastitis case? Check this one closely, because a cow with chronic mastitis is producing below her capability and, in addition, could be spreading mastitis to other cows in the herd through the milking equipment.
3. Will she be dry four months or more? Long dry periods are costly to the dairyman and may indicate the cow has a problem of becoming pregnant, a trait not desired.
4. Is she a hard milker? Is her udder shape or teat structure such that she is a nuisance to milk?
5. Does she have a history of calving difficulties or post calving illnesses such as retained placenta, metritis, or milk fever? Cows that cause problems at calving time are not pleasant to have and are costly to keep in the herd.
6. Does she have an undesirable disposition?
7. Is she a nervous cow or does she kicks whenever her udder is touched? These are undesirable traits that should be noted along with production and calving problems.
8. Is she below the herd's average body type? Check body confirmation to see if it comes up to specifications for the herd.
9. Is she a timid cow? With the type of dry lot housing systems most dairymen have today, timid cows usually will not get the amount of feed required to be high producing animals.
10. Is she an old cow, and is the available barn space needed for freshening heifers? Fresh heifers usually have a higher genetic potential for milk production than older cows, especially if a progressive A.I. program is used in the herd.

A yes answer should probably be given to at least two questions before making the cow a strong candidate for culling. In many cases, though, one reason may be enough justification to base a culling decision. Besides using a checklist in making culling decisions, other facts should be considered.

Culling should be based on the evaluation of the following

1. First-calf heifers

In evaluating first calf heifers, consider the size of the heifers. Undersized heifers will probably produce less milk the first lactation because of their size.

This situation is an indictment of the dairyman's heifer feeding program and not necessarily the producing potential of the heifer. So, among possible culls of equal performance, preference should probably be given to the younger, undersized heifer, especially if she improved during her lactation.

2. Stage of gestation

Extremely long calving intervals can be costly. With other factors being equal, cows in mid-lactation with several months to go before freshening are better prospects for culling than cows that will freshen sooner and return to peak production sooner.

3. Mastitis

Mastitis CMT (California Mastitis Test) scores, somatic cell counts should be checked carefully. Cows with CMT scores of 2, somatic cell counts of 1.2 million or greater, should be culled before other potential culls because they are potential sources of intra-mammary infections of other cows.

4. Age

Other factors being equal, cull older cows before younger cows of comparable relative value. The genetic potential of younger animals should be greater than that of older animals, so keeping the younger cows in the herd longer should be a sound practice.

5. Past performance

Given two cows with the same relative value and other factors equal, cull the cow first that has the lowest previous production records. Past performance can be suggestive of future potential. Management errors in the current lactation could adversely affect a cow's performance.

24

Milking

Milk

Importance

Milk contains approximately 86% water, 4.7% sugar (lactose), 4.1% fat, 4.2% protein and 1% minerals. It supports the growth of micro-organisms and thus is prone to contamination. The purpose of milking a dairy cow is to obtain milk that is fit for human consumption. Milk from the udder of a healthy cow contains very few bacteria and to ensure that it remains fresh for long it should be handled under conditions of good hygiene. Unclean milk can be a source of disease to the consumer, rejected at the market and so is a loss to the farmer, does not keep for long and is not good for processing.

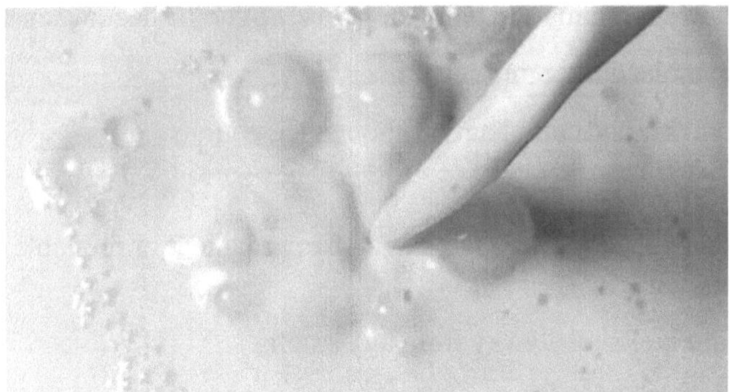

Characteristic color of milk

Milking

The milking procedure is the first step in obtaining clean milk. At the farm this starts with ensuring the cow to be milked is healthy.

The cow

- The cow should be well fed with a diet well balanced with forage and concentrates to ensure high production of good quality milk. Feeding very high amount of concentrates and low amount of forages result in milk with low butter fat. On the other hand feeding too little concentrates leads to low milk yield.

- An unhealthy cow will feed less and produce less milk. Cows should always be kept healthy and clean as sick animals can transmit diseases like tuberculosis and brucellosis to milk consumers. If a cow is suspected to be sick, a qualified veterinary practitioner should be contacted immediately. Milk from a cow that is being treated with antibiotics should not be consumed or sold until the withdrawal period is over.
- Farmers are encouraged to vaccinate their animals against brucellosis. Animals should also be checked periodically for all types of contagious diseases and treated promptly in case they are infected.
- Mastitis is an inflammation of the mammary glands in the udder caused by infection with disease-causing bacteria which can be controlled by observing general hygiene and proper milking procedure.

Guidelines for clean milk production

The milker

Should:

- be healthy and clean.
- Maintain short nails and hair (for ladies, cover the head when milking).
- Never smoke during milking time.
- Milk quickly and completely without interruptions.

The environment

- A milking shed (parlor) which can be permanent or movable should be constructed.
- It should be located away from any smells.
- The floor of shed should be clean and dry and if possible have a cement floor for ease of cleaning.
- The shed should be cleaned after every milking and animals kept off outside milking time.

Equipments

- Use seamless aluminum or stainless steel cans for milking and storing milk. Plastic container is difficult to clean.
- Clean utensils immediately after milking or after emptying milk: rinse with cold water, scrub with a brush using hot water with detergent then rinse with cold water.

- Place upside down on a rack and dry in the sun.
- Store utensils in a safe, clean and well ventilated room.

Milking Methods for Clean Milk Production

What is clean milk?

'Clean Milk' is defined as milk drawn from the udder of healthy animals, which is collected in clean dry milking pails and free from extraneous matters like dust, dirt, flies, hay, manure etc. Clean milk has a normal composition, possesses a natural milk flavour with low bacterial count and is safe for human consumption.

Need for clean milk production

1. Clean milk is safe for human consumption and free from disease producing microorganisms.
2. Has a high keeping quality.
3. Has a high commercial value.
4. Longer self-life- Can be transported over long distances.
5. Clean milk production avoids unnecessary financial losses through spoilage of milk.

Measures for clean milk production

I. The Cow

The source of pure and wholesome milk is the clean and healthy cow.

The Animal Health

1. The herd should be free from pathogens that may be spread to human beings through the milk like tuberculosis, brucellosis, etc and all bacterial and viral diseases which can be transmitted from animal to man through milk. The animals should periodically be checked for all types of contagious diseases
2. Check all the animals for mastitis once in 15 days
3. Vaccinate the animals against diseases like FMD, HS, etc.
4. Regular deworming.

Body and Udder Hygiene

1. Clip the long hairs from the flank and udder.
2. Prevent dirt from falling into the milking pail by brushing the flank and udder and by wiping the udder with clean damp cloth prior to milking.
3. Buffaloes should be invariably washed before milking as they wallow in dirty ponds and carry mud and filth on their body
4. While beginning to milk, the udder should be properly wiped with a clean moist cloth dipped in disinfect solution (1% potassium permanganate solution) and squeezed. It is advisable to change the cloth from animal to animal. If not possible, at least dip the cloth in disinfectant while going to the next animal. During winter the cloth may be dipped in warm antiseptic solution.

II. The Barn

The cleanliness of the barn reflects the cleanliness of milk production.

1. Separate premises located far away from human living quarters, sewage, manure pits and stagnant water pools are advisable for housing and milking of animals.
2. The barn should be at a well-elevated place.
3. The barn should be well lighted and ventilated
4. Where possible provide a cement floor for easy and proper cleaning.
5. There should be good drainage. Floor and gutters should have adequate slope for easy drainage and removal of dung.
6. Provide a clean feed trough, water trough and protected store
7. The manure should be removed daily to a sufficient distance from the barn so that the odour will not drift back into milk room. Keep the shed clean and dry,
8. Wash floor everyday
9. Remove dung more than once a day
10. Milking barn should be thoroughly washed and scrubbed after each milking and kept clean and dry before the next milking starts.
11. Fly control measures are important since they can carry germs of typhoid, dysentery and other contagious diseases.

III. Feeding

1. Feeding of the animals should be made an hour before milking. At the time of milking for the purpose of keeping milking cows busy, provide only concentrates which will be less dusty.
2. Hay carries a large amount of bacteria bearing dust, so, should not be fed during milking
3. Silages should not be fed until after milking because of the possibility of silage flavour carrying over into the milk.

IV. The Milker

1. The milker should be free from any infectious diseases as this may be carried and transmitted though the milk.
2. Milkers should wear clean clothes and cover their heads with suitable cap so as to prevent loose hair falling in the milk
3. The nails should be periodically trimmed and made smooth.
4. Hands should be thoroughly washed with soap and dried with clean towel or washed with antiseptic solutions before milking.

V. The Milking Utensils

1. Milking utensils should be as clean and free from pathogens as possible. Best way to achieve this is to rinse the utensils immediately after use. Following washing with ordinary water the utensils should be washed with warm water – containing a suitable detergent. Soap should not be used as it leaves a greasy film.
2. The type of milk pan - Sanitary milking pails with dome- shaped top should be used instead of open buckets or vessels during milking.

VI. Storage of milk

Aluminum or stainless steel cans with tight lids are good for storing and transporting milk. When tin or chrome-plated iron cans are used, see that there are no rust spots.

i. Milk should be covered with lids to avoid dust, dirt, entry hot, or cold, day light or strong artificial light, all at which tend to decrease milk quality.

ii. Don’t keep the milk in direct sunlight as the taste of the milk changes and some vitamins are destroyed.

iii. To keep milk cool, place milk cans in a tub containing cold water.

iv. Don't mix fresh milk with old milk.

v. Empty milk vessels should be washed and cleaned immediately.

VII. Collection and transport of milk

1. The milk collection room should be maintained absolutely clean to prevent contamination.
2. Store milk in cool and clean place.

VIII. Marketing or disposal

1. Milk should be delivered to market as soon as possible
2. It is advisable to deliver milk early in the morning and evening to avoid the hot period of the day

Prerequisites for milking

1. Milking should be done gently, quietly, quickly, cleanly and completely.
2. Do not excite the animal. Cows remaining comfortably yield more milk than a roughly handled and excited cow.
3. Maintenance of clean conditions in the milking barn results in better udder health and producing milk that remains wholesome for longer period.
4. The milking process should be completed within 5 to 7 minutes.
5. Complete milking has to be done. If any residual milk is left it may act as nidus for mastitis causing organism and the overall yield will be reduced.
6. Regularise milking interval.
7. Dispose fore-milk as it has high bacterial count.
8. If calf is used for let down of milk, wash udder after suckling by the calf.
9. Isolate sick animals and milk them last (Their milk should not be mixed with good milk).
10. Tie tails of troublesome animals when milking.
11. If cloth is used for straining it should be washed after every collection and sanitised by using bleaching powder.
12. Always keep the milk covered
13. Disinfect the teat by teat dip (Iodophor) after milking to avoid entry of micro-organisms to the teat canal.

Methods of milking

1. Hand milking
2. Machine milking

1. Hand milking

Cows are milked usually from left side. Milking can be done either cross wise or forequarters together and then hind quarters together or teats appearing most distended milked first. The first few strips of milk from each quarter should be discarded as it contains highest number of bacteria.

Methods of Hand milking

I. Stripping
II. Full hand method.

I. **Stripping-** Stripping is done by firmly holding the teat between the thumb and fore finger and drawing it down the length of the teat and pressing it to cause the milk to flow down in a stream.

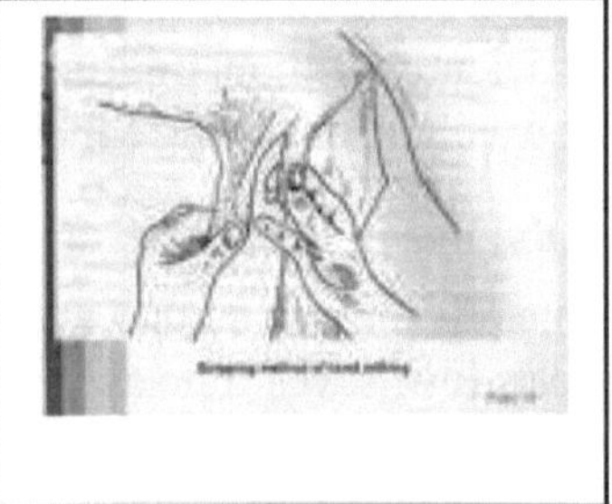

II. **Full Hand method**- Grasping the teat with all the five fingers and pressing it against the palm. The teat is compressed and relaxed alternatively in quick succession. The method removes milk much quicker than stripping as there is no loss of time in changing the position of the hand. Full hand milking should be followed by stripping to remove the residual milk.

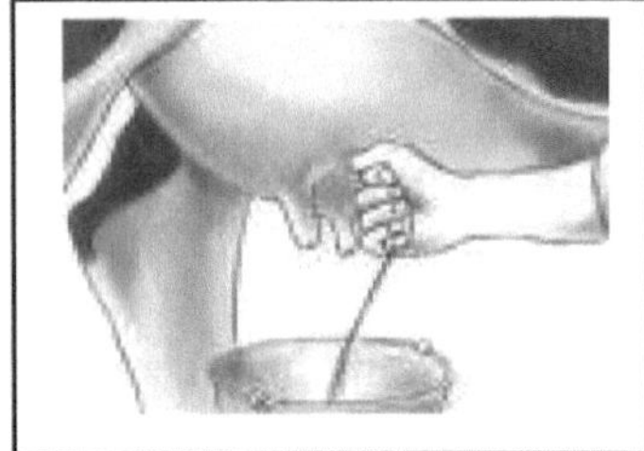

Full hand method is superior to stripping because it stimulates the natural suckling process by calf and this method exerts an equal pressure on the large teats of cows and buffaloes.

Many milkers during milking tend to bend their thumb against the teat. The method is known as **knuckling** which should always be avoided to prevent injuries of the teat tissues.

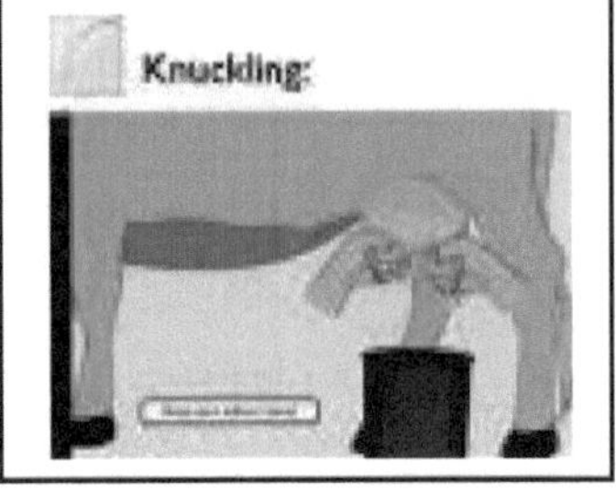

Thus milking should always be done with full hand unless the teats are too small or towards the completion of milking.

In hand milking two methods are there

Wet hand milking

Dry hand milking

Wet hand milking: It is done by lubricating the milker's hand and teat either with water or oil. These make the teats dry and chaffed. Crack and sores may appear which will cause pain to the animal

Dry hand milking: In this method, the milking operation is practised without lubrication of the milker's hand and teats. It is considered to be the best method as it doesn't cause any chaffing/sore on the teats

2. Machine milking: Milking machines are used to harvest milk from cows instead of manual milking for milking more cows using fewer people and less effort. Modern milking machines are capable of milking cows quickly and efficiently, without injuring the udder, if they are properly installed, maintained in excellent operating conditions, and used properly.

Advantage

The advantages of this milking machine are manifold. It is easy to operate, costs low, saves time as it milks 1.5 litre to 2 litres per minute. It is also very hygienic and energy-conserving as electricity is not required. All the milk from the udder can be removed. The machine is also easily adaptable and gives a suckling feeling to the cow and avoids pain in the udder as well as leakage of milk.

Milking Hygiene

Good Practice

- Washing hands with soap and water before milking each cow. Washing of hands thoroughly between finishing milking one cow and beginning the milking of the next.
- Washing the udder and each teat vigorously with soap and water and dry them with a clean cloth.
- Direct the first milk outside the milking bucket into separate container and throw away.
- Have a clean, dry, floor preferably of rough surfaced concrete without sharp points for the milking area.

- Keep calves where cows can see them during milking.
- Use clean containers for milking and before re-using the milk container, rinse it, scrub it with warm water and detergent or soap, rinse it again leave it to air-dry.
- After milking, cover the milk to avoid contamination and place in a clean and cool area.
- Keep the area clean and safe for animals.

Bad Practice

- Using Milk from sick cows can transmit diseases to humans.
- Using unclean plastic containers.
- Leaving milk uncovered.
- Keeping the milk in the sun or outdoors.

Types of Hand Milking

Hand milking is done by 3 ways

1. Full hand milking

In this type, the force on the teat is applied from all the sides equally and full hand is used for handling the teat during milking.

It is the most useful method of hand milking and many diseases related to udder and teats can be prevented by using this method of milking.

2. Stripping

It is used to drain last few drops of milk from the udder and the teat is pressed between the thumb and the four fingers.

3. Knuckling

In this case, the teat is pressed by using the force of thumb and the fingers. It is different from stripping in such a way that the thumb is crushed in the teat forcefully which may lead to injuries of teat canal and hence mastitis.

Practical Aspects of Milking

Milk synthesis and secretion is continuous unless interfered with by pressure from the filling of the gland cistern (this explains why more milk is extracted by frequent emptying (milking) to ensure pressure does not built up). The ejection of milk from alveolar lumen is under influence of oxytocin (hormone).

Steps

The cow is brought to the milking parlor as calmly as possible. Frightening the animal at this stage has a negative effect on milk let down due to release of adrenaline (hormone) which has a negative effect on milk letdown.

1. Feed the cow its production ration (this is optional depending on the feeding system). This calms the animal and stimulates milk letdown.
2. Restrain animal - tie hind legs above hock joint in the form of a figure 8. A loose knot should be used to safeguard both animal and man (applicable only for hand milking).
3. Wash hands with soap and clean water before milking. Dry hands with towel.
4. Test for mastitis using a strip cup - strip first few rays of milk into strip cup from each quarter and observe for any abnormalities. If mastitis is detected, the cow should be milked last.
5. Wash udder with warm clean water with disinfectant using a clean towel.
6. Warm water also stimulates milk let down. Dry udder using a dry towel.
7. Apply milking jelly - prevents cracking of teats and eases milking (for hand milking only)
8. Milk quickly and completely by squeezing the teat, do not pull. Milking each cow should take 5-6 minutes at most.
9. Use clean containers for milking.
10. After milking: Strip the animal - getting last drops of milk from udder to avoid incomplete milking (can lead to mastitis).
11. After milking dip the teats in a teat dip (disinfectant to ensure that bacteria do not gain entry through the teat sphincter which is loose immediately after milking).
12. It is recommended that the animal remain in a standing position for at least one hour to ensure the teat does not come into contact with the ground while the sphincter is still loose.

Note

- Routine milking procedures stimulate milk letdown and should therefore not be changed unnecessarily.
- After cow has been maximally stimulated for milk let down, it should be milked immediately since the stimulus reduces over time. Oxytocin effects

are maximum between **5-6 minutes**, thus milking should be completed during this time.

- Don't harass animal since adrenaline (hormone produced due to fright) has opposite effect of oxytocin (milk let down hormone).

Comparison of cow and buffalo milk

Trait	Cow	Buffalo
Total solids (%)	13.10	16.30
Fat (%)	4.30	7.90
Protein (%)	3.60	4.20
Lactose (%)	4.80	5.00
Tocopherol (mg/g)	0.31	0.33
Cholesterol (mg/g)	3.14	0.65
Calcium, Ca (mg/100 g)	165	264
Phosphorus, P (mg/100 g)	213	268
Magnesium, Mg (mg/100 g)	23	30
Potassium, K (mg/100 g)	185	107
Sodium, Na (mg/100 g)	73	65
Vitamin A, incl. carotene (I.U.)	30.30	33
Vitamin C (mg/100 g)	1.90	6.70

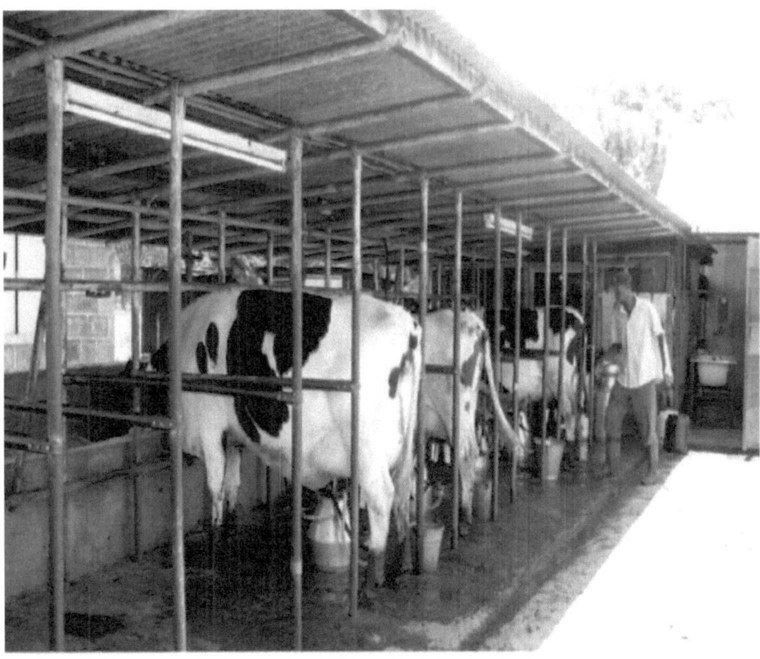

Milking parlor

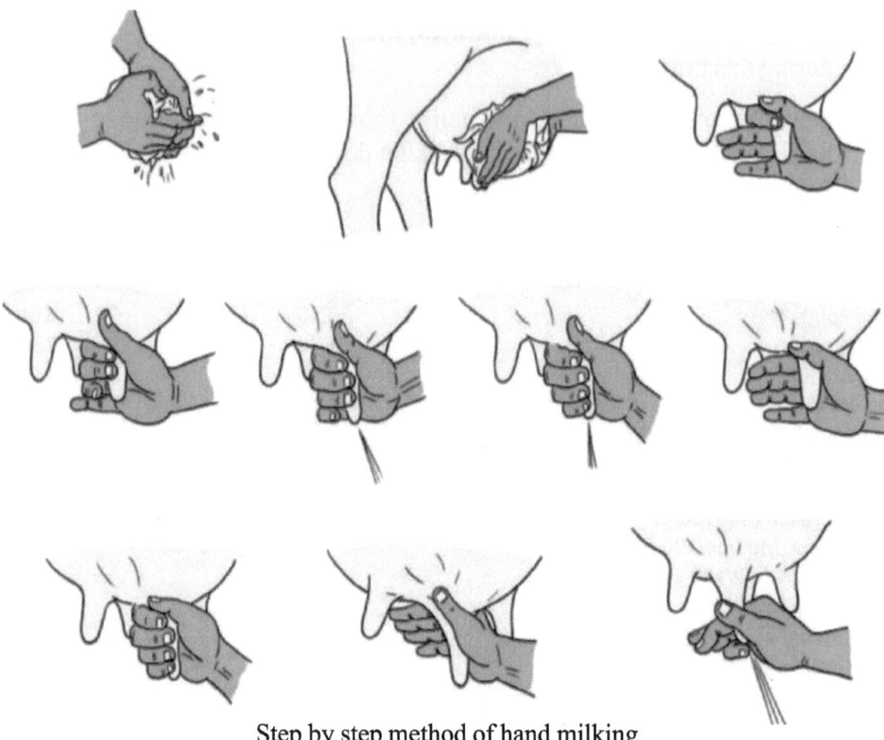

Step by step method of hand milking

Handling the Milk

The following guidelines should be followed to avoid milk spoilage:

- **Filter milk immediately after milking:** Use a white filter cloth or strainer. Disinfect, wash and dry the cloth/strainer after use.
- Always handle milk in clean, preferably metal, containers.
- When transferring milk between containers, pour the milk instead of scooping since scooping may introduce spoilage bacteria.
- Do not store milk at high temperatures.
- **Do not handle milk if you are sick:** Seek medical treatment and resume work only when the doctor says you are fit to do so.
- Store milk in a cool clean place preferably lockable room set aside for milk only. If storing overnight, keep the milk in cold/ chilled water.
- Deliver milk to the market as soon as possible preferably in the cool morning or evening.

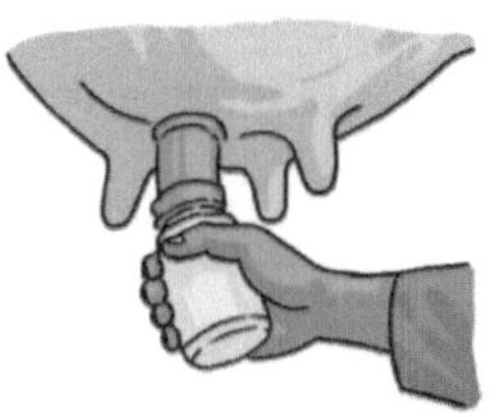
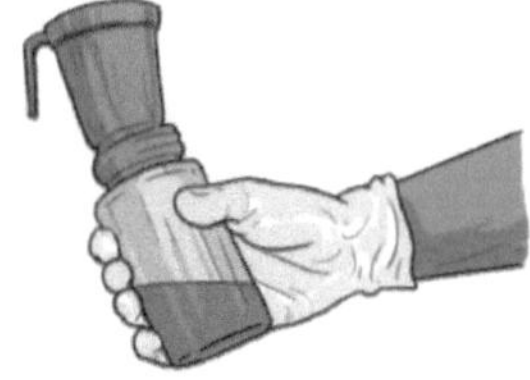

Dipping cow teats in disinfectant

Proper cleaning of milk equipments

Milk cans

Immediately cans are emptied of milk they should be cleaned as follows:

- Rinse with cold water.
- Scrubbing with brush and warm detergent (any un-perfumed liquid soap will do).
- Rinse with cold water.
- Sterilize (sanitize) with boiling water or steam if available or use dairy sanitizing solution such hypochlorite or commercial brand preparations in accordance with manufacturer's instructions.
- Dry cans on a drying rack. Exposure to sunlight will enhance killing off bacteria during drip drying of cans.

Milking machines

Milking machines should be cleaned according to recommended practice:

- Rinse with cold water.
- Use the "cleaning-in-place" (CIP) method where detergent in hot water is circulated in the system.
- Rinse with hot water.

25

Health and Diseases

General Signs of Healthy and Ill Animals

Health

It is a state of freedom from disease. It may also be stated as a condition of an animal in which all the body organs are normal and are functioning to their optimum capacity in relation to animal's age, sex, work, and production with optimum pulse, temperature and respiration rates appropriate to the species, sex and environment.

Disease

Disease may be any deterioration from normal health or normal functioning of any or all the tissues or organs of animal body. Thus, it shuns animal to perform its normal physiological functions though the nutritional and environmental parameters are maintained normal.

Signs of Healthy Animal

1. wet muzzle.
2. Shining skin and eyes.
3. Rosette pink mucous membranes.
4. Normal rumination (Ruminal movements: 3 per 2.5 minutes).
5. Normal gait and eating behavior.
6. Active reflexes.
7. Urination and defecation normal.
8. Well kept head.
9. No abnormal discharge from any natural orifice.
10. No abnormality in milk and milk composition.

Signs of Illness in Animals

- General posture of animals, its behavior, movements and expressions change.
- Animal show dull dejected appearance and stands in isolation with head downwards.
- Loss of appetite and cessation of ruminal movements.
- Skin becomes dry, hair coat becomes dull, and hair may become brittle and fall off.
- Muzzle becomes dry.
- Sunken, glued eyes, staring look, discharge from eyes.
- Any abnormal discharge from natural orifices, pus from the organ involved shows septic changes.
- Blood or dark colored urine with repulsive odor.
- Change in color and consistency of feces.
- Change in quality and quantity of milk production.
- Change in voice of animal i.e. grunting, groaning or grinding of teeth by animal shows that animal is in pain.
- Nervous signs, edema of any body part, abnormal gait, inflammatory conditions.
- Change in respiration, body temperature, and pulse rate. Normal data is given as:

S.no.	Species	Body temperature (°F)	Pulse rate (per minute)	Respiration rate (per minute)
1.	Cattle :			
	1. Calf	101.3-104.4	90-120	27-50
	2. Adult	101.5	50-60	20-25
2.	Buffalo	98.3 (winter) 103 (summer)	40-50	15-20

Diseases

A. Production Diseases

A. Mastitis

Mastitis or inflammation of mammary gland or udder is an economically important condition in milking animals. Mastitis is a disease that affects a large number of dairy cattle throughout the world. It may affect one or all quarters of the udder. It is manifested in the form of swelling of the affected quarters, change in milk color and composition.

Pathogenesis

Development of mastitis is complex and involves three stages: invasion, infection and inflammation. The factors which contribute to the causation of mastitis include:

- Contamination with milker's hands, contaminated floors, utensils and clothes.
- Presence of high population density of the causative bacteria in milking shed.
- Damage to the teat sphincter.
- Udder infected with FMD, Pox virus.
- Physical trauma that may accelerate the growth of these causative bacteria.
- Sawdust and shaving used as bedding, which are harboring *E. coli* and *Klebsiella pneumoniae.*
- Edema and congestion of udder during parturition.
- Poorly designed housing, uneven faulty surface.
- Dirty milking machine.

How to diagnose?

Clinical signs, palpation of udder, monitoring the milk consistency may give clue about causation of mastitis. Diagnosis of mastitis is based on bacteriological and cytological methods of examination. Subclinical cases may go unnoticed and therefore testing of milk with California mastitis test (CMT) or any other spot test is necessary. Bacteriological examination of CMT positive samples should be carried out.

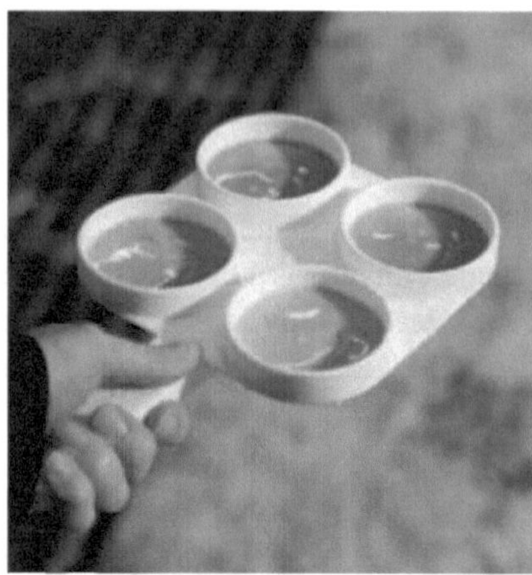

California Mastitis Test Cups

Impact of the problem

If one quarter is affected by mastitis, 25% milk yield is lost permanently. It may also spread to other quarters; hence it causes major economic losses to the farmer. High yielding animals are more prone to this condition, if not milked properly. The milk from infected udders contributes to high microbial counts of milk, which in turn is not suitable for preparation of milk products. Mastitic organisms are also pathogenic for human beings. Mastitis control is prerequisite to any of the clean milk production programmes.

Treatment

a. **Udder infusion:** Disposable tubes with water soluble ointment base need to be used. Emptying of udder is essential before infusion. For animal with clinical mastitis manual removal of congestion in the gland and inflammatory debris from the duct system should be done.

b. Parental treatment is advisable. Before antibiotic therapy, the sensitivity of the pathogens to particular antibiotics should be carried out.

c. The use of preparations containing disinfecting ingredients and added emollients is effective which promote the healing of teat lesions and prevent new infections.

   Iodophors are important teat dips. Application of preparations containing 3-5000 mg. available iodine per kg, depending on the glycerin concentration, leads to reduction in bacterial numbers.

d. Culling of cows with therapy resistant udder diseases.

e. If machine milking is practiced then rinsing of the teat cups and dipping them in the disinfectant wash water between cows, by dipping a pair of each cluster in turn or hot water (170°-180°) for 10 sec. is effective.

In case of dry cows, infusion at the time of the last milking or at the beginning or end of the dry period is recommended.

Control and Prevention

- Mastitis control also entails a good understanding of the factors that encourage its incidence and the microorganisms that cause it.
- Mastitis control must be concentrated on the prevention aspects, which depends mainly on the whole hygienic management and absence of stress conditions.
- Estrogenic compound in foods should be reduced. Young animals should be milked before older. Newly introduced animal should milked separately.
- Specific control measures need to be taken according to the respective cause and the extent of losses. Specific control measures include:
- Correction of milking technique.
- Teat disinfection (e.g. teat dipping) following milking.
- Antibiotic treatment at drying off.
- Culling of animals with therapy - resistant mastitis.

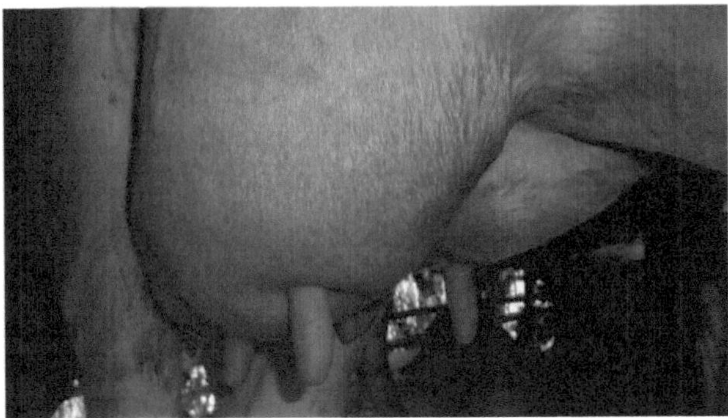

Mastitis

B. Milk Fever

- Milk fever is a common metabolic disorder in dairy cattle that generally affects older, high producing cows. It may also be referred to as parturient paresis or hypocalcaemia.

- At the beginning of lactation high yielding cows experience a sudden rise in demand for calcium to replace the large amount lost through milk. This may result in great decrease in blood calcium if the cow is not able to replenish the calcium fast enough, causing a disease called milk fever.
- The majority of milk fever cases occur within 48 to 72 hours of calving when demand for calcium for milk production exceeds the body's ability to mobilize calcium reserves.
- Fever is a misnomer as body temperature is usually below normal. Low blood calcium interferes with muscle function throughout the body causing general weakness, loss of appetite and eventually heart failure.

Signs of Milk Fever

At first, cow experiences muscle tremors, lack of appetite, and unsteadiness. Eventually, cow is unable to rise, body temperature falls, and constipation occurs. Cows go down to a sitting position often with a kink in her neck. Death can occur if the cow is not treated promptly.

Causes of Milk Fever

The onset of milk production drains on the animal's blood calcium levels. If the cow is unable to replace this calcium quickly enough due to loss of its ability to mobilize reserves of calcium in bone and absorb calcium from the gastrointestinal tract, milk fever occurs. Older cows are more susceptible as they produce more milk and are unable to replenish calcium quickly.

Prevention of Milk Fever

- Management of the diet can be a valuable aid in preventing milk fever.
- The key to prevention of milk fever is management of a close-up dry cow which should be kept on a low calcium diet. This stimulates their calcium regulatory system to keep the blood levels normal by mobilizing the body stores from the bone.
- When the demand for calcium increases at calving, calcium can be mobilized much more rapidly thus preventing milk fever.
- Lucerne, a feed high in calcium and potassium, should not be a major ingredient in close-up dry cows' diets.
- In early lactation, high yielding cows should receive as much calcium as possible.
- High risk cows can be injected with Vitamin D3 2-8 days prior to calving.

- Diets providing less than 15gcalcium/cow/day and fed for at least 10 days before calving will reduce the incidence of milk fever.

C. Ketosis

- Ketosis, or acetonaemia, is a metabolic disorder in cattle associated with an inadequate supply of the nutrients necessary for the normal carbohydrate and fat metabolism that is seen mainly in times of high milk production in early lactation.
- Hypoglycemia (low blood sugar) is the major factor involved in the onset and development of clinical signs of ketosis.
- Ketosis affects high producing cows during the first 6-8 weeks of lactation when cows are in negative energy balance.
- The excessive ketone bodies in the bloodstream come from the breakdown of fat when the animal is forced to draw on its bodily reserves for energy.
- The excess ketone bodies are eliminated in the urine, milk and breath of the animal.

Predisposing factors

- Cows of any age may be affected but the disease appears more common in later lactations peaking at about the 4th lactation.
- Over conditioning at calving has been associated with increased incidence of ketosis.
- A reduction in the production of propionic acid, the main precursor of glucose in ruminants, will result in hypoglycaemia. Hypoglycaemia leads to a mobilization of free fatty acids and glycerol from the fat stores.
- The reduction of propionic acid production is usually the result of underfeeding or a reduced feed intake caused by in-appetence. The in-appetence may be caused by poor feed quality, sudden changes in diet or excessive fatness at calving.

Clinical signs of Ketosis

- The clinical signs of ketosis include lack of appetite (refusal to eat even concentrates) and a sudden drop in milk output.
- There is a sweet smell of acetone in the urine, breath and milk.
- Cows will have raised blood ketone levels and may excrete ketones in urine and milk.
- There is a gradual loss of body condition over several days or even weeks.

Prevention of Ketosis

Ketosis causes financial loss through lost production and treatment. It may be prevented by management strategies that maintain a good appetite and supply adequate feed to meet this appetite during the late dry period and immediately after calving. These strategies include;

- Avoid sudden changes in feed type to newly calved animals.
- Ensure that any health problems that may cause reduced feed intake are treated as early as possible.

Infectious Diseases

A. Foot and mouth disease

It is a highly infectious and contagious viral disease of all cloven footed domesticated and wild animals. The infection imposes a high spread during the cooler season when the air remains in damp condition.

Vaccination is the only means to control the disease.

Vaccine	Age	Dose	Booster	Interval	Season
FMD	6-8 wks	10 ml s/c	6, 9 or 12 months	Annual	Preferably November, December

B. Black Quarter

Black Quarter is one of the deadly bacterial diseases of cattle. The disease spreads rapidly after heavy rainfall by contamination of soil with spores of the organism. Areas where previous death occurs from Clostridium infection have a higher incidence or risk of disease because of increased environmental contamination. Treatment of the disease with specific antibiotic is useful if the diagnosis of the disease can be made at the early stage.

The disease can be controlled by regular vaccination.

Vaccine	Age	Dose	Booster	Interval	Season
Polyvalent B.Q. Vaccine	All age	5 ml s/c	6 months	Annual	Before onset of monsoon, all season in endemic areas

C. Haemorrhagic septicaemia (HS)

Haemorrhagic septicaemia, as the name implies is a poisoning of the blood accompanied by internal haemorrhages, is an acute septicaemic disease caused by a bacterium, *Pasteurella multocida.* The incidence of H.S. is throughout the year. The outbreak is not only in the period of high humidity or monsoon but also in winter season. Highest number of outbreaks during high humid and rainy season as compare to winter season. Although antibiotics are available for the treatment, there may not be any time for treatment in most cases.

The disease may be controlled by regular vaccination.

Vaccine	Age	Dose	Booster	Interval	Season
H.S. adjuvant vaccine	All ages	3 ml i/m	6 months	Annual	Preferably in May/June

D. Rabies

Agent

Lyssavirus is a genus of viruses belonging to the family Rhabdoviridae.

Reservoir

Warm-blooded mammals and bats are responsible for maintenance of the virus – urban rabies primarily by dogs, and sylvatic rabies by wild animals.

Transmission

Dog bite.

Clinical signs and symptoms

The incubation period is usually 4–8 weeks, but may extend to several years.

Once clinical symptoms develop in a person who has been bitten by a rabid animal, the disease is almost always fatal. Symptoms appear in phases and include:

- initial pain or a tingling sensation at the site of the bite;
- fear of water (hydrophobia);
- restlessness;
- excess salivation;
- convulsions; and finally
- death.

Treatment

- Post-bite anti rabies vaccination at 0, 3, 7, 14, 28 days respectively.
- Local dressing is not preferred.
- Give antibiotics and anti-inflammatory drugs supportively.

Parasitic Diseases

The incidence of parasitic diseases varies greatly. Poorly fed animals suffer more, but optimum nutrition does not offer complete protection.

- Poor Nutrition - Trichostrongylosis is more in calves. Excellent nutrition but favorable environmental conditions favor Haemonchosis in calves.
- Specific nutritional deficiency such as cobalt, copper, phosphourus, or protein reduces animal resistance.
- Dung pat can act as reservoir for larvae, for 5 months in summer and 7-8 months in winter and when the outer covering softens by rain. Larvae come out. Breaking up of dung pat and introduction of suitable dung beetles help in worm control.
- Feed contaminated with stools in the bran spreads infestation. Because of the possibility of the cross infection, different species of animals should not be grouped together.
- Larvae can remain alive for 6 to 8 weeks under favorable conditions of warmth and moisture. Areas with severe winter and dry summer the load is low, but when winter is mild and summer is wet, serious outbreaks come up. Insect vectors also play a part (in Filiroidea).
- Immunity to helminths is transient and is less efficient to the immunity to micro-organisms (may be because they do not reproduce in the host).

Specific signs include

- The animal appears pale around the eyes (anaemia) has a dry, dull coat.
- Animal may appear to be swollen around the jaws owing to accumulation of body fluid (referred to as 'bottle jaw').
- In some cases, adult worms or tapeworm segments may be seen in the feces.
- Diarrhea (may be bloody), loss of weight, and death may occur.

Treating worms

- If worm infestation is suspected all animals should be treated with broad-spectrum dewormers (antihelmintics). For advice on which type of dewormer to use and the method of administration, one should consult a veterinarian.

Control Measures

Control of parasites is a group treatment. Presence of one clinical case needs whole herd to be treated.

1. Have balanced nutrition.
2. If there is pasture, have rotational system for grazing.
3. In housed animals, feed and water should not get contaminated with dung.
4. Do not group young and old animals together.
5. Give broad spectrum anthelmintics having 90% efficacy. Give medication twice per year for whole herd.
6. Have timely diagnosis; by fecal examination.
7. In order to find out a clinical case, examination of fecal samples of the herd, at regular intervals is necessary (in calves at the interval of 15 days, before and after monsoon, for 3 to 4 times in a year). Mere presence of an egg in the stools does not indicate medication. Clinical symptoms, eggs per gram (of stools) will indicate extent of infestation.
8. The control measures mainly depend upon knowledge of live cycle of parasite in relation to climatic and biological factors like:
    - Immunological competence of animal to particular parasite.
    - Relationship of anti-parasitic drug to parasitic immunity.
    - Efficacy of drug on different stages of parasites.
    - Anti-parasitic drugs should reduce worm burdens to a tolerable level (95% efficacy of drug). It should be safe for the host, and have a broad spectrum.
    - We do not get strong immunity in case of parasites. For tapeworms, certain nematodes and flukes there is very little evidence of passive immunity.
    - In the animals varieties of drugs are available for different types of worms.

Zoonotic Diseases

1. Brucellosis

Brucellosis is one of the major zoonotic diseases and causes great economic losses due to loss of milk production, abortion at late pregnancy and high rate of infertility in females and varying degree of sterility in males. There is no seasonal variation for occurrence of the disease. **Regular screening of serum samples for detection of the disease is required.** Incidence of brucellosis can be reduced by elimination of infected bull, isolation and treatment of positive reactors and **calfhood vaccination.** *Brucella* is one of the world's major zoonotic pathogens, and is responsible for enormous economic losses as well as considerable human morbidity in endemic areas.

How to diagnose?

Diagnosis can only be confirmed by laboratory tests. The RBPT, tube agglutination and ELISA procedures are recommended.

Treatment

Treatment for brucellosis in animals is neither advisable nor practicable.

In humans

Treatment of uncomplicated cases in adults and children eight years of age and older: doxycycline 100 mg twice a day for six weeks + streptomycin 1g daily for two to three weeks.

OR

Doxycycline 100 mg twice a day for six weeks + rifampicin 600–900 mg daily for six weeks.

Control and Prevention

- Animal brucellosis is best prevented by careful herd management and hygiene.
- Vaccination is useful for prevention and control of infection.
- *B. abortus* strains 19 and RB 51 are recommended for prevention of bovine brucellosis.
- *B. melitensis* Rev 1 is recommended for prevention of B. melitensis infection in sheep and goats.
- Control and prevention schemes require effective collaboration between all sections of the community.

- Education and information programmes are essential to ensure cooperation at all levels in the community.
- Effective preventive measures and control of animal movements are essential.

2. Anthrax

Anthrax is a bacterial disease that usually affects herbivorous animals, but outbreaks involving humans are increasingly being reported.

However, case-fatality estimates for inhalation of anthrax spores, although based on incomplete information, are extremely high (75–100%, even with all possible supportive care, including appropriate antibiotics). The case-fatality rate for cutaneous anthrax, which accounts for the vast majority of cases, is usually low (about 20%, if untreated).

Agent: The bacteria Bacillus anthracis.

Reservoir: Reservoir hosts include domestic and wild animals such as cattle, buffalo, sheep, goats, pigs and horses.

Human infection

Risk factors

Although anthrax spores can live in the soil for many years, anthrax infection in humans is rare. Skin contact with, or inhalation of, aerosolized spores and consumption of undercooked or raw meat or dairy products from infected animals can cause the disease.

Mode of transmission

People can become infected in four main ways: by the cutaneous route, e.g. direct skin contact of anthrax spores with a cut or abrasion; by contact with infected animals or animal products (usually related to occupational exposure); through consumption of undercooked or raw meat or dairy products from infected animals (gastrointestinal form); and by inhaling a large number of anthrax spores suspended in the air (the pulmonary form of anthrax, which is the rarest and most severe).

Clinical signs and symptoms: Incubation period: 1–7 days for the cutaneous form; 12 hours–5 days for the gastrointestinal form; and 1–5 days for the pulmonary form. Clinical symptoms are listed below:

- Cutaneous form: red marks on the exposed area of skin, which swells and forms blisters. The skin tissue then dies, leaving a black central scar. These signs are accompanied by fever and malaise. The vast majority of anthrax cases (up to 95%) are cutaneous.
- Gastrointestinal form: loss of appetite, fever, vomiting and diarrhoea.
- Pulmonary form: fever, cough, difficulty in breathing, respiratory failure and, in severe forms, death within 24 hours.

(Animals exhibit sudden acute illness, high fever, localized swelling, bleeding from natural orifices (nose, mouth, ear, anus), or death. Tonsillitis is seen in pigs, and colic in horses.)

Treatment

Anthrax responds well to antibiotic treatment. Antibiotics must be prescribed and taken with medical advice. Treating the pneumonic form of anthrax is very difficult.

Prevention and control

- Avoid examination of (suspected) infected carcasses.
- Dispose of carcasses by deep burial or burning.

3. Tuberculosis (TB)

Tuberculosis is a chronic bacterial disease of animals caused by *Mycobacterium* sp. and characterized by presence of tubercle nodules in lungs, spleen and lymph nodes.

Etiology:

Mycobacterium tuberculosis

M. bovis

Characteristic symptoms

- Low grade fever
- Progressive wasting/ weakness, loss of production
- Coughing

Diagnosis

- Symptoms and lesions
- Tuberculin testing of animals

- Immunodiagnostic tests- ELISA
- Demonstration of acid fast bacilli

Treatment

Long term treatment with antibiotics for 2-3 months.

4. Pseudo-cowpox

Also called as milker's nodule.

Zoonoses through milking the infected teats.

Disease caused by parapox virus.

Disease can be cured.

Symptomatic and palliative treatments are to be followed using antibacterial agents.

Managemental Diseases

1. Acidosis

Acidosis is a syndrome related to a fermentative disorder of the rumen resulting in overproduction of acid resulting in lowering of rumen pH below pH 5.5.

- The problem is related to feeding management, where the ration has high levels digestible carbohydrates and low effective fiber.
- Acidosis commonly occurs when switching from a high fiber to high concentrate diet (that is rich in fermentable carbohydrates (starches and sugars).
- Large amounts of starch and sugar stimulate bacteria that make lactic acid. In a normal, healthy rumen, lactic acid production equals lactic acid use. Large amounts of starch and sugar stimulate bacteria that make lactic acid. In this instance, bacteria that normally use lactic acid cannot keep up with production.
- Lactic acid is about ten times a stronger acid than the other rumen acids and causes the rumen pH to decrease. As the rumen pH drops below 6.0, bacteria that digest fiber begin to die depressing fiber digestion.

Causes of Acidosis

- Diets very high in readily fermentable carbohydrates and low in roughage.
- Very fast switch from high forage to high concentrate.
- Excessive particle size reduction by feeding finely chopped forage.

Signs of Acidosis

- **Low milk fat test** (one of the end products of fiber digestion (acetate) is a precursor of milk fat synthesis).
- Diarrhea (Accumulation of acid causes an influx of water from the tissues into the gut resulting in diarrhea. The feces are foamy with gas bubbles. There is an appearance of mucin/fibrin casts in feces).

2. Sore hooves-laminitis

Endo-toxins resulting from high acid production in the rumen also affect blood capillaries in the hoof, causing them to constrict resulting in laminitis. High levels of acid in the rumen also cause ulcers in the rumen resulting in infiltration of bacteria into the blood causing liver abscesses, which are seen at post mortem.

Prevention Sore hooves-laminitis

Good management practices are needed to prevent the predisposing situations from occurring. The root problem must be found and corrected. Buffers can also be used to prevent drop in rumen pH when high concentrate diets are fed. Ensuring presence of effective fiber in the diet promotes production of saliva which is a buffer.

3. Bloat

Bloat is the abnormal accumulation of gas in the rumen. There are three categories of bloat:

a. Frothy bloat which occurs when diets that lead to the formation of a stable froth or foam in the rumen are fed.

b. Free gas bloat caused by diets that lead to excessive gas production

c. Free gas bloat caused by failure to eructate rumen gases leading to accumulation (e.g. esophageal obstruction).

When bloat occurs, gases cannot escape and they continue to build up causing severe distention of the abdomen, compression of the heart and lungs, and eventually death.

Predisposing factors

- Bloat is a risk when animals are grazing young, lush pasture, particularly if the pasture has high legume content (clover or lucerne).
- Ruminant animals produce large volumes of gas during the normal process of digestion which is either belched or passes through the gastrointestinal

tract. If anything interferes with the gas escape from the rumen, bloat occurs.

- Natural foaming agents in legumes and some rapidly growing grasses cause a stable foam to form in the rumen. Gas is trapped in small bubbles in this foam in the rumen and the animal cannot belch up the gas. Pressure builds up in the rumen causing an obvious swelling on the left side of the body.

Signs of Bloat

- Animal stops grazing and is reluctant to walk.
- The left side of abdomen is distended.
- The animal strains to urinate and defecate.
- Rapid breathing — mouth may be open with tongue protruding.
- Staggering.

Prevention of Bloat

a. **Pasture management**: Legumes should be introduced into the diet gradually over several days. Avoid cows gorging on new pastures by feeding them on other feeds before letting them out to graze. Silage, hay or more mature pasture can be used to reduce the cow's appetite.

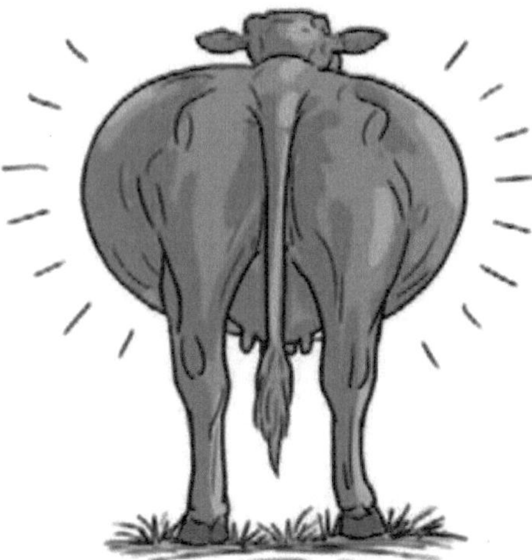

Staggering: a sign of bloat in cow

Initially, cows should only be allowed access to the pasture for short periods (one hour or so) and monitored closely during grazing and immediately after removal. Cutting and wilting the pasture for 2-3 hours prior to feeding reduces the risk of bloat.

b. **Preventative medication:** Detergents and anti-foaming agents can be drenched prior to grazing.

c. **Treatment:** A sharp knife can be used to puncture the rumen on the left side of the animal (at the farm level as an emergency).

   Puncturing the rumen with the standard trocar and canula is a quickest way to release the gas which cannot be expelled with a stomach tube. The trocar is used to puncture while the canula is left in place to release the gas.

4. Indigestion

There are many reasons which may cause indigestion. These include:

a. Change of feed.

b. Acidosis.

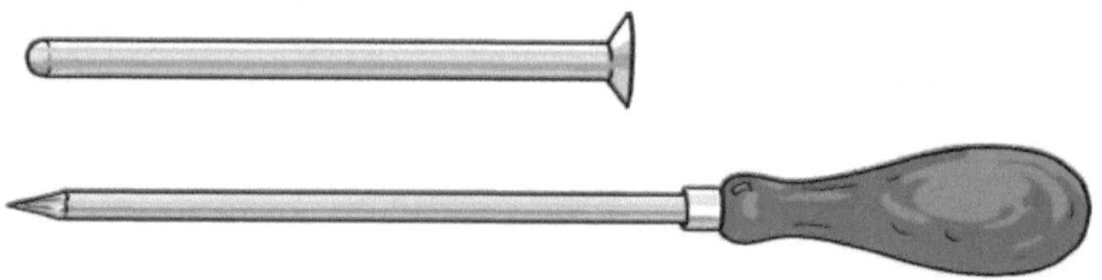

Trochar and canula

Treatment: giving normal saline and DNS as a supportive treatment. Give rumenotorics and fermentation enhancers consisting of yeast cultures.

Other Disorders

- **Foot rot** – this is caused by a break in the skin or hoof, usually between the toes, allowing bacteria to enter. Symptoms are a rapid, progressive lameness; swollen foot; and a characteristic foul odor. Infection often gets into joints, spreads up the leg, and may kill the cow. To avoid this problem, yards should be cleaned of any materials that might cause a break in the skin or hoof. Soft, non-callused feet are highly susceptible to injury. Small stones lodging between the toes can also be a problem. Animals should be provided with the recommended iodine and zinc levels. Use a footbath with copper sulfate (2%).

- **Grass tetany** (hypomagnesemia) – this is likely to be observed in cows grazing on lush grass pasture that is high in nitrogen, resulting in low absorption of magnesium. Cows will suddenly develop tetany, walk with a stiff gait, fall, go into convulsions, and die. Cattle grazing on grass fields fertilized heavily with nitrogen should be carefully monitored and supplemented with 60gm of magnesium oxide daily during this period.
- **Hardware disease**- this results from a puncturing of the reticulum if a cow swallows a sharp object. The animal will have a sudden lack of appetite, a reluctance to move, and a careful gait. Respiration is frequently rapid, pulse rate is fast, and rectal temperature is 40°C or higher. Give magnets to cows when a herd problem exists.
- **Moldy feed toxicity** (aflatoxins) - The fungus, *Aspergillus flavus*, and certain other molds, may produce toxic substances when feed grains are stored under high moisture and poor ventilation conditions. Cows fed on such feed develop fatty liver degeneration, large adrenal glands and oversized bile ducts. They reduce feed intake, reduce milk production, and may have a poor reproductive performance. Death in adult animals is rare. Feeds suspected to be contaminated should be tested in a laboratory.
- **Poisonous plants** - Several hundred plants are known to be toxic to livestock under certain conditions. Bracken fern, algae, and nightshade are common poisonous plants. Cattle will eat whatever is available when feed is scarce, and consuming enough of a toxic plant can have toxic or fatal effects. Fortunately, cattle that consume adequate amounts of other feeds will seldom eat enough of a poisonous plant to do any harm.
- **Udder edema** - Edema is an excessive accumulation of fluid in the udder under the skin. This condition usually occurs at calving and is more severe in first lactation cows. Prevention is by limiting access to either sodium or potassium salts during the dry period. Also avoid excess grain. Treatment includes stimulating circulation by massaging the udder. Diuretics (drugs that promote the formation of urine) should be used with care and direction of a veterinarian.
- **Urea toxicity** (ammonia toxicity) - Too much urea at one time or insufficient carbohydrate intake results in excessive ammonia in the rumen. Animals show uneasiness, muscle and skin tremors, excessive salivation, labored breathing, Inco-ordination, and bloat. Animal urinates excessively. No more than 0.2 kg of urea should be fed per cow per day.

Animal Health Strategies

Adequate preventive health coverage to minimize incidence of disease in livestock concentrations like milk sheds, poultry breeding areas, sheep flock, etc.

1. The preventive coverage should be especially against diseases like F.M.D., Rinderpest, Haemorrhagic Septicaemia, Black Quarter, Clostridial infections, Brucellosis (wherever present).
2. **Efficient vaccines** are available and what is needed is the systematic time bound programme of preventive vaccination, where larger coverage to susceptible population is a must to reduce the focus of infection and survival of infectious agents.
3. Diseases of economic importance like Brucellosis, Tuberculosis, Johne's disease and Mastitis need to be diagnosed and suitable policy for isolation, sexual test, controlled breeding, elimination (where must), quarantine, vaccination should be adopted.
4. An important disease problem arises due to parasitic infestation(s). These can be tackled by diagnosis and availability of various new generation economic anti-parasitic drugs given as per the recommendations. This is very important and relevant as parasitic load reduces productivity of animals as well as capacity of resistance to infection. This problem gets enhanced due to irrigated lands as in the tropics where the available water resources are conserved to last upto the next monsoon. There is no perennial rainfall which can provide feed stuffs and irrigated lands spread infectious larvae on a wider scale.
5. The planned health coverage against viral, bacterial, parasitic diseases can reduce health hazards, mortality and morbidity by 80% to 90% and will be able to increase productivity.

Overall health control in buffaloes

- Buffalo should be checked daily for injuries and illnesses. Wounds and open sores are a perfect growing place for all kinds of bacteria. It is easy to keep control over milking buffalo since they are studied closely twice a day. But apart from looking at the udder at milking the farmer or milker should observe the whole animal. Heifers, calves and bulls should be checked too, not just milking animals.
- Lameness and large injuries are easier to detect than small scratches. Lameness can be caused by injuries in the hooves and legs as well as back pains. Touch the animal carefully all over the body, to locate the injury.

- Large as well as small injuries must be taken care of. Bleeding sores may require veterinary attention although this is quite rare.
- Wounds should be carefully cleaned, and the best way is to use clean water and mild soap. Cleaning should be done very gently with clean hands and cloths. Chemicals such as ethanol and iodine might hurt. **Never** attend to wounds during milking. It is best to take the animal to a sick box or undisturbed area to attend to any wounds.
- Looking at the faeces is an easy way to detect internal defects. This is easy in the milking place when one pail of faeces can be related to one buffalo. If the feces look different from usual, the milker/farmer should be observant. If the buffalo is not eating properly or otherwise seems dull and unfit it might be a sign of some kind of illness. If an animal has some or all of the above mentioned symptoms it is advisable to measure the rectal temperature.
- Normal rectal temperature is 38° to 39°C. If it is above that, the animal may have some sort of infection and a veterinarian should be called. The quicker a wound or an infection is taken care of, the less likely the risk of more buffalo becoming ill.

Parasitism in case of buffaloes

- In the tropics and subtropics, parasites, ticks and mosquitoes can be a big problem. Internal parasites may cause malfunction of the digestive tract and thereby decrease feed utilization. Ticks and mosquitoes cause discomfort and damage to the skin that in turn can lead to inflammatory processes.
- Chemicals and drugs to fight parasites should be used both to prevent disease and to treat it. A disadvantage with chemicals and drugs is that they often leave traces in the milk. Some may be harmless and undetectable, yet others may influence processing of the milk and/or leave traces dangerous for human consumption.
- Chemicals against parasites should be sprayed on the animals. Care must be taken not to spray in the eyes or genital area. The chemical should be applied with a sponge on the face and around the genitals.
- Dip baths, which are used for sheep, are most unsuitable for buffalo. The buffalo will see the dip baths as wallows and this has at least two disadvantages:

    1. They may enjoy wallowing in the dip, and be difficult to get out. This prolonged immersion in the dip may harm their skin.

2. Buffalo natural behavior is to defecate in their wallow, which would make the dip bath extremely unhygienic.

Deworming and Vaccination

Deworming schedule for cattle and buffaloes

S.No.	Type of worm	Deworming Schedule
1.	Roundworms	First dose at 3 days of age and thereafter at monthly interval upto 6 months.Thrice a year in animals above 6 months of age.
2.	Liver flukes	Twice a year in endemic areas (before and after monsoon).
3.	Tapeworms	Twice a year i.e. in January and June in calves in problematic herds.

Vaccination

Vaccines are present to prevent many diseases. No vaccination should be without the disposal of veterinarian. Veterinarian should make a suitable card for the vaccination of individual animals. The following is list of some common vaccinations:

Disease	Initial immunization	Booster
Rhinotracheitis	4-6 month old single injection with modified live vaccine	Booster with killed product 1-2 months before breeding. Yearly booster.
Parainfluenza	4-6 month old single injection	Booster with killed product 1-2 months before breeding. Yearly booster.
Bovine viral diarrhea	4-6 month old single injection with modified live vaccine	Booster with killed product 1-2 months before breeding. Yearly booster.
BRSV	4-6 month old single injection	Booster with killed product 1-2 months before breeding. Yearly booster.
Brucellosis	Heifers, 6-10 months. Calfhood vaccine	None.
Black quarter	Single injection or combined vaccine	Repeat after 3 weeks, booster yearly.
Leptospirosis	Single injection or vaccine containing 5 species	Repeat after 3 weeks, booster yearly.
Calf scours rota virus	Calves, orally at birth	Cows, 1 month before calving
E.coli	Oral vaccine for calves at birth. Cows, 3 months before calving.	Booster at 30 days in milk.
Pink eye.	Heifers, beginning of fly season.	Repeat in 3 weeks to one month. Repeat again in middle of fly season.

Vaccination programmes in buffaloes

- There are a number of vaccines available for common diseases. Most vaccination programmes are more efficient if applied to young calves, with boosters given at regular intervals. This is further evidence of the advantage of recruiting calves at the farm.
- Buffalo are sensitive to the same diseases as cattle. Diseases strike harder on animals in poor condition.
- In order to protect the animals, they should be properly vaccinated and de-wormed at regular intervals.
- It is important to include all animals at the farm in a veterinary control programme in order to minimize risks of disease outbreaks.

Ectoparasitic Management

The ectoparasites i.e. ticks, fleas, mites, flies, etc serve as major carrier of various life threatening diseases to dairy cows and buffaloes. Various measures which should be taken to curb the problem of ectoparasites include:

1. Better housing facilities which should include filling of cracks and crevices in the walls of the animal shed, construction of *pucca* floor, shed should be well ventilated and lightened, the corners of the shed should be rounded, mangers and water troughs should be cleansed regularly and the water logging should be prevented.
2. The surrounding should be kept clean, the litter should be dumped away from the animal shed, marshy and damp areas should not surround the animal shed.
3. Treatment of animals suffering from ectoparasites should be done away from the animal sheds and milking parlor.
4. Treatment of all the animals in a herd should be done at same time and at regular intervals.
5. Before treating the animal with any anti-ectoparasitic drug the animal should be given enough water for drinking and the mouth of the animal should be restrained by application of muzzle.

Treatment of ectoparasites include

1. Deltamethrin @ 2-3ml/liter of water should be used for spraying or dusting on animal body and 5ml/liter for spraying in animal shed.
2. Amitraz: 2ml/liter (for spraying on animal body), and 4ml/liter (for spraying in animal shed).
3. Ivermectin: 1ml for 50 kg weight of the animal through subcutaneous route.

26

Miscellanous

A. First Aid

1. Abscess

What to Do

- Abscesses should be examined by a veterinarian as soon as possible and within 24 hours.
- Fluid may normally drain from the site of an abscess. An abscess does not drain through the tube, but rather around the latex tubing. Therefore, it is important for you to clean the area around the drain twice daily with warm water.
- Apply a hot compress to the affected site at least two times daily for 3 to 5 days after the animal leaves the hospital. Wet a clean washcloth with very warm water and place it directly over the affected site, and then apply gentle pressure ideally for 5 to 10 minutes.
- Be sure you and/or other family members wash your hands thoroughly after contacting any fluids draining from the abscess site.
- Be sure to administer all prescribed medications exactly and completely as detailed by your veterinarian. Some patients may appear to feel better after only a few days of treatment; however, it is crucial for medications to be administered according to schedule to prevent the infection from recurring.
- Notify your vet doctor should your animal experience any of the following:
  - Increased redness and/or heat from the site of abscess
  - Failure of abscess to heal
  - Worsening of your animal's general health
  - Loss of apanimalite lasting longer than 24 hours

What NOT to Do

- Do not attempt to open the abscess yourself.
- Do not attempt compressing the wounds of an animal. Your safety is of utmost importance to us. Contact your veterinarian for assistance should this situation arise.
- Do not apply medicines, potions, or home remedies unless directed by a veterinarian.

2. Burns

What to Do

- Extinguish all flames.
- Avoid touching any animal that has been electrocuted until the power has been turned off.
- For thermal or electrical burns, immediately apply cool water compresses with a clean cloth to the site of the injury, changing them frequently as necessary to keep the site cool and wet. Continue this for at least 30 minutes.
- Transport your animal to a veterinary facility as soon as possible for further care. Burns can become worse before they get better, and may require several weeks of therapy, multiple surgeries and possibly skin grafting.

What NOT to Do

- Do not apply ointments or butter.
- Do not delay seeking veterinary attention.
- Do not attempt to remove burned hair or skin yourself.

3. Wounds

A wound is a break in the skin, usually caused by a sharp object. Wounds are caused accidentally or by parasites and other animals (e.g. fights and bites). When left untreated, the exposed tissues may become infected. Treating a wound involves the following steps:

a. Stop any bleeding.

b. Clip hair or wool way from the edges of the wound.

c. Remove all foreign objects. Wash the wound thoroughly with plenty of clean water (the water should have been boiled, cooled and salt or a mild antiseptic added).

d. Dry the wound with a clean cloth.

e. Put a wound dressing or antibiotic powder on the wound.

f. When there are a lot of flies about, use a wound dressing that repels flies or kills fly eggs and larvae.

g. Encourage wounds to drain and pus to come out by pressure and incision if necessary.

h. If the wound does not heal, becomes black and smells bad, the dead flesh must be cut away. Wash the wound with antiseptic and treat with antibiotic powder.

4. Fractures

Fractures (usually to the legs) result from falling into holes, falling over heavy farm implements or jumping over fences. For large, heavy animals or fractures where the bone breaks high up in the leg it is better to slaughter the animal for meat. For young and light animals:

a. Keep the animal quiet and stop it from moving around.

b. Stop any bleeding.

c. If the bone has come through the skin, clean the wound and give local anesthesia by injection.

d. Arrange the leg so that the broken ends of the bone touch in their normal positions as far as possible.

e. Tie a piece of wood (a splint) to the leg to keep the bones in position.

f. Confine the animal to reduce movement during the healing period.

Splints can be also made by dipping strips of cloth in mud and egg white and wrapping around the leg. Cover with a strip of tree bark and a fresh goatskin. As it dries, the splint will harden and shrink, holding the broken bones together. Check every day that the fixing is not too tight. If the leg below the splint is cold or very swollen, loosen the fixing and then tighten again carefully, keeping the leg in the same position. Leave the splint on for at least 10 –14 days for a young animal or 21–28 days for an adult animal.

5. Snake Bite

What to Do

- Muzzle your animal to avoid being bitten – snakebites can be painful, and your animal may try to protect itself.

- Immobilize the part of the animal that has been bitten by the snake, if this can be done safely. Try to keep it at or below the level of the heart.
- Keep the animal calm and immobile.
- Seek veterinary attention as soon as possible.
- Try to identify the snake if it can be done without risk: Do not Attempt to capture or kill the Snake. It is helpful to identify the type of snake to aid your veterinarian with treatment. Do not bring the snake into the veterinarian's office – a photograph will do.

What NOT to Do

- Do not cut over the fang marks.
- Do not attempt to capture or kill the snake
- Do not manipulate the bitten area any more than needed.
- Do not allow the animal to move about freely.
- Do not ice pack or tourniquet the area.
- Do not administer any medications except on a veterinarian's advice.

B. Sanitation in Dairy Farm

Sanitation is necessary in the dairy farm houses for elimination of all micro-organism that are capable of causing disease in the animals. The presence of organisms in the animal shed contaminates the milk produced thus reducing its shelf life, milk produced in an unclean environment is likely to transmit diseases which affect human health. Dry floorings keeps the houses dry and protects from foot injury. Similarly the presence of flies and other insects in the dairy farm area are not only disturbs the animals but also spreads deadly diseases to the animals e.g. Babesiosis, Theileriosis.

Cleaning of animal sheds

The easy and quick method of cleaning animal house is with liberal use of tap water, proper lifting and disposes all of dung and used straw bedding, providing drainage, to the animal house for complete removal of liquid waste and urine. The daily removal of feed and fodder left over in the manger, reduces the fly nuisance. Periodical cleaning of water through eliminates the growth of algae, bacterial and viral contamination and thus keeps the animal healthy.

Sanitizers

Sunlight is the most potent and powerful sanitizer which destroy most of the disease producing organism. Disinfection of animal sheds means making these free from disease producing bacteria and is mainly-carried out by sprinkling chemical agents such as Bleaching Powder, Iodine and Iodophore, sodium carbonate, Washing soda, Slaked Lime (Calcium hydroxide), Quick Lime (Calcium oxide) and Phenol.

1. **Bleaching powder:** This is also called calcium hypochloride. It contains upto 39 % available chlorine which has high disinfecting activity.
2. **Iodine & iodophores:** This is commercially available as iodophores and contains between 1 and 2 % available Iodine which is an effective germicide.
3. **Sodium carbonate:** A hot 4 % solution of washing soda is a powerful disinfectant against many viruses and certain bacteria.
4. **Slaked lime and quick lime:** White washing with these agents makes the walls of the sheds and the water troughs free from bacteria.
5. **Phenol:** Phenol or carbolic acid is a very potent disinfectant which destroys bacteria as well as fungus.
6. **Insecticides:** Insecticides are the substances or preparations used for killing insects. In order to control flies and disease transmitting ticks, insecticides are used in dairy farms. Ticks usually hide in cracks and crevices of the walls and mangers. Smaller quantities of insecticide solutions are required for spraying. Liquid insecticides can be applied with a powerful sprayer- hand sprayer, a sponge or brush, commonly used insecticides are BHC, DDT, Gamaxane wettable powders, malathion, surriithion, Sevin 50 % emusifying concentration solutions.

These are highly poisonous and need to be handled carefully and should not come in contact with food material, drinking, water, milk etc.

Precautions while using disinfection Insecticide.

- Remove dung and used bedding completely.
- Avoid spilling of dung and used bedding while carrying it out.
- Avoid the use of dirty water in cleaning the sheds.
- Never put the fresh fodder over the previous day's left over fodder in the manger.

- Prevent algae to grow in the water troughs.
- Use proper concentration of disinfectant / insecticide solutions to avoid any toxic effects poisoning.
- Avoid of the mat the milking time as milk absorbs these quickly.

Procedure

- Remove the dung from the floor and urine channel with the help of a shovel and basket (iron) and transfer it to the wheel - barrow. Remove the used bedding and leftovers from the mangers in a similar way.
- Empty the water trough and scrape its sides and bottom with the help of a floor brush.
- Wash the water trough with clean water and white wash it with the help of lime mixture once a week.
- Scrape the floor with a brush and broom and wash with water.
- Clean and disinfect the splashes of dung on the side walls, railing and stanchions.
- Remove the cobwebs periodically with the help of a wall brush.
- Sprinkle one of the available disinfecting agents in the following concentration. Bleaching powder should have more than 30% available chlorine. Phenol 1-2% solution. Washing Soda (4% solution).
- Allow adequate sunlight to enter in to the shed.
- Spray insecticides at regular intervals especially during the rainy season (Fly season).
- Whitewash the walls periodically by mixing insecticides init to eliminate ticks and mites living in cracks and crevices.

Detergents and disinfectants

- Detergents increase the 'wetting' potential over the surfaces to be cleaned, displace milk deposits, dissolve milk protein, emulsify the fat and aid the removal of dirt.
- Detergent effectiveness is usually increased with increasing water temperature, and by using the correct concentration and time of application.
- Detergents contain inorganic alkalis (e.g. sodium carbonate and silicates and tri-sodium phosphate), surface-active agents (or wetting agents), sequestering (water-softening) agents (e.g. polyphosphates) and acids for de-scaling.

- An inexpensive mixture can be made to give a concentration in solution of 0.25% sodium carbonate (washing soda) and 0.05% polyphosphate (Calgon).
- Disinfectants are required to destroy the bacteria remaining and subsequently multiplying on the cleaned surfaces.
- The alternatives are either heat applied as hot water or chemicals. Heat penetrates deposits and crevices and kills bacteria, providing that correct temperatures are maintained during the process of disinfection.
- When hot water alone is used, it is best to begin the routine with water at not less than 85°C, so that a temperature of at least 77°C can be maintained for at least 2 minutes.
- If any concentrated detergent and/or disinfectant come in contact with the skin or eyes the affected area should be washed immediately with copious amounts of clean water.

Milking premises

The milking premises should have a dairy or suitable place equipped with a piped hot and cold water supply, a wash trough, brushes, a work surface, storage racks and cupboards and, if necessary, a vacuum pipeline connection. In addition, it is advisable to have a dairy thermometer (0°C - 100°C), rubber gloves and goggles for use when handling chemicals.

Daily routines

- Coolers, either the corrugated surface or the turbine in-can, can best be cleaned and disinfected manually and stored in the dairy to drain.
- Refrigerated bulk milk tanks can be cleaned either manually using cold or warm detergent/disinfectant solutions, or for the larger tanks, by automatic, programmed equipment. In either case, cold water chlorinated (50ppm) rinse proceeds and follows the washing solution.
- Foremilk cups can be a potent source of bacterial contamination and need to be cleaned and disinfected after each milking. They should then be stored in the dairy to drain.
- It is important with any method of cleaning that the equipment is drained as soon as possible after washing for storage between milking. Bacteria will not multiply in dry conditions but water lodged in milking equipment will, in suitable temperatures, provide conditions for massive bacterial multiplication.

- Equipment with poor milk contact surfaces, crevices and large number of joints, remaining wet between milking in ambient temperatures above 20°C, should receive a disinfectant rinse (50ppm available chlorine) before milking begins.

C. Dentition of Cattle and Buffalo

Dental formula

Temporary of deciduous dentition: 2 (DI 0/4, DC 0/0, DPM 3/3, DM 0/0) = 20

Permanent dentition: 2 (I 0/4, C 0/0, PM 3/3, M 0/3) = 32

Age and eruption pattern of teeth in cattle

Time of eruption	Incisors	Cheek teeth
Birth to 1 month	All temporary incisors	First 3 pairs of temporary cheek teeth.
6 months	-	4th pair permanent cheek teeth
1 ½ years	-	5th pair permanent cheek teeth
2 years	Central permanent pair	1st, 2nd pair of permanent cheek teeth
2 ½ years	-	3rd pair of permanent cheek teeth
3 years	Medial permanent pair	-
4 years	Lateral permanent pair	-
5 years	Corner permanent pair	-

D, Common Vices of Animals, Their Prevention and Cure

A vice is an undesirable quality or the faulty bad habit of an animal. It adversely affects the health and performance of other animals of the herd too. Some vices are dangerous and some are injurious to the owner, animal or both and make the animals almost useless.

E. Record Keeping

Record keeping is an important activity in any dairy enterprises. Farmers should therefore ensure that all farm activities are recorded promptly. Records are important to farmers because they can help farmers in many ways such as in making:

- Management decisions.
- Financial accounting.
- Identifying problems.
- Planning for the future.
- Determining whether targets are met.

S.no.	Vice	Meaning	Reason	Prevention & cure
1.	Kicking	Striking others with a foot.	Lack of floor space, fear, irritation, mischievousness, estrous, faulty milking.	1. Application of anti-kicking straps. 2. Holding tail vertically high. 3. Apply 'anti-cow kicker' above hocks.
2.	Self-sucking	Sucking their own udder	Bad management and deficiency of feeding	1. Separate the cows. 2. Apply muzzle. 3. Apply anti-sucking plate.
3.	Butting	Hurting other animals or humans with horns	Lack of feeding, insecurity, irritation to a particular thing.	1. By judicious management. 2. By dehorning. 3. Isolating animal from rest of the herd.
4.	Coprophagia	Eating its own feces	Bad weather, indigestion, half starved condition, mineral deficiency.	1. Providing sufficient feed both in quality and quantity. 2. Proper disposal of manure.
5.	Pica	Eating of unusual materials	Deficiency of phosphorous and worm infestations.	1. Well balanced ration. 2. Mineral mixture in ration.
6.	Licking or gnawing.	Cattle licking each other, walls, urine, etc.	Deficiency of sodium, chlorine, calcium. Worm infestations.	1. Provide adequate ration containing sufficient amount of minerals and vitamins. 2. Provide salt licks to affected animals. 3. Following routine deworming programmes.
7.	Inter sucking in calves	Problem of presence of animals above average size in herds.	When calves are grouped shortly after their birth or when they are bucket fed.	1. Separate the calf after feeding. 2. Do not group the calves until they are more than 4 weeks of age. 3. Provide good feed.

In the dairy enterprise, several types of records are kept by the farmer. For a successful operation of a dairy enterprise the following records should be kept by the farmer. Pedigree and numbers of each animal kept on the farm, dates of heat periods, breeding, pregnancy checks, bulls used, animal health records deworming, vaccinations, performance records milk production, growth rates.

Good records should have the following characteristics:

a. Easy to update.

b. Easy to understand.

c. Up to date i.e. include the latest event (current).

d. Easy to access.

e. Easily summarized.

Several types of records are kept which include:

a. Ancestry or genetic records. These include the maternal and paternal records

b. Breeding records -sire, date of breeding, pregnancy confirmation, date of calving, and particulars of calf.

c. Veterinary records - disease type, date and treatment

d. Production - amount of milk (daily, weekly or monthly), butter fat, drying date.

e. Feed records - these could be amount of concentrate fed for pasture grazed animals or the totals amount fed for zero grazed animals.

f. Financial records - all financial transactions should be recorded.

Recording

- Records are important because they give the animal's ancestry and hence prove quality and increase the value of the animal.
- Records also help farmers in making management decisions. Farmers keep mainly two types of records; pedigree records which show the ancestry of the animals and performance records. Ancestry records are kept by the stud book while performance records for dairy cattle are kept by Dairy recording services of Department of Animal Husbandry, Dairying & Fisheries (DAHDF), Department of Agriculture, Government of India.

The following are some sample recording tables:

a. Record card for daily milk yield:

Record card for daily milk yield:

1	2	3	4	5	6	7	Total milk	Average per day	Comment
Jan	AM								
	PM								
Feb	AM								
	PM								
Mar	AM								
	PM								
Apr	AM								
	PM								
……									

b. Cow identification and health card

Cow identification and health card:					
Cow identification				Health record	
Cow name Number Breed Birth date Date animal received Source	Sire	Dam Number Breed Sire name Number Breed	Date born	Illness/event	Outcome

c. Breeding/reproduction card

Breeding/reproduction card:
Lactation No........................ Date of last calving...................

Date on heat
Service dates
Bull /AI
Breed and owner
Pregnancy check
Date and result
Date to dry
Date to calve

d. Calving record

Calving record:

ID				Birth		Weaning		12 months		Remarks
Number	Name	Sex	ID	Date	Weight	Date	Weight	Date	Weight	

F. Organic Dairy Farming: Entrepreneurship and Alternatives

Organic Dairy farming means raising animals on organic feed (i.e. pastures cultivated without the use of fertilizers or pesticides), have access to pasture or outside, along with the restricted usage of antibiotics and hormones. Products obtained from Organic dairy farm are the organic dairy products. Organic farming is a system of production, a set of goal-based regulations that allow farmers to manage their own particular situations individually, while maintaining organic integrity. In this chapter, the benefits, conditions required, constraints involved, SWOT analysis and managemental practices of organic dairying along with information about the regulatory authorities concerned with the organic dairy farming are discussed in brief to make students and farmers aware of organic dairy farming.

Traditionally, Indians love "Nature" and every component of our civilization, style of living endeavors to bring us near to the nature. To elucidate in our music we have ragas for each season. With growth in population everything changed. Pressure on cultivated land increased and food production system became intensively input oriented with increasing use of chemical fertilizers, pesticides, and lately use of genetically modified food items. However, now with rising disposable income, effective mass communication, growing awareness about health environmental and food safety, is picking up which has pushed the community to use costlier organic foods including organic milk.

Definition and Origin

Organic milk means the milk derived from organic disease-free animals, reared under natural conditions on pesticide-free feed and fodder produced organically on natural fertility of soil, treated by herbal or homeopathic medicines. According to Dr. T. Nissen of "The Organic Service Centre Denmark", organic farming in real term is bio-dyanamic farming which was founded by philosopher Rudolf Striver in Germany in 1924. Organic movement, in real effective way got started in 60s based on experience of biodynamic farming. In 1981, organic farmers coordinated internationally and established the International Federation of Organic Agriculture Movements (IFOAM) (Banerjee, 2001).

The philosophy of organic farming emphasizes the need to produce food or milk in an, "integrated, humane, environmentally and economically sustainable agricultural production system" Organic products have characteristics which differentiate them from conventional farm produces, viz.:

- Integrated animal & crop production.
- Safer products devoid of chemical residences of pesticides, antibiotics, etc.
- More nutritious and natural products.
- Higher quality and natural appearance, and
- Environment friendly.

Organic production systcms, unlikc traditional systems of production, are governed by a set of standards, (organic standards) to be followed strictly by producers of organic foods. Compliance of these standards is verified by certification agencies authorized by the respective governments. Organic certification guarantees not only the quality of product but also the quality of production method or system. In the conventional products, there is no way to guarantee the production procedure.

Requirements or Standard for Organic Livestock Production

Standards for organic livestock keeping are meant to assure both an organic product to the consumer and living conditions for the animals which limit stress and promote good health. These address substances used in health care and feeding and herd management and housing

Animal Management

Must fulfill the basic behavioral needs health and welfare of the livestock. Livestock farming cannot be done in isolation from crop farming. Ample provision should be made for free involvement, open fresh air, water, feed and grazing opportunities for the animals.

Conversion Period

The time between the start of organic management and certification of animals is known as the conversion period, which is fixed as 12 months for dairy animals.

Brought in Animals

Animals should be born and raised on organic holding and not on conventional holdings, brought-in-conventional animals are allowed when organic livestock is not available.

When organic livestock is not available

For this situation, calves upto 4-weeks-old that have received colostrum and are fed a diet consisting mainly of full milk. Time limit for certification of these animals is 5 years and yearly 10 percent of the animals of the same species can be replaced.

Breeds and Breeding

Breeds which remain well adapted to local conditions should be selected. Breeding should be natural. Artificial insemination not allowed unless it is a veterinary necessity.

Mutilations

Mutilations are not permitted. Following exceptions are, however, allowed viz, castration, dethroning, ringing in dairy animals and should be done with minimum suffering to the animal.

Animal Nutrition

Dairy stock should receive 100% organically grown feeds of good quality from the farm itself. Force feeding is forbidden. In a situation, when it proves impossible to obtain feeds from organic farming the accredited certification programme may allow 15% of dry matter intake to be procured from conventional sources. Synthetic growth promoters appetizers preservatives, all types of excreta feeds supplied to solvent extraction, other chemical agents, pure amino acids, genetically engineered substances are not to be added. Vikamius, trace elements and supplements shall be used from natural origin.

Veterinary Medicines

For preventive health care and treatment only herbal, homeopathic medicines, acupuncture or local techniques should be used. Allopathic medicines are not permitted.

Transport of Animals

Journey time should not exceed 8 hours and ample water and feed should be available during the course.

Record Keeping

Producer should keep written records concerning production and processing. Input used, sources of inputs, medicines given, sources of feeds and fodder given and welfare measures taken are to be recorded. Besides, the records should contain (i) Third party certification (ii) Audit trails (iii) annual inspection (iv) material list (iv) conversion periods (vii) sustainable farm plan.

Labour

No child labour to be used in production, processing and marketing of dairy products.

Scope for Organic Milk Production

One can witness people daily going in the morning to nearby dairy/ *Khatals* in their localities to fetch clean and unadulterated milk in their presence. They want to ensure that the milk their family consumes is unadulterated and are ready to pay premium price. Right now, they fail to notice what is fed to the animals, under what conditions the milking of the animal is done and the milk is containing antibiotics etc. However awareness is growing; and sooner demand for organic milk will appear as is already there for vegetables, fruits and food products. A 'SWOT analyses" can throw better light about the unfolding market for Organic milk.

SWOT Analysis

Strength

Indigenous Cattle and Buffalo Wealth

India is enriched with an enormous bovine population (273.3 million) with 26 native cattle breeds (10% of worlds) all breeds (8 breeds) of riverine buffaloes producing over 84 million tonnes of milk annually making number one milk producer in the globe.

Milk production is predominately the domain of small holding farmer in a mixed farming system of which 70% constitute dry land or rain fed areas. As such use of chemical fertilizer and agrochemical is very low. Indigenous breeds have unique characteristics like endurance, docility, resistance to tropical diseases, ability, resistance to tropical diseases, ability to utilize coarse fodder and heat tolerance. This is why these have attracted attention of foreign countries particularly South America. Programmes have been taken up to develop these (Chander & Kumar, 2002). Energy efficiency of desi Cattle is 17% as compared to 4% of American beef breeds (Chander & Kumar). As such these are most suited for organic farming. Enough dung an important component of organic farming is manuring. Yearly Cattle dung, in India has a fuel value equivalent to 35 million tonnes of coal. An estimated 1/3 of this or 300 million tonnes of dung is used as fuel which can be diverted for manuring if bottled methane gas from bio-gas plants is made available to such families (Anon, 2005)

Expanding Market

With growing awareness for environment, chemical free foods, health and nutrition, market for organic foods is opening up.

Rising Income

Per capita income is continuously showing an upward trend. Consequently, the quality consciousness and willingness to pay more for good quality products including organic items would definitely go up in coming years.

Export Potential

The market for organic dairy products in Austria, U.K. and Denmark is annually growing @ 30 per cent whereas in Sweden, Germany and France @ 15 per cent. Besides, organic dairy products are fetching 60% greater price than conventional dairy products (Banerjee, 2001). Organic dairy farming add up greatly to the export item list of Indian dairy products.

Contract Farming System

Land holding are small. With the introduction of contract farming system, this bottle neck can be removed. Larger organic dairy farms will not remain a distant dream.

India being the treasure of herbal, Ayurvedic & Homeopathic medicines, which an important prerequisites for producing organic milk.

Milks is Cost Competitive

Indian milk, cost-wise is quite competitive being stands fourth lowest in the world and fortunately there are no subsides in the Indian dairy industry (Jain, 2002). This is a great plus point.

Weakness

- Seventy percent of the milk producers are landless. Most of them are illiterate. These will be major bottleneck for organic farming. But contract farming and large number of educated unemployed, put together promise a bright ray of hope to face it.
- Lack of training in organic farming. In due course facilities will be created to take care of this.
- Herbal and homeopathic remedies: available at present are of unreliable efficacy.
- Long gestaion period required for start ups.
- Use of child labour: No child labour is permitted in organic dairy farming. This may be yet a newer constraint for India where children share a lot of work relative to livestock production. As incomes grow in rural areas, this handicap will be nullified.
- Clean drinking water & green fodder: are to be supplied to animals in organic milk production. Both these requirements appear difficult to be met. Adoption of contract organic dairy farming will certainly erase these limitations. Moreover our breeds have strong survival potential and can maintain themselves on crop residues.
- Shrinking land and grazing area: Due to population growth land and grazing areas are shrinking due diversion for crop farming. Looking to the potential and to efforts underway to maximize production of food crops, in near future requirement for grazing area certainly can be fulfilled.

Opportunities

High profit margin

On average organic milk producers are charging 60 percent higher price than the milk produced by the conventional method. (Banerjee, 2001).

Export Potential

Export of livestock products is fast growing.

Value Addition and Diversification

As in the conventional milk production and processing, organic milk processing and manufacturing also offers a great scope in this respect. Add to the equipment line and increase your organic milk product lines. With value addition, profits will move faster

Threats

Multi agencies involvement: For certifications and labeling, organic diary production has to face several agencies. Process becomes slow and the path becomes difficult to tread and tackle.

Lack of Infrastructure and Bureaucratic Slow Action

Different committees and agencies for certification and accreditation's are to be formed for different regions and stages by the government. This remains slow and tiring for the organic producer. However, as the things get moving, the process will catch up. Successful implementation and efficient guidelines can remove these constraints.

Looking to the aforesaid 'SWOT' analysis, it is not difficult to conclude that 'strength' and opportunities outweights 'weakness' and 'threats'. The scope for organic milk industry is great.

Opportunities & Challenges

Having established the scope of organic dairying in the country let us briefly look to the opportunities it offers:

- Opportunities in production of Organic feed & fodder.
- Opportunities in raising organic replacement of livestocks.
- Opportunities for cultivation & processing of herbal and ayurvedic medicinal plants.
- Opportunities in preparation of homeopathic, ayurvedic and herbal medicines for livestock. Besides local market big export market is true for these.
- Opportunities in processing & production of organic dairy products.
- Opportunities in promotion & presentation of organic dairy products.

G. Disposal of waste and carcasses

Before handling a carcass, consider the diseases that can be passed to humans (anthrax, brucellosis, rabies, ringworm and mange are the most common ones). If the animal died unexpectedly, a post-mortem will reveal the cause of death and guide the means of disposal.

How to burn a carcass:

- Dig two trenches (2 m long, 40 cm wide and 40 cm deep) in the form of a cross. The trenches will provide oxygen to the fire.

- Place two iron bars so they lie across one of the trenches.
- Place strong wooden posts across the bars.
- Place the carcass and a heap of fuel (wood and straw soaked in waste oil) on the wooden posts.
- Light the fire and burn the carcass.

Disposal by burying

1. Dig a hole 2 m long by 1.5 m wide and 2 m deep.
2. Put the carcass in the hole and cover with soil and logs or large stones to stop wild animals or dogs digging it up again.

H. Disbudding in calves

Disbudding means removing the horn buds in calves before any horn material can be seen. It is preferable to dehorning as it is less stressful to the animal.

Why disbudding is performed

- For better managemental practices
- To prevent injuries to handlers or other cattle.
- To house more animals in less space as horned livestock take up more space.
- To avoid the need of separate equipment, such as feeders and cattle crushes for individual animal.
- To avoid many conditions associated with horns like overgrown horns eventually causing injury to the animal itself, broken horn causing blood loss and infection of sinuses, horn cancer etc.
- To avoid trapping of animals in fences or vegetation.

Age

Golden rule says the earlier the better. Preferably should be done at the age of 10-15 days.

Methods

- Hot iron method
- Chemical method

Anaesthesia and control

Keys to ensure that disbudding has the least impact on the calf are proper restraint and the effective anaesthesia.

Animal can be restrained either in standing position or in lateral recumbency Effective anaesthesia can be obtained by blocking cornual nerve halfway between the base of the ear and the corner of the eye

1. Hot iron method

Materials required

Lox 2% (Lignocine HCl), Syringe (10 ml), Razor, Shaving blade, Cotton, Betadine lotion, Hot iron rod or electric dehorner

Procedure

- Shave, clean and dry the area of horn bud
- Restrain the animal in proper position (either standing position or lateral recumbency) and give cornual nerve block using 3-5 ml of local anaesthetic.
- After 2-3 minutes check for loss of sensation using needle pricks
- Preheat the dehorning iron rod to a red colour
- Hold the calf's ear out of the way to keep it from being burned.
- Apply the iron straight onto the horn bud for 2 - 3 seconds, then move the iron rod through 360^0 around the bud .
- Continue the application of heat for 10-15 seconds. Do not leave the dehorner in place for much longer, especially in young calve as heat can be transferred through the thin bones of the skull and damage the calf's brain.
- Then push the iron underneath the bud to scoop it out.
- Make sure that the horn-producing tissue is destroyed by looking for the 'copper ring' around the edge of the burnt area.
- If there are still white areas apply the iron to those sites again for not more than 2-3 seconds
- Place a betadine soaked gauge piece on the wound and turn the animal on the other side to repeat the procedure for the second bud.

Precautions

- After disbudding apply some antibiotic ointment
- Keep the wound dry
- Keep flies off using fly repellants e.g. topicure or himax ointment

Advantages

- less painful
- No chances of bleeding
- No postoperative pain or complications
- Rapid healing and less scar tissue formation

2. Chemical method

Caustic chemicals will prevent the growth of horns when properly applied to the horn buds of new-born (less than one to three weeks of age) calves by destroying the horn-producing cells around the horn bud.

Materials required

Lox 2% (Lignocine HCl), Syringe (10 ml), Razor, Shaving blade, Cotton, Betadine lotion, Vaseline petroleum jelly, KOH or NaOH sticks or tablets

Procedure

- Restrain the animal in lateral recumbency
- Clip and shave the area of horn bud
- Clean and dry the area
- Apply a layer of vaseline around the periphery of horn bud
- Hold the caustic (NaOH or KOH) with some artery forecep and rub over the area of horn bud very gently
- Keep rubbing till the blood vessels starts appearing beneath the bud
- Once the blood vessels are visible and whole horn bud tissue is destroyed cover the area with an antiseptic soaked gauge
- Turn the animal on the other side and repeat the same for the second horn bud

Precautions

- To protect yourself, wear gloves while applying the chemicals.
- To protect the calf, avoid application near its eyes.
- Avoid use of caustics in rainy weather
- If bleeding results during the procedure apply potassium permanganate crystal directly over the bleeding vessels

Disadvantages

- Postoperative pain and itching
- Bleeding may result during the procedure
- Caustics can cause damage to the surrounding tissue in case of accidental spillage

Sterilization of equipments under field conditions

Sterilization is the complete elimination of microbial viability, including both the vegetative forms and spores. To assure complete freedom from the danger of implanting pathogenic bacteria into the tissues through the medium of instrument and surgical accessories during operations these must be made aseptic.

Sterilization can be achieved with one or more of the following methods:

1. Heat 2. Chemicals 3. Irradiation and 4. Mechanical (Filtration)

Only first two methods can be used at field level.

A. HEAT

Heat can be used as dry heat or moist heat. Moist heat has more penetration power and can sterilise instruments earlier than dry heat.

1. DRY HEAT

Direct flaming

- Clean and dry the instrument properly (there should be no dust , dirt or any organic material adhered to the instruments)
- Place them in a large stainless steel tray
- Pour 5-10 ml of methylated spirit over the instruments and ignite them.
- If any instrument is large it should be tilted while flaming
- Do not touch the instrument anywhere after flaming except the site to be used

or

- Make instruments red hot immediately before use

Used for: wire loops, probes, teat dilators, teat canula, small tray, any metallic instrument etc.

2. MOIST HEAT

a. Boiling b. Pressure cooker

A. Boiling

- Boiling of instruments at 100ÚC for 10 -15 minutes is sufficient to destroy most vegetative forms of bacteria and if used longer can kill spores also.
- Addition of 2% Na_2CO_3 or 0.1% NaOH enhance destruction of spores and prevent rusting of the metal wares.

Used for: Syringes, needles, surgical instruments, i/v infusion sets, canulas, probes, teat instruments etc.

b. Pressure cooker

Surgical instruments can be sterilized in a pressure cooker under field conditions.

Procedure

- Clean and dry the equipments to be sterilized
- Wrap them in a clean piece of cloth
- Put some water in a pressure cooker and place a steel stand in it.
- Place the wrapped instruments on the stand and close the lid.
- Keep heating for about 15-20 minutes after the first steam for complete sterilization.

Chemical Sterilization (Cold sterilization)

Chemicals are also used for sterilization. They are used to sterilize heat-sensitive materials such as biological materials, rubber and plastic materials etc. Chemicals, either as gases or in liquid form, can be used as sterilants. While using chemical sterilants, one must ensure that article to be sterilized is chemically compatible with the sterilant being used.

Commonly used chemicals are:

a. **Formalin**-as gas sterilization and in solution as formaldehyde-paraformaldehyde tablets are placed in an air tight chamber for sterilization of catheters, endoscopic bulbs or other delicate articles which cannot be boiled.

Borax and formaldehyde solution (borax 15gm, Formaldehyde 25ml and water 1000ml) kills ordinary micro-organisms in 30 minutes and 24 hr immersion produces complete sterility

b. **Iodine and its compounds** (Tr. iodine and povidone iodine) – effective in both aqueous and alcoholic solutions. Water soluble povidone iodine is available for sterilization.

c. Quarternary ammonium compounds (zephiran chloride) –zephiran chloride 1: 1000 is commonly used.

d. Chlorinated compounds (Hypochloride solution, Dakin solution -diluted hypochloride solution)- 2.5%sodium hypochlorite solution is effective. A 3% solution of chloride of lime (bleaching powder) is used for sterilizing utensils.

e. Coal tar derivatives (phenol and cresol)- phenol 1% for 5-10 minutes and cresols (Lysol or eusol) 2% for 5 minutes are commonly used.

f. Chlorxylenol solution (dettol): It is used as 5% solution for 30 minutes for sterilization of utensils

g. Detergents (cetrimide, chlorhexidine)- 1% chlorhexidine and 2% cetrimide in alcohol in combination is good for skin preparation.

h. Alcohol (70% ethyl alcohol and isopropyl alcohol) – 70% ethyl alcohol is sufficient to kill any micro-organism but has no action on spores.

i. Mercurials (Bichloride of mercury)- bichloride of mercury 1:1000 or 1:2000 is used for disinfection of glass and rubber articles and thermometers.

j. Oxidising agent (hydrogen oxide and potassium permanganate) -0.5 to 1% for hand scrubbing and 1:3000 for wound irrigation.

Note: Instruments sterilized with chemical sterilization must be washed with normal saline before their use.

ITKs for treating minor ailments in dairy animals

1) Stomach Disorder

S. No	Condition	Remedies / Plant name (Hindi name in brackets)	Portion used and preparation mode	Dose and amount
1	Bloat (mild)	Ginger (Adrak), garlic Cardamom (elachi), clove(laung) and jaggery (gud)	50 gm ginger, 1 full garlic, 3 Cardamoms, 5 to 6 cloves, all to be boiled in half liter of water, put a little jaggery and prepare a decoction.	Give once a day for 2 days. Prepare Give half the quantity to calves fresh d daily.
2	Diarrhoea	(1) Tea leaves, Ginger	Boil handful of Tea leaves in one lit. of water. Strain & add half handful of ground ginger.	Drench twice a day for 3 to 4 days. Prepare freshly every day.
		(2) Guava (Amrut)	Boil half kg of fresh Amrut leaves in three glass of water.	Drench twice a day.
		(3) Potassium permanganate	Mix 5 to 10 crystals of Potassium in 1 liter of water.	Drench twice a day.
3	Stomach disorder	(1) Ginger (Adrak), Drum Stick (Soanjana), Honey	Take 500 ml each of juice of Ginger, Drum stick leaves, and 200 ml of Honey. Mix thoroughly to make a single dose.	Give twice a day for 2 days.

Tea leaves

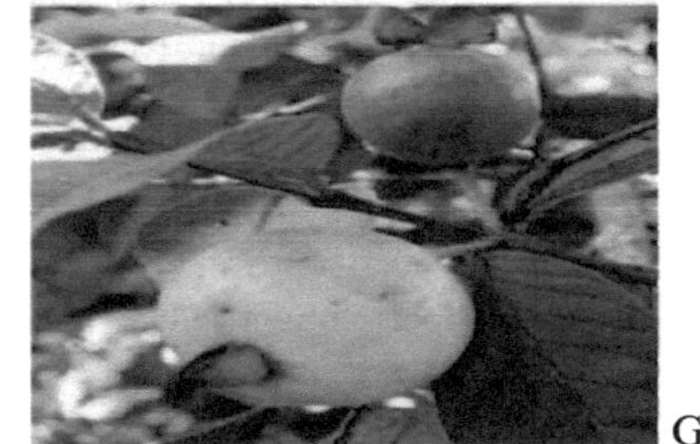

Guava

2) Repeat Breeding

S.no	Condition	Remedies / Plant name (Hindi namein brackets)	Portion used and preparation mode	Dose and amount
1	Infertility	(1) Brinjal (Bengan), Horse gram	Ripened fruit– 1 Kg (either alone or with horse gram) Horse gram– 250 gm soak and grind.	Give brinjal first followed by horse gram daily for one week.
		(2) Coconut tree	Extract the juice from the newly opened inflorenscence and mix with tender coconut water.	Drench once a day for 3 to 4 days.
2	Repeat Breeding	(1) Curry leaves (Kari patti)	Take 2 handful of Curry leaves.	After insemination for 10 days.
		(2) Mimosa pudica (Chuimui)	200 gm of the plant and prepare decoction.	Give for 2-3 days.

Jatropha

Datura metel plant

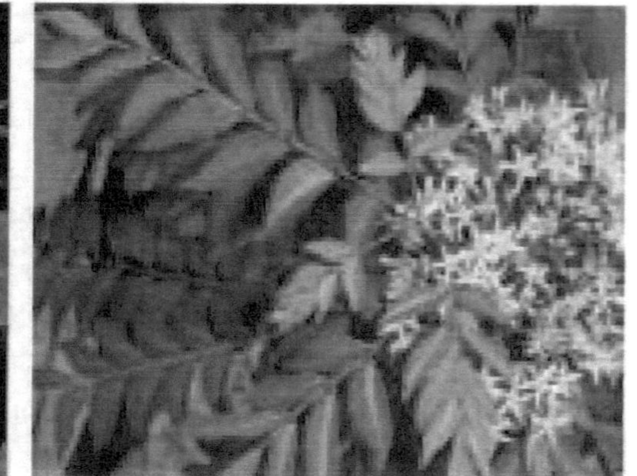
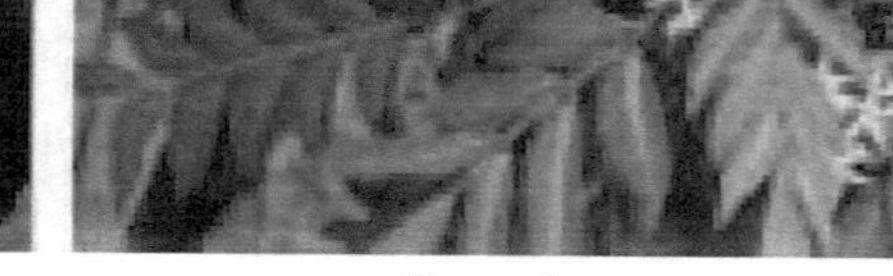

Curry leaves

3) Milk Production Related Conditions

S.no	Condition	Remedies / Plant name (Hindi name in brackets)	Portion used and preparation mode	Dose and amount
1	Failure to produce milk	(1) Asparagus racemosus (Satavari, Shahakul)	Grind 250 gm. of Asparagus root.	Give orally for 3 to 5 days.
		(2) Leptadenia reticulata (Jivanti)	Leaf and stem of Leptadenia to be given along with feed.	50 gm. Twice a day for 30 days.
2	Blood in milk	Mimosa pudica (Touch me not plant)	Half to one kg of plant made into paste.	Feed as such for 3-5 days, twice daily.
3	Improper milk let down	(1) Jatropha curcas (Jangali arandi)	Leaves	2-3 handful of leaves
		(2) Datura metel (Sadah datura)	Take one datura fruit, warm it in hot ash and crush along with rice polish.	Feed only once. Do not allow animal to stray after giving medicine.
		(3) Asparagus racemous (Shatavari)	Asperagus tuber or its extract	Twice a day for 4 days.

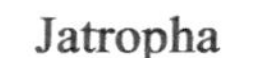

Jatropha

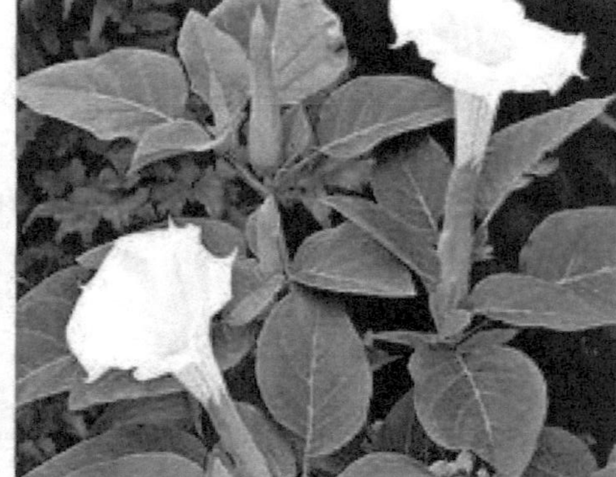

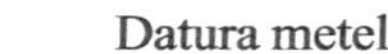

Datura metel plant

4) Post Calving Conditions

S.no	Condition	Remedies / Plant name (Hindi name in brackets)	Portion used and preparation mode	Dose and amount
1	Udder oedema	Aloe vera, Lime or mimosa leaves	Take 2 to 3 leaves of Aloe alone or; mix with 50 gm of Lime or; 2-3 handfuls of mimosa leaves and prepare a paste.	Apply twice a day for 4 to 5 days (Mix the Lime with Aloe before 2 to 3 days). Apply after milking.
2	Prolapse	Mimosa pudica (Chuimui)	Crush two handful of leaves and give. Also extract juice of the Leaves.	Give thrice a day and apply the juice to the prolapsed portion of Uterus.
3	Retention of Placenta	(1) Mimosa pudica (Chuimui)	1 Kg to leaves	Once a day for 2 days.
		(2) Aegle marmelos (Bael), Pepper, Garlic & Onion	Bael leaves—handful; garlic – 6 cloves; pepper –10 corns; onions-2. Make a paste and mix in butter milk.	Give once daily.
		(3) Gossypium herbaceum (Kapas)	Prepare a decoction from 2 to 3 handfuls of root & shell.	Give once daily.

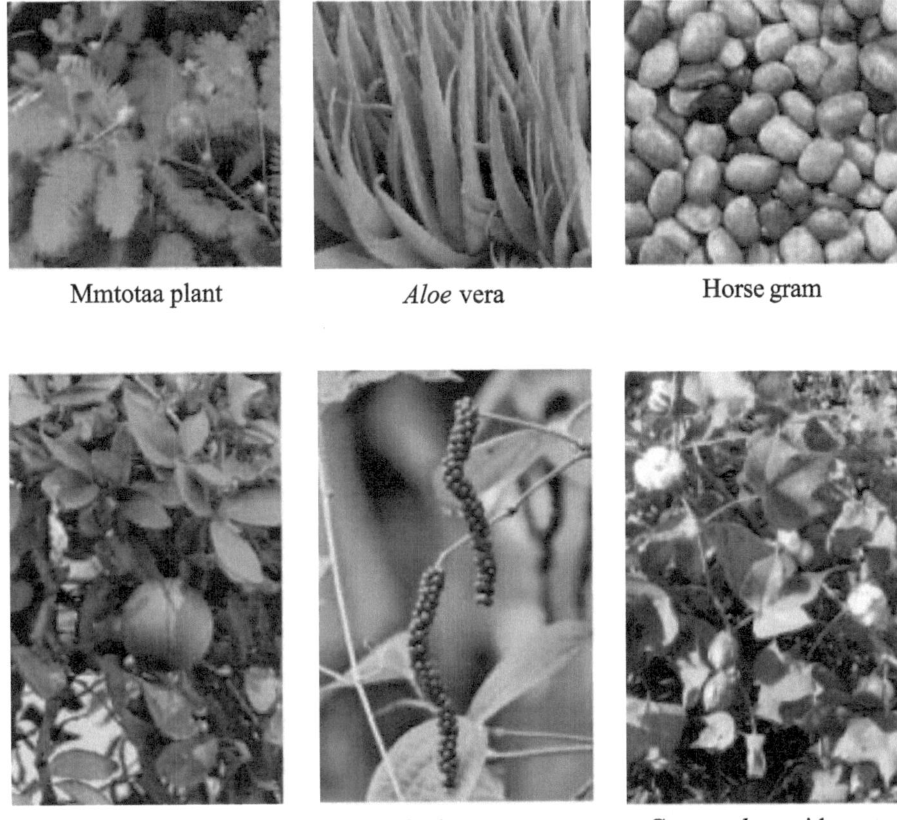

Mmtotaa plant

Aloe vera

Horse gram

Mimosa plant

Black pepper

Catron *plant* with port

5) Skin Conditions

S.no	Condition	Remedies / Plant name (Hindi name in brackets)	Portion used and preparation mode	Dose and amount
1	Fungal infection	(1) Garlic (Lussan)	Make a paste	Apply on the affected part till it recovers.
		(2) Neem	Bark, flower, seed oil or tender twig–make a paste	Apply on the affected part till it recovers.
2	Skin diseases	(1) Neem	Make paste of bark, flower, tender twig or use seed oil.	Apply on affected part.
		(2) Brinjal	Crush brinjal and mix with Jowar powder.	Apply on affected part

6) Maggot Wound

S.no	Condition	Remedies / Plant name (Hindi name in brackets)	Portion used and preparation mode	Dose and amount
1	Maggot wound	(1) Marigold, Garlic and Tulsi	Handful of leaves of both leaves and 1 garlic is crushed with lime to get the paste.	Apply paste twice daily on the wound.
		(2) Custard apple, Neem	Crush leaves (either one or both) to a paste.	Once a day for 5 to 6 days.

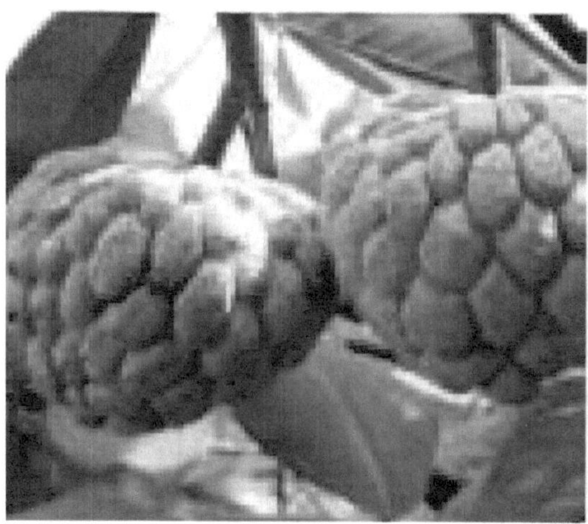

Custard apple

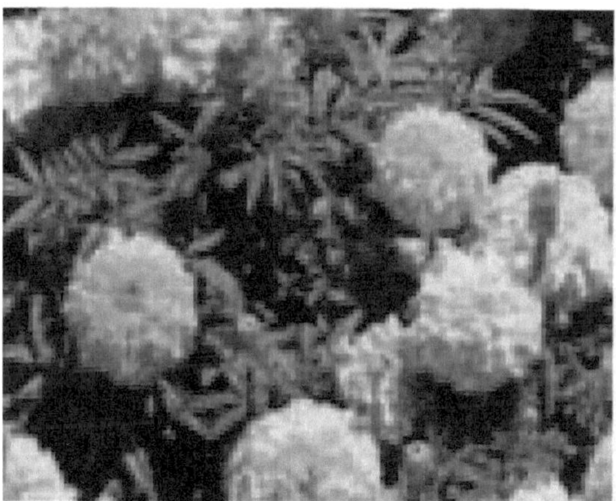

Marigold

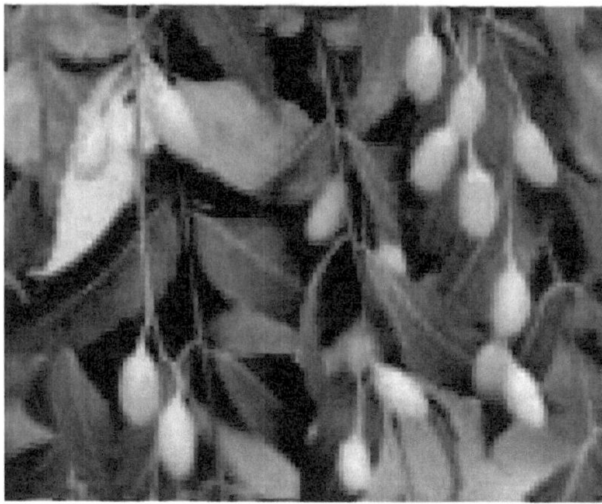

Neem leaf with seeds

7) Dehydration

S.no	Condition	Remedies / Plant name (Hindi name in brackets)	Portion used and preparation mode	Dose and amount
1	Dehydration	Salt, baking soda & sugar	Dissolve 2 teaspoons of Salt, half teaspoon of baking soda & 4 teaspoons of sugar in 1 Liter of water.	Adult animals - 2 - 3 ltrs 2 - 3 times/ day. Calves-1/2 to 1 liter till recovery.

8) Poisoning

S.no	Condition	Remedies / Plant name (Hindi name in brackets)	Portion used and preparation mode	Dose and amount
1	Poisoning	(1) Paraffin Oil/ Raw linseed Oil/ Natural Vegetable Oil.	One litre of any oil	Drench once a day
		(2) Milk/ Coconut water/ Charcoal	One litre of milk or coconut water; 200 gm charcoal in 800 ml water	Drench once a day

9. Warts

S.no	Condition	Remedies / Plant name (Hindi name in brackets)	Portion used and preparation mode	Dose and amount
1	Warts	(1) Euphorbia neriifolia (Barki-thohar)	Apply drops of Latex of Euphorbia on the wart.	Apply twice a day until the wart falls off.
		(2) Papaya (Papita)	Apply one or several drops of Latex of Papita trunk, fruit or leaves on the wart.	Apply twice a day until the wart falls off.

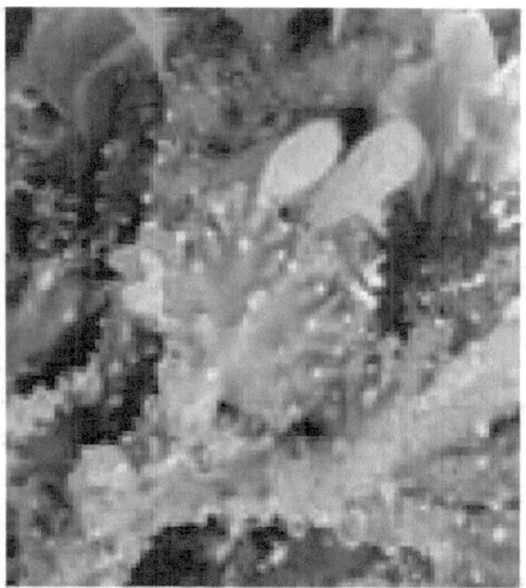
Euphorbia

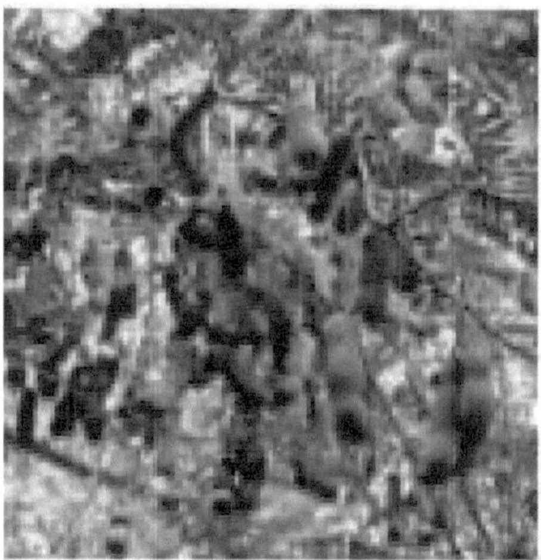
Tamarind Tree

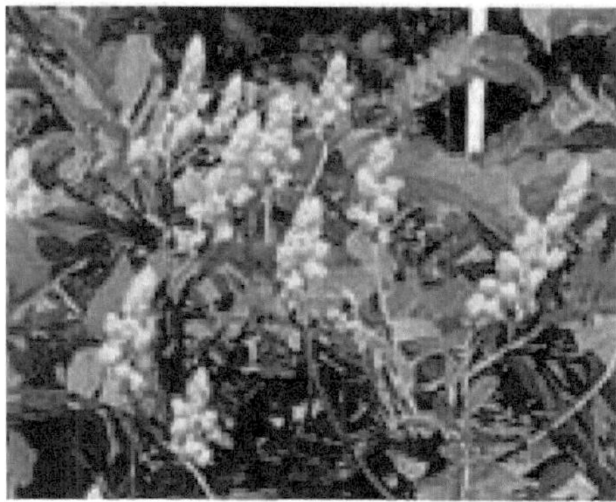
Cassia alata plant and flower

10) Tongue Ulcer

S.no	Condition	Remedies / Plant name (Hindi name in brackets)	Portion used and preparation mode	Dose and amount
1	Tongue ulcers	Tamarind (Imli)+ Gingely oil (Til oil)	Tamarind- 100 gms; Gingely oil- 200 ml. Mix thoroughly to make a paste.	Apply on mouth and tongue 3 - 4 times a day.

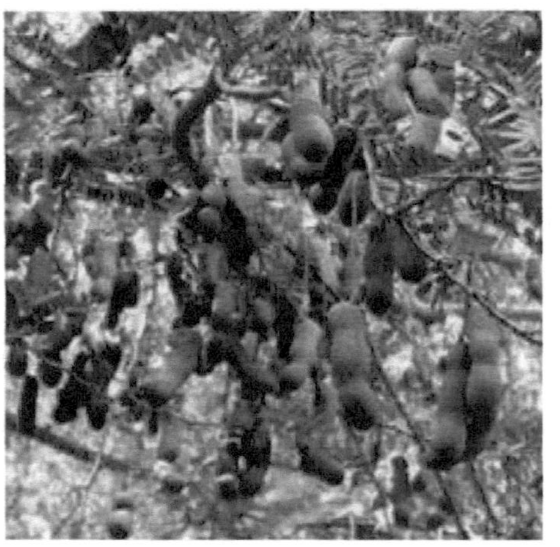

Tamarind

11. External Parasites

S.no	Condition	Remedies / Plant name (Hindi name in brackets)	Portion used and preparation mode	Dose and amount
1	Mange Infestation	Cassia alata (Dadmurdan)	Grind a handful of fresh/air dried leaves to make a paste with water or lemon juice	Apply on the infected skin daily using a brush or coconut husk till the infection has been cured.
2	External parasites	(1) Custard Apple (Sitaphal)	Seed and leaf extract diluted up to 50% in oil base in any cheap vegetable oil.	Apply over the body for 5 days, twice a day.
		(2) Neem	Leaf pulp	Apply over the body
		(3) Custard apple,	Custard apple seeds- 1 part; Neem seeds-1part tobacco leaves– 1/5th part. Make paste and allow to soak in 2 litres of water.	Apply over the body.

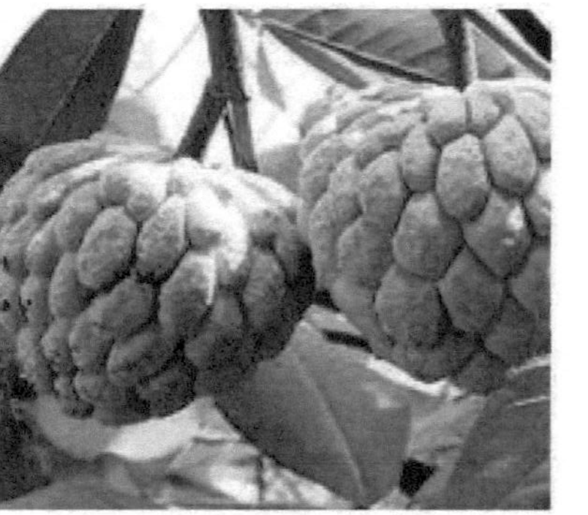

Custard apple

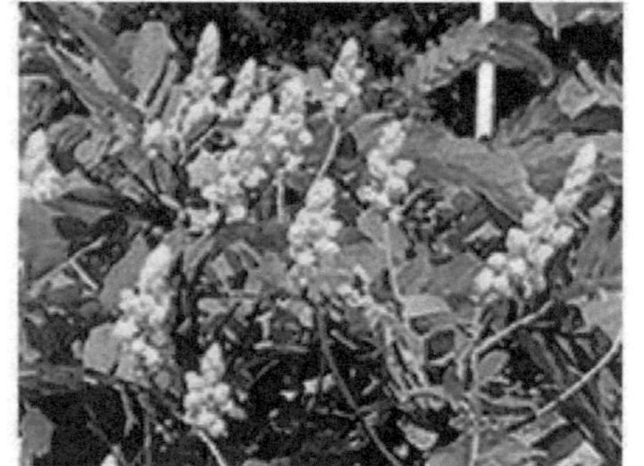

Cassia alata

12) Fly Repellent

S.no	Condition	Remedies / Plant name (Hindi name in brackets)	Portion used and preparation mode	Dose and amount
1	Fly Repellent	Aloe vera (Ghilkanvar)	Grind and extract juice of aloe leaves	Apply on the cow's body and also sprinkle in the surroundings.

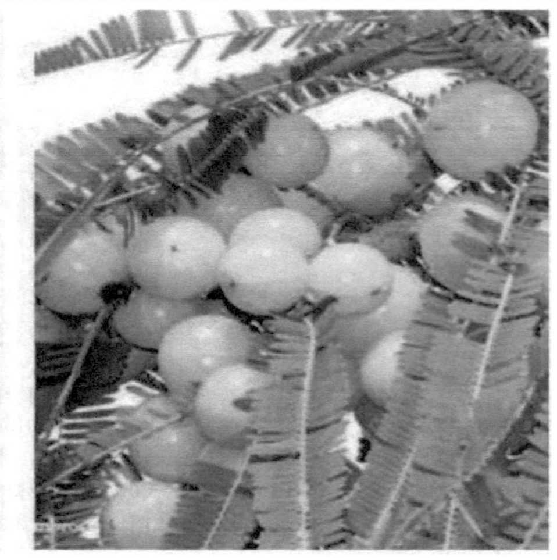

Aloe vera

Amla

13) Anaemia

S.no	Condition	Remedies / Plant name (Hindi name in brackets)	Portion used and preparation mode	Dose and amount
1	Anaemia	Phyllanthus embelica (Amla)	Grind around 50 gm of fruit /bark.	Give daily.

J. Synthetic Milk

As the name suggests, *synthetic milk* is not milk but it is entirely a different component with a high degree of adulteration to increase the volume of milk and thereby the profit. Generally it is a mixture of water, pulverized detergent or soap, sodium hydroxide, vegetable oil, salt and urea.

The simplicity and rapidity with which milk can be adulterated always tempted the unscrupulous milk vendors to indulge in fraudulent practices and adulterate the milk. The ever-rising greed has given way to the development of a new type of adulterated milk known as synthetic milk.

Similar to genuine milk production, the practice of preparing the synthetic milk too starts at the village level. The places notorious for the production of synthetic milk include parts of Rajasthan, Haryana, and Uttar Pradesh in India. Slowly but steadily the practice is spreading to other parts of India.

How synthetic milk is produced?

Vegetable refined oil (any brand) whose butyro-refractometer reading is less than 42 is taken in a wide mouthed container along with a suitable emulsifier and thoroughly mixed so that the entire content is made in to a thick white paste. After this is achieved, water is slowly added to the paste until the density of the liquid is similar to that of milk. Then it is added with urea or sodium sulphate or glucose or maltose or sometimes any one of the commonly available fertilizers is added. These substances are usually dissolved in hot water and then added to the seemingly milk like solution.

The refined oil in synthetic milk acts as a source of fat where as the hot solution of any one of the substances above mentioned acts as a source of solids not fat (SNF). The ingredients that go in to the making of synthetic milk are calculated in such a way that the fat and SNF percentage is similar to mixed milk. Hence it easily passes the platform tests carried out at the village level dairy co-operative society (fat and lactometer reading etc.) but from the health point of view of the consumers, it is highly dangerous. The taste is highly objectionable.

Comparison Between Genuine And Synthetic Milk

Differentiating tests	Genuine Milk	Synthetic Milk
Physical tests		
Colour	White	White
Storage	On storage, it remains white	It turns pale yellow after some time
Texture	When rubbed on the palm, it doesn't form foam	When rubbed on the palm, foam formation noticed.
pH	6.6 to 6.8	10 – 11 (Highly alkaline)
Fat	4.5 – 5.0%	4.5 – 5.0%
Solids Not Fat	8 – 9%	8 – 9%
Chemical tests		
Heat	No change in color on heating	It turns yellow on boiling
Urea test	Pale yellow color develops	Dark yellow color develops

Tests to Detect Adulteration in Milk

There are many methods known for detection of adulteration in *milk* but the methods discussed below are simple but rapid and sensitive methods to detect *adulteration.*

I. Detection of Neutralizers in milk

1) Rosalic acid test (Soda Test)

In milk neutralizers like hydrated lime, sodium hydroxide, sodium carbonate or sodium bicarbonate are added which are generally prohibited.

How to detect?

Take 5 ml of milk in a test tube and add 5 ml alcohol followed by 4-5 drops of rosalic acid. If the colour of milk changes to pinkish red, then it is inferred that the milk is adulterated with sodium carbonate / sodium bicarbonate and hence unfit for human consumption.

This test will be effective only if the neutralizers are present in milk. If the added neutralizers are nullified by the developed acidity, then this test will be negative. In that case, the alkaline condition of the milk for the presence of soda ash has to be estimated.

How to proceed?

2) Take 20 ml of milk in a silica crucible and then the water is evaporated and the contents are burnt in a muffle furnace. The ash is dispersed in 10 ml distilled water and it is titrated against decinormal (N/10) hydrochloric acid using phenolphthalein as an indicator. If the titre value exceeds 1.2 ml, then it is construed that the milk is*adulterated* with neutralizers.

II. Test for detection of hydrogen peroxide

Take 5 ml milk in a test tube and then add 5 drops of paraphenylene diamine and shake it well. Change of the colour of milk to blue confirms that the milk is added with hydrogen peroxide.

III. Test for detection of formalin

Formalin (40%) is poisonous though it can preserve milk for a long time.

How to detect?

Take 10 ml of milk in test tube and 5 ml of conc. sulphuric acid is added on the sides of the test tube with out shaking. If a violet or blue ring appears at the intersection of the two layers, then it shows the presence of formalin.

IV. Test for detection of sugar in milk

Generally sugar is mixed in the milk to increase the solids not fat content of milk i.e. to increase the lactometer reading of milk, which was already diluted with water.

How to detect?

Take 10 ml of milk in a test tube and add 5 ml of hydrochloric acid along with 0.1 g of resorcinol. Then shake the test tube well and place the test tube in a boiling water bath for 5 min. Appearance of red colour indicates the presence of added sugar in milk.

V. Test for detection of starch

Addition of starch also increases the SNF content of milk. Apart from the starch, wheat flour, arrowroot, rice flour are also added.

How to detect?

Take 3 ml milk in a test tube and boil it thoroughly. Then milk is cooled to room temperature and added with 2 to 3 drops of 1% iodine solution. Change of colour to blue indicates that the milk is *adulterated* with starch.

VI. Test for detection of glucose

Usually poor quality glucose is added to milk to increase the lactometer reading. There are two tests available to detect the **adulteration** of milk with glucose.

How to proceed?

1. Phosphomolybdic or Barford Test

Take 3 ml of milk in a test tube and add 3 ml Barford's reagent and mix it thoroughly. Then keep it in a boiling water bath for 3 min and then cool it for 2 min by immersing in tap water with out disturbance. Then add 1ml of phosphomolybdic acid and shake. If blue colour is visible, then glucose is present in the milk sample.

2. Diacetic test

Take a strip of diacetic strip and dip it in the milk for 30 sec to 1 min. If the strip changes colour, then it shows that the sample of milk contains glucose. If there is no change in the colour of the strip, then glucose is absent. In this method the presence of glucose in milk can be quantified by comparing the colour developed with the chart strip.

VII. Test for detection of urea

1. Urea is generally added in the preparation of synthetic milk to raise the SNF value.

   Five ml of milk is mixed well with 5 ml paradimethyl amino benzaldehyde (16%). If the solution turns yellow in colour, then the given sample of milk is added with urea.

2. Take 5 ml of milk in a test tube and add 0.2 ml of urease (20 mg/ml). Shake well at room temperature and then add 0.1 ml of bromothymol blue solution (0.5%). Appearance of blue colour after 10-15 min indicates the *adulteration* milk with urea.

VIII. Test for detection of ammonium sulphate

The presence of sulphate in milk increases the lactometer reading.

How to proceed?

5 ml of hot milk is taken in a test tube and added with a suitable acid for e.g. citric acid and the whey thus separated is filtered. Collect the whey in another test tube and add 0.5 ml of 5% barium chloride. Appearance of precipitate indicates the presence of ammonium sulphate in milk.

IX. Test for detection of salt

Addition of salt in milk is mainly resorted to with the aim of increasing the corrected lactometer reading.

How to detect?

Five ml of silver nitrate (0.8%) is taken in a test tube and added with 2 to 3 drops of 1% potassium dichromate and 1 ml of milk and thoroughly mixed. If the contents of the test tube turn yellow in colour, then milk contains salt in it. If it is chocolate coloured, then the milk is free from salt.

X. Test for detection of pulverized soap

Take 10 ml of milk in a test tube and dilute it with equal quantity of hot water and then add 1 – 2 drops of phenolphthalein indicator. Development of pink colour indicates that the milk is adulterated with soap.

XI. Detection of detergents in milk

Take 5 ml of milk in a test tube and add 0.1 ml of bromocresol purple solution. Appearance of violet colour indicates the presence of detergent in milk. Unadulterated milk samples show a faint violet colour.

XII. Detection of water in milk

Though the adulteration of milk with water can be checked by lactometer reading, other adulterations too affect the lactometer reading. Hence freezing point depression, recognized by AOAC, is usually adopted.

Percentage of water added = Normal freezing point – Observed freezing point X 100

Normal freezing point

Normal freezing point of milk is taken as –0.55°C. A tolerance level of 3% is given which is equivalent to specifying a minimum freezing point depression for authentic milk of –0.55°C.

XIII. Detection of skim milk powder in milk

If the addition of nitric acid drop by drop in to the test milk sample results in the development of orange colour, it indicates the milk is adulterated with skim milk powder. Samples with out skim milk powder shows yellow colour.

XIV. Detection of vegetable fat in milk

The characteristic feature of milk is its fatty acid composition, which mainly consists of short chain fatty acids such as butyric, caproic, caprylic acid; whereas the vegetable fats consist mainly of long chain fatty acids and hence adulteration of vegetable fat in milk can be easily found out by analyzing the fatty acid profile by gas chromatography.

XV. Detection of buffalo milk in cow milk

The presence of buffalo milk in cow milk is tested by Hansa test. It is based on immunological assay. One ml of milk is diluted with 4 ml of water and then it is treated with 1 ml of antiserum. The characteristic precipitation reaction indicates the presence of buffalo milk in the sample taken. (The antiserum is developed by injecting buffalo milk proteins into rabbits).

XVI. Detection of benzoic and salicylic acid in milk

Five ml of milk is taken in a test tube and acidified with concentrated sulphuric acid. 0.5% ferric chloride solution is added drop by drop and mixed well. Development of buff colour indicates presence of benzoic acid and violet colour indicates salicylic acid.

XVII. Detection of borax and boric acid in milk

Five ml of milk is taken in a test tube to which 1 ml of concentrated hydrochloric acid is added and mixed well. Tip of a turmeric paper is dipped into the acidified milk and it is dried in a watch glass at 100°C or over a small flame. If the turmeric paper turns red, it indicates the presence of borax or boric acid.

Confirmation can be made by adding a drop of ammonia solution on the turmeric paper and if the red colour changes to green, it shows the presence of boric acid.

27

Images

I. Dairy Farm Equipments

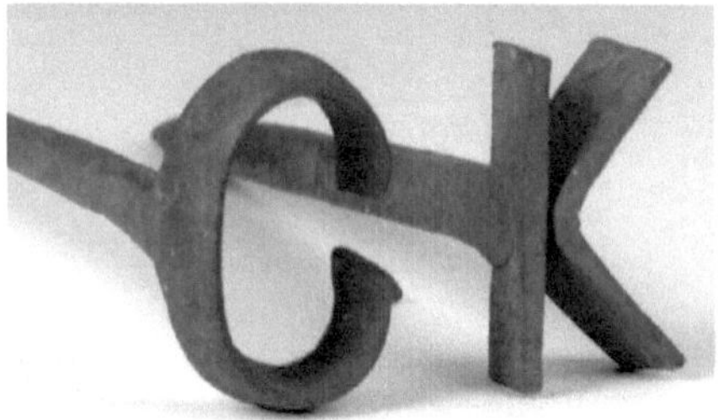

Branding Rods

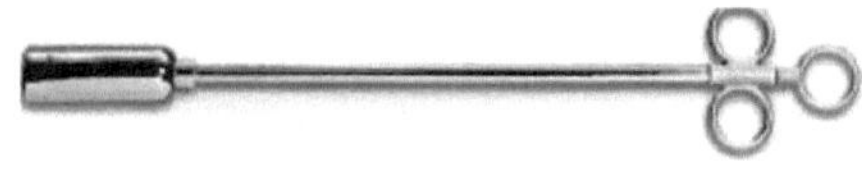

Balling Gun

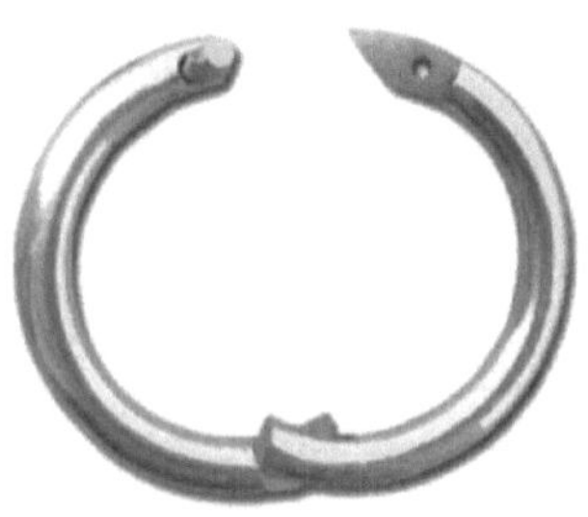

Bull Nose Ring

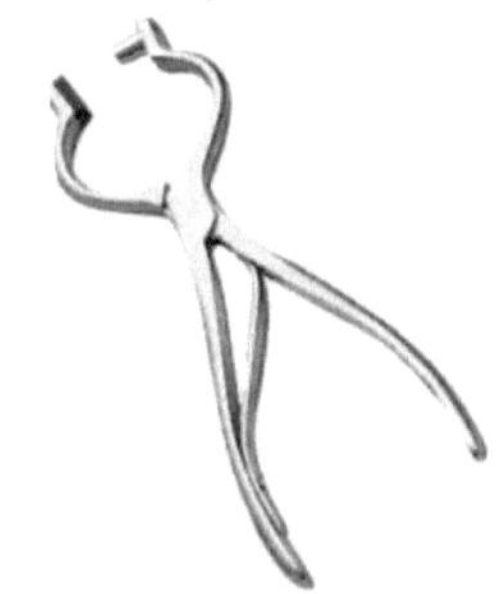

Bull Nose Punch

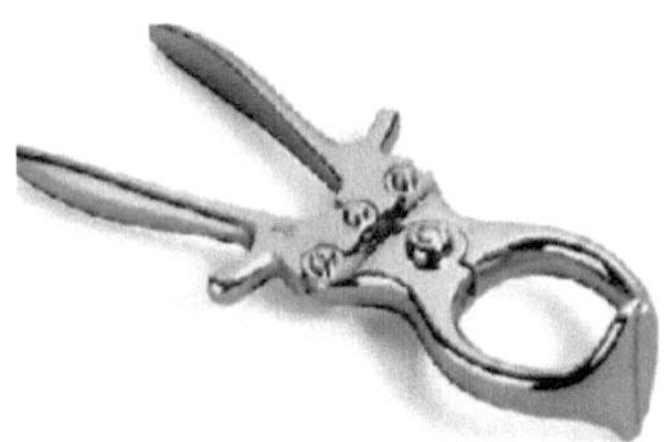

Burdizzo Castrator

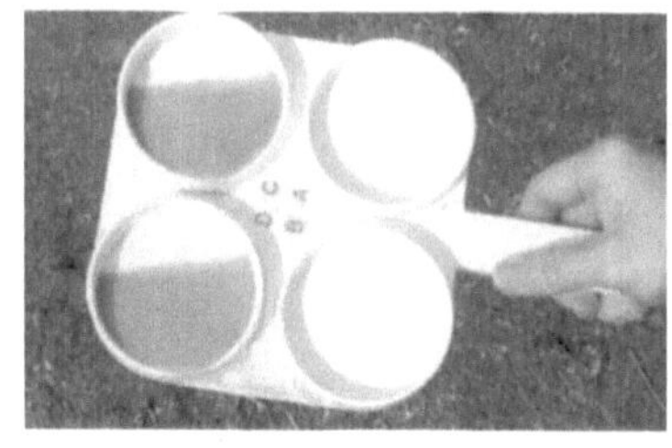

California Mastitis Cup

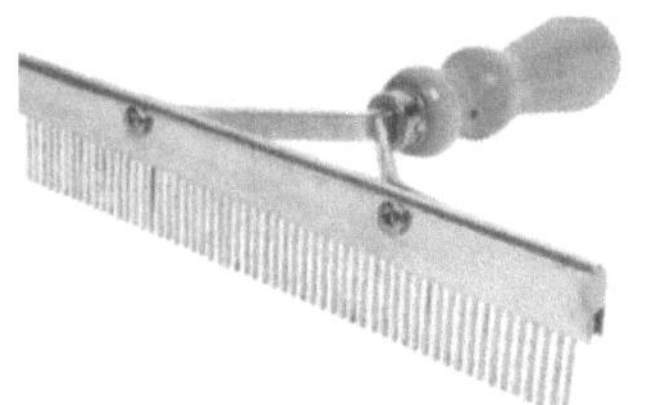

Curry Comb

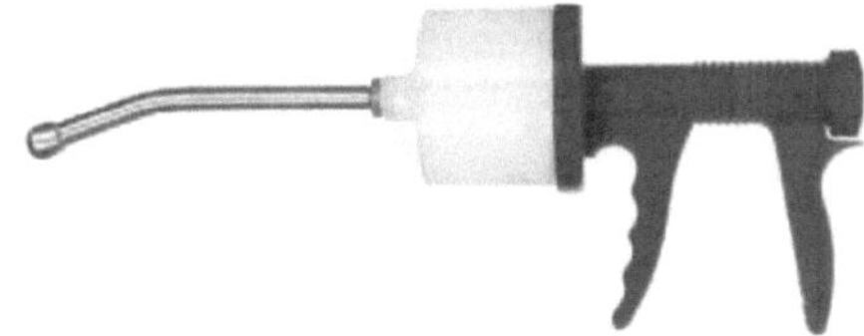

Drenching Gun

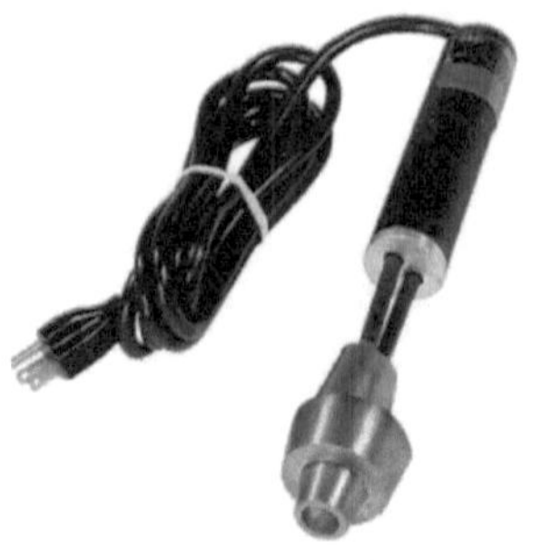

Electric Disbudder

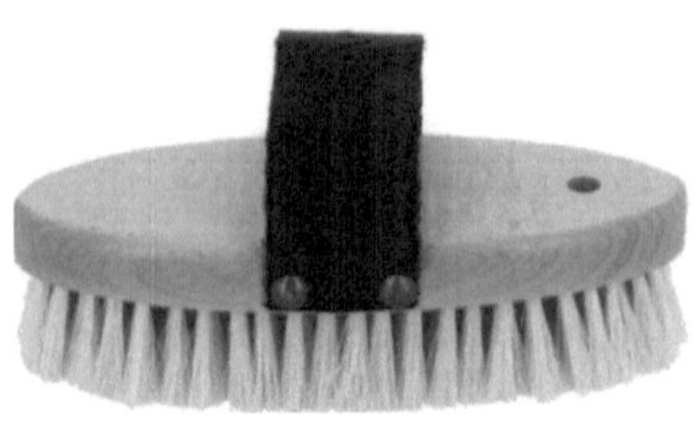

Grooming Brush

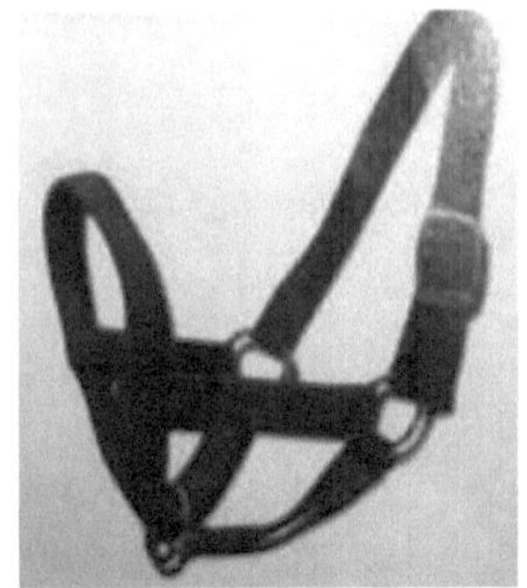

Halter

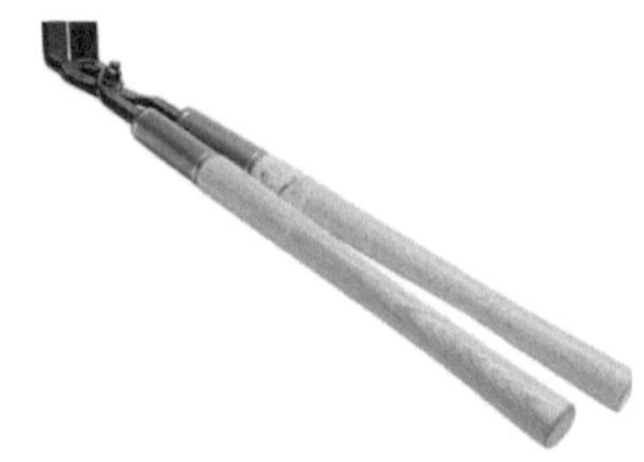

Hoof Trimmer

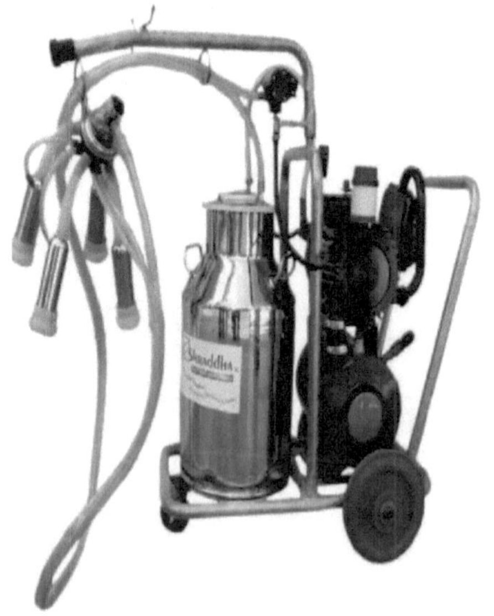

Milking Machine

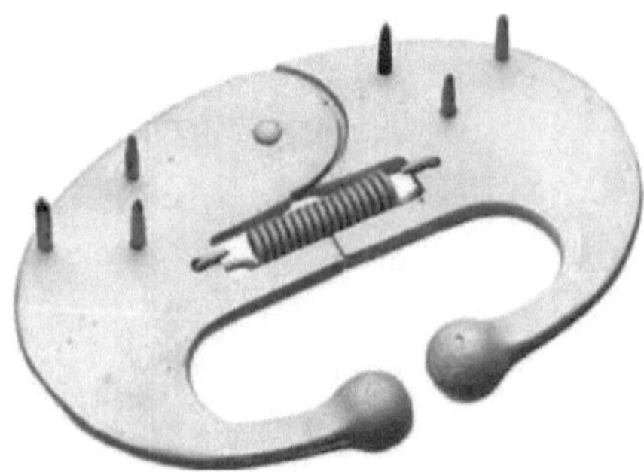

Milk Sucking Preventer

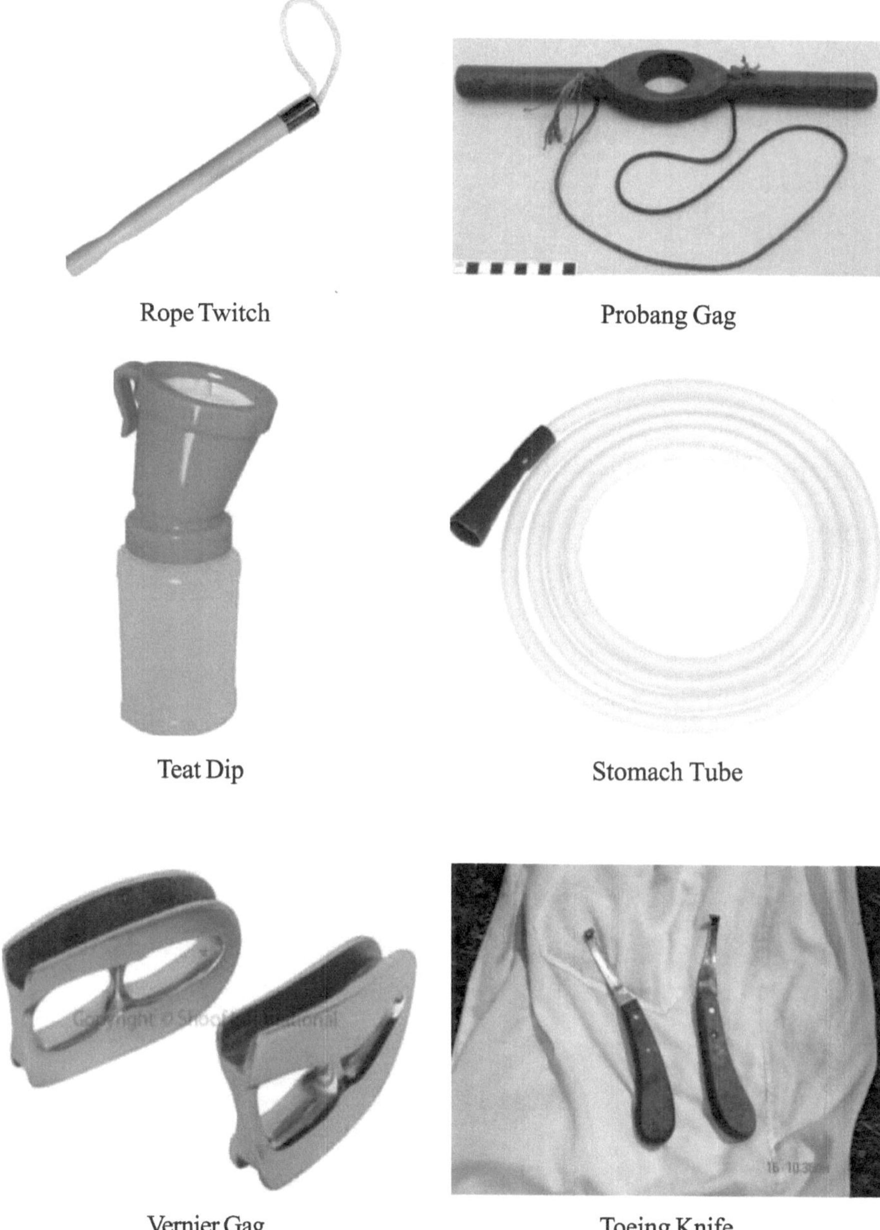

Rope Twitch

Probang Gag

Teat Dip

Stomach Tube

Vernier Gag

Toeing Knife

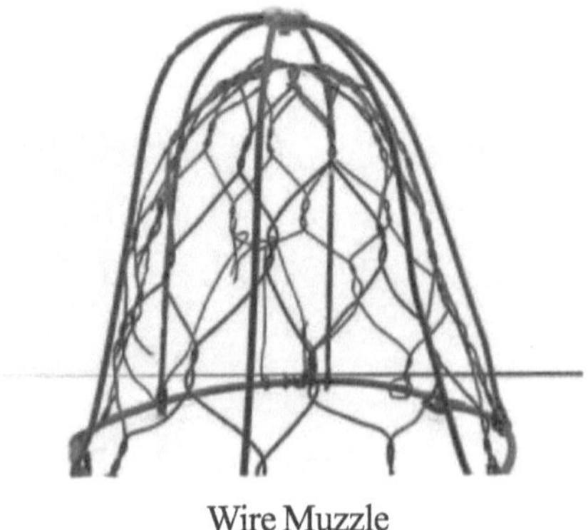

Wire Muzzle

Artificial Insemination Gun

II. Major Diseases of Dairy Animals

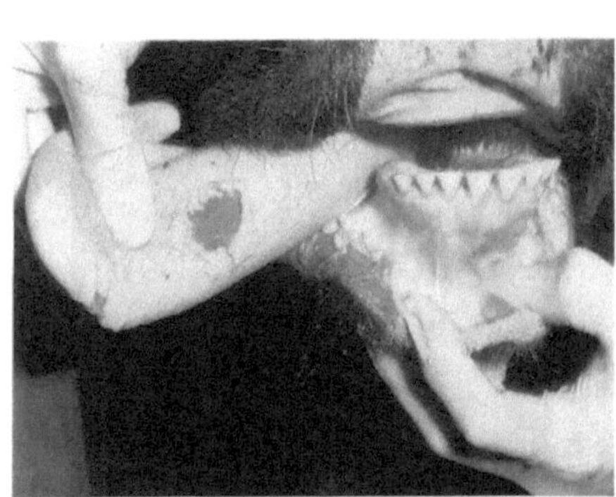

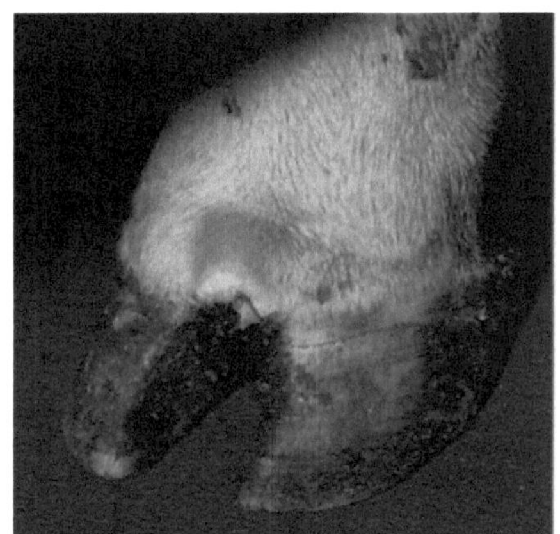

Foot & Mouth Disease

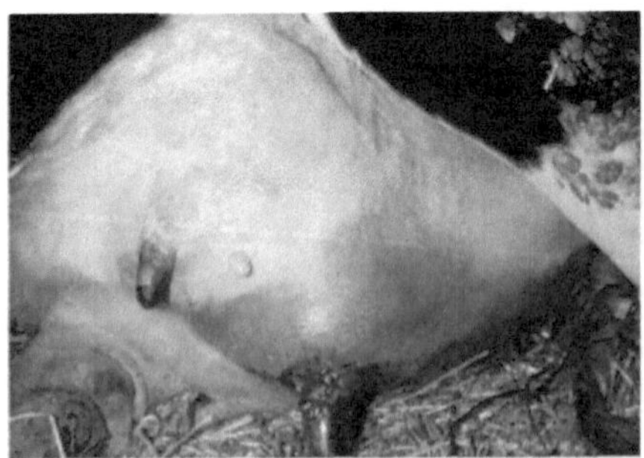

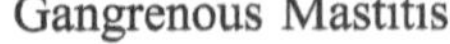

Gangrenous Mastitis

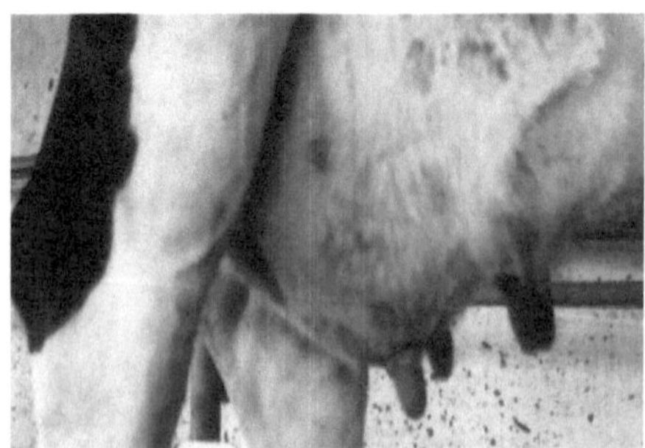

Mastitis

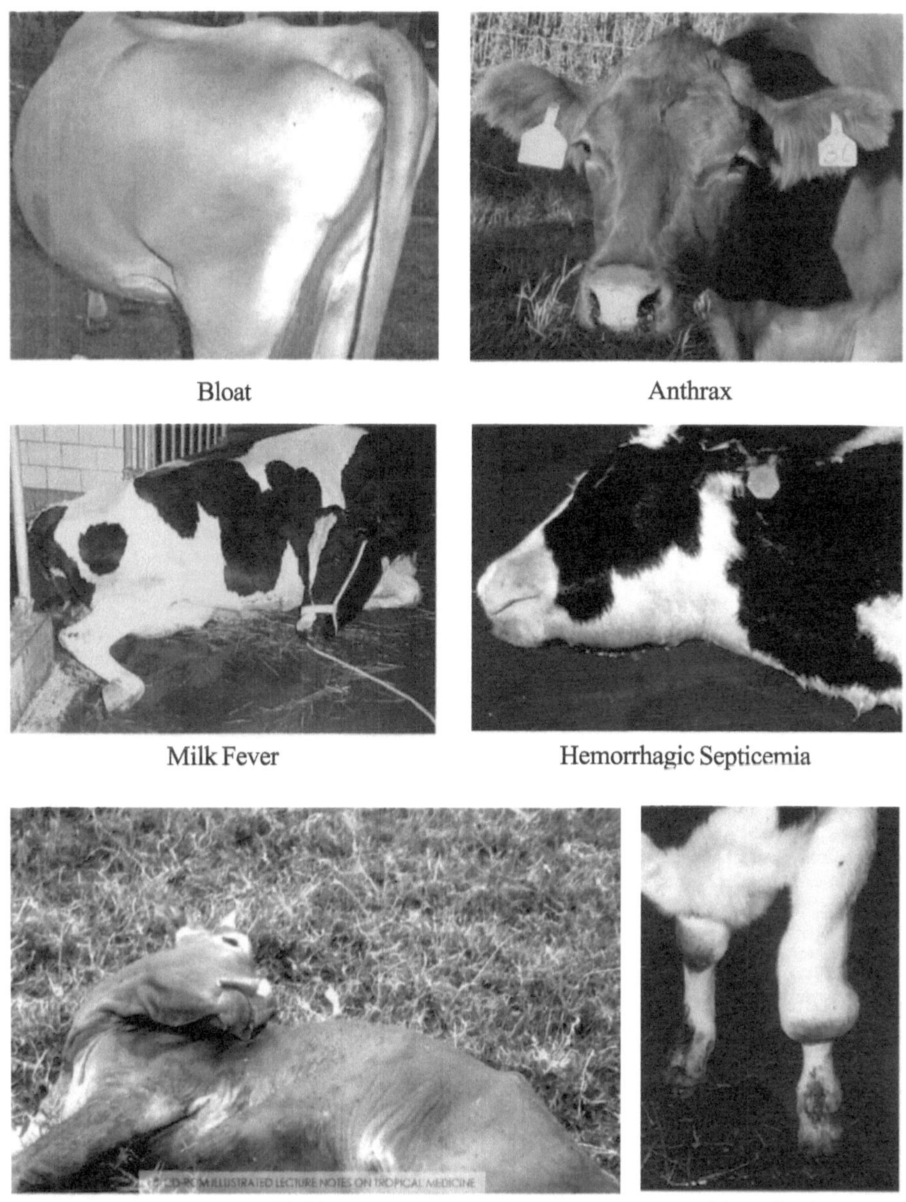

Bloat

Anthrax

Milk Fever

Hemorrhagic Septicemia

Rabies

Brucellosis

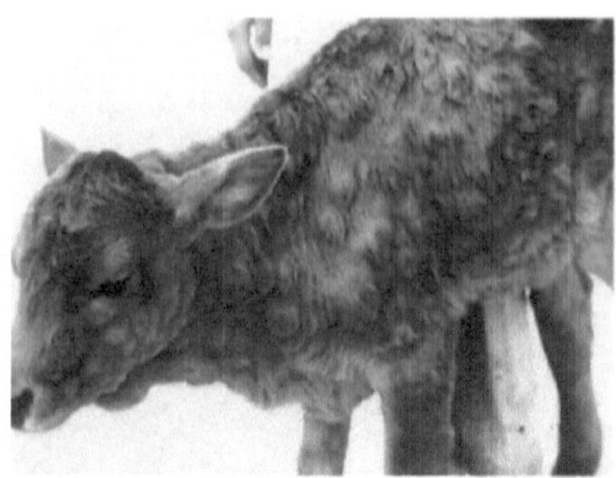

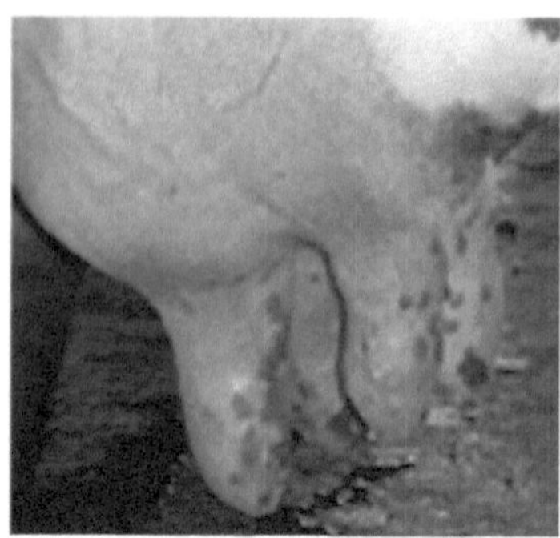

Pseudo Cow-pox

III. Major Parasitic Diseases of Dairy Animals

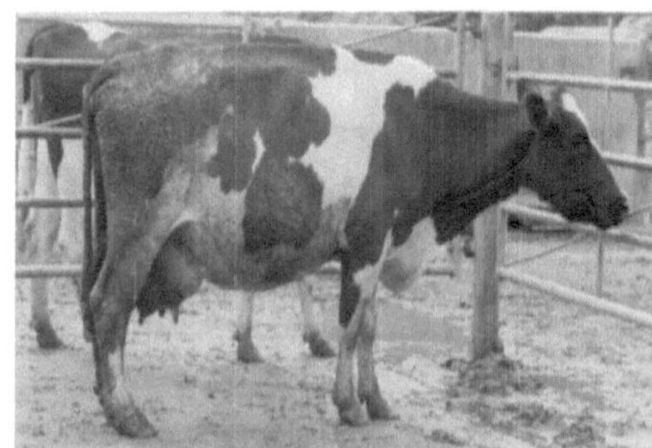

Fascioliasis in cattle

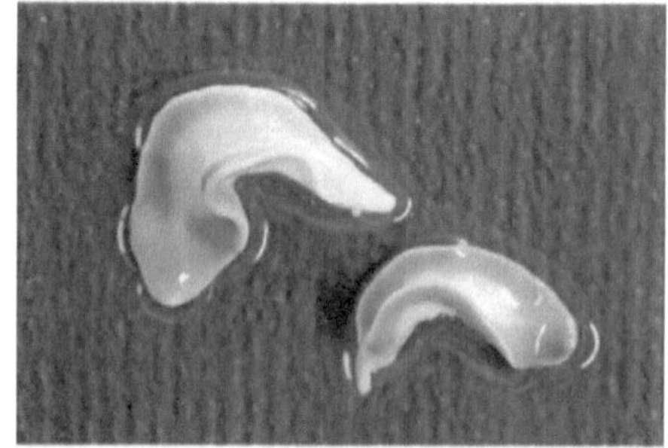

Liver flukes

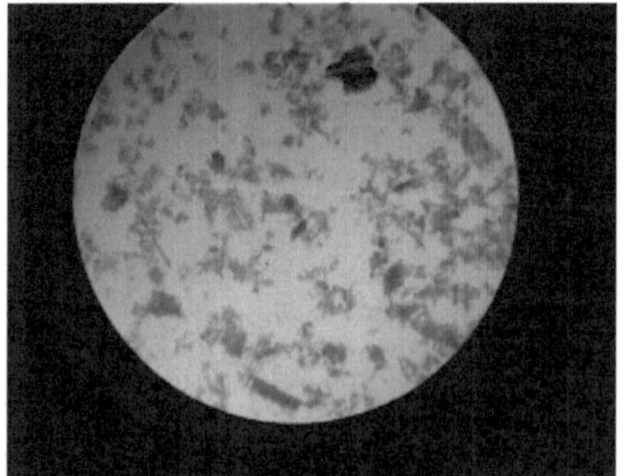

Toxocara vitulorum egg

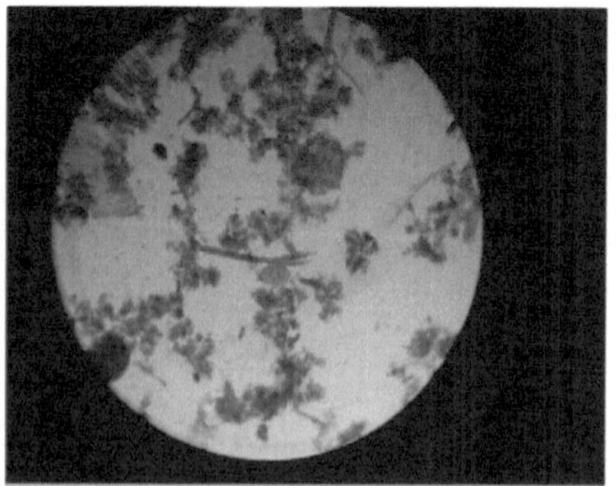

Strongyle egg

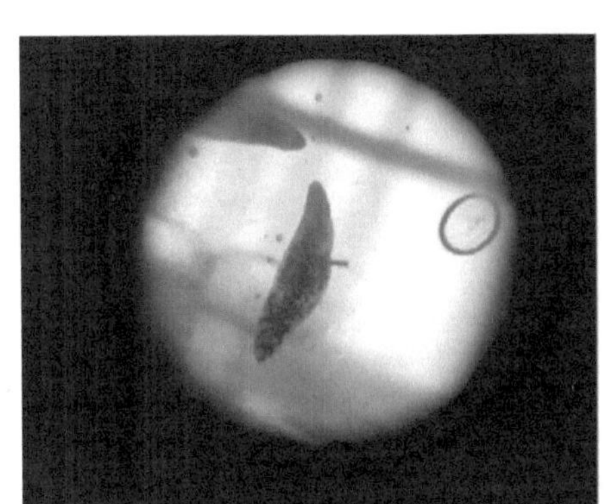

Dicrocoelium

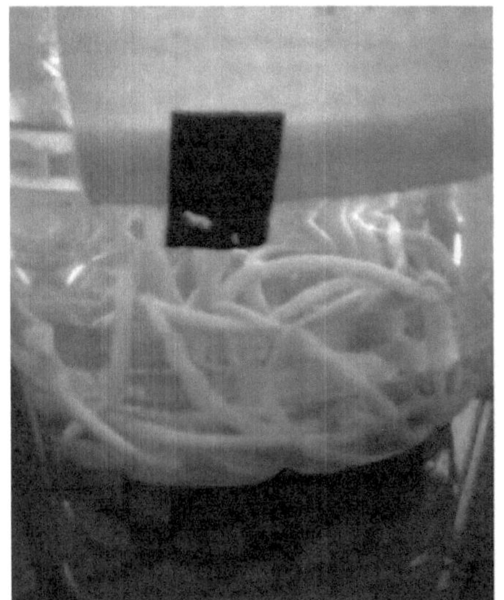

Ascarid worms

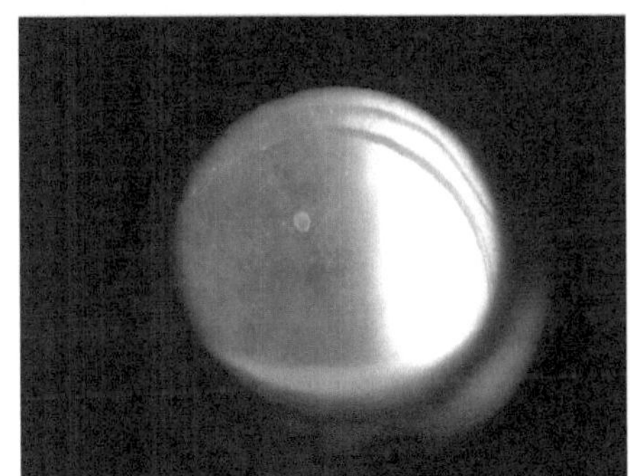

Boophilus

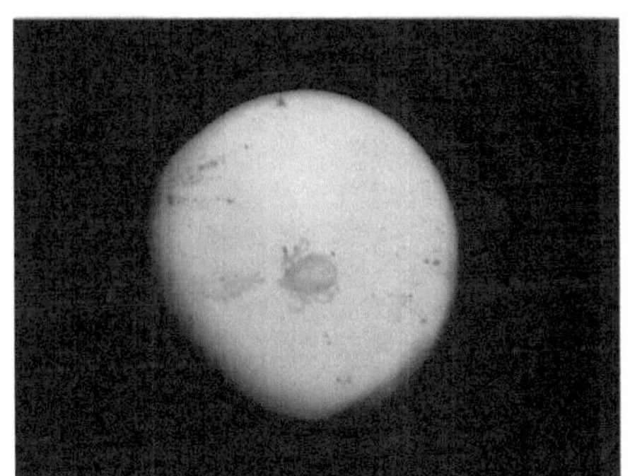

Rhipicephalus

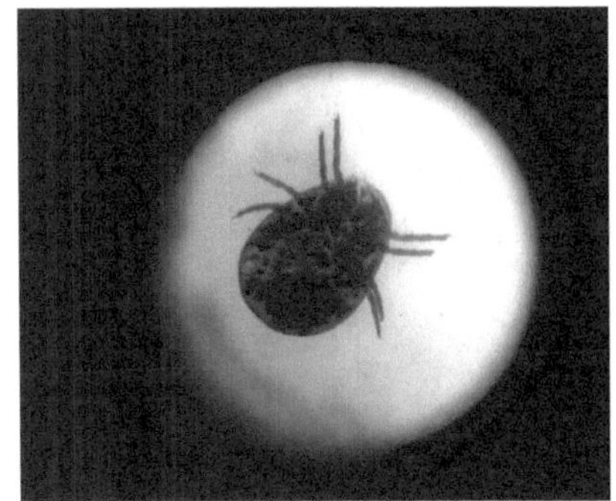

Argas

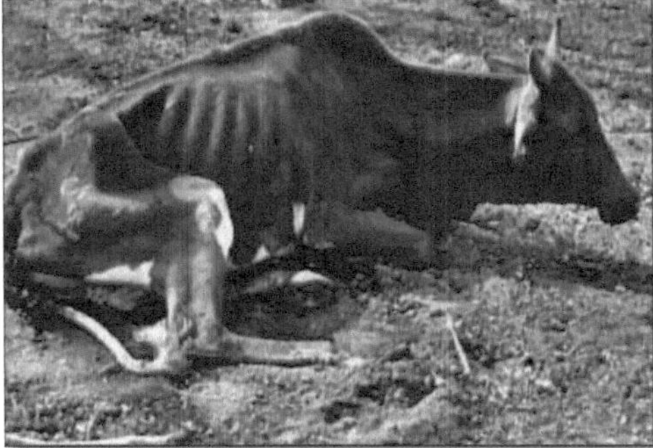

Trypanosomiasis

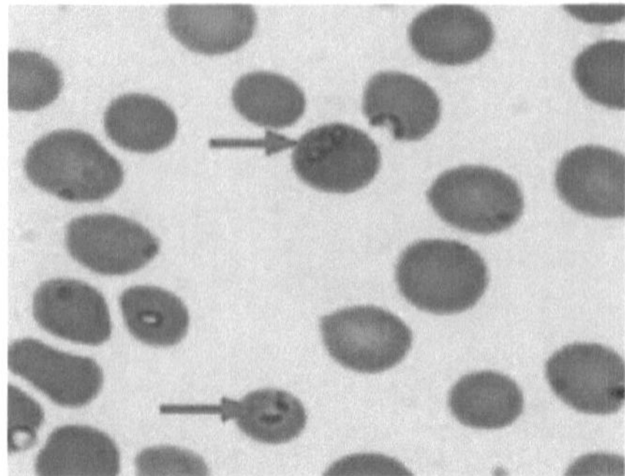

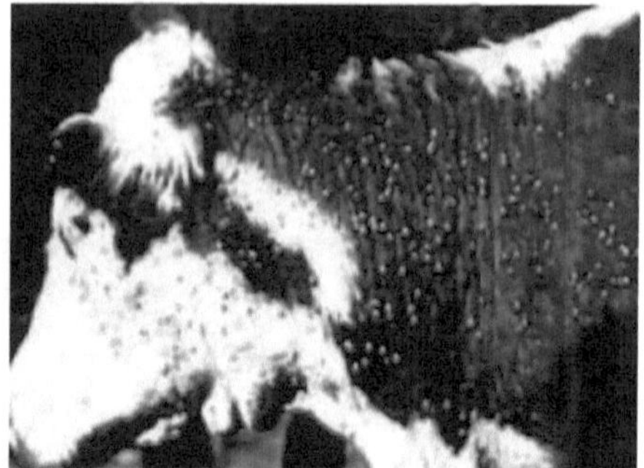

Babesiosis, a tick borne disease

IV. Gynaecological Disorders in Dairy Animals

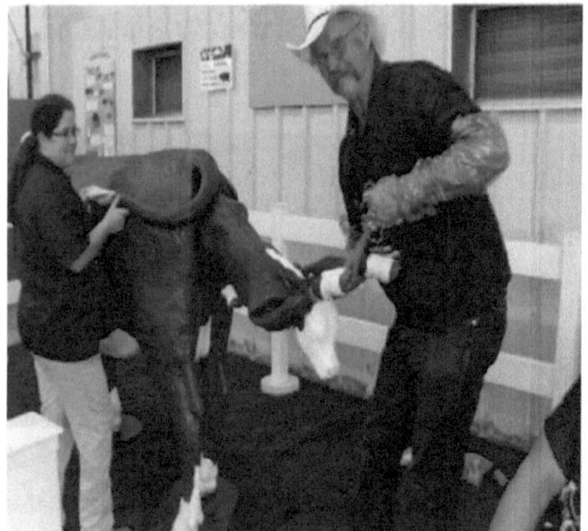

Dystocia

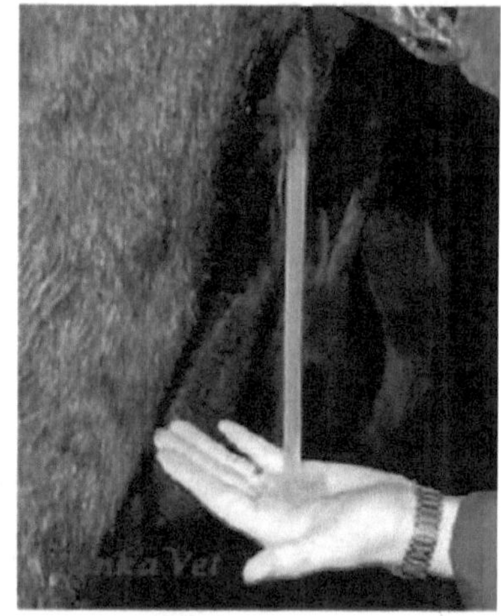

Pyometra (open)

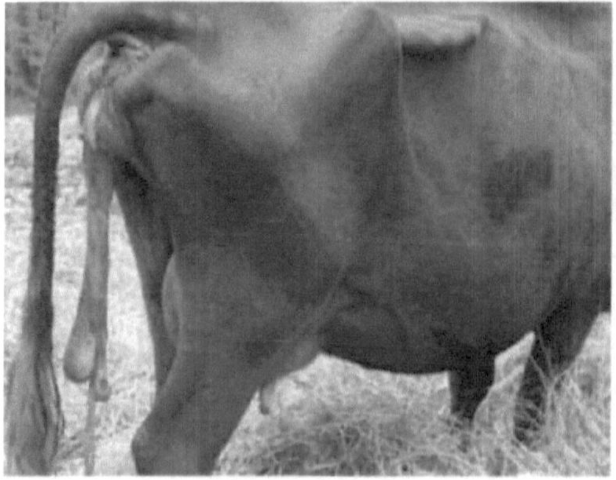

Retention of Placenta

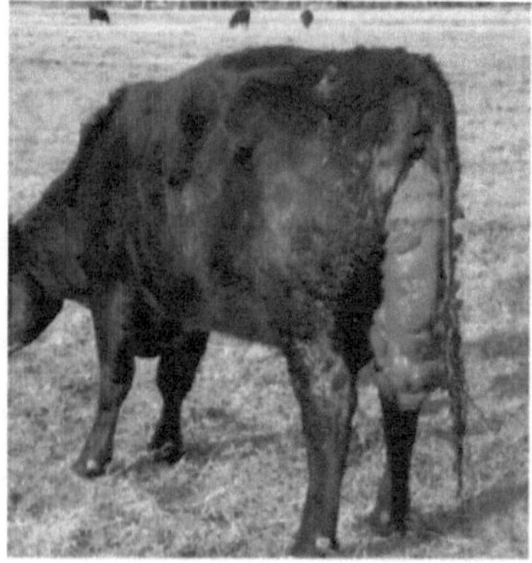

Cervico-Vaginal Prolapse

Suggested Readings

A Brief Guide to Emerging Infectious Diseases and Zoonoses by World Health Organization.

A draft on 'Selection of Dairy Cattle'.

A textbook of Animal Husbandry by G.C. Banerjee, Eighth Edition.

A.K. Sah, B.S. Malik, Nishi and Vikram Singh (2005) Entrepreneurship as Critical Input for Dairy Development. Lead paper presented in National Workshop on Entrepreneurship Development in Dairy and Food Industry held at NDRI, Karnal, December 23, 2005.

A.K. Thiruvenkadan, S. Panneerselvam and R. Rajendran; Non-genetic and genetic factors influencing growth performance in Murrah Buffaloes.

Anil Chauhan (2005) Organic Dairy & Foods Entrepreneurship and Alternatives. Lead paper presented in National Workshop on Entrepreneurship Development in Dairy and Food Industry held at NDRI, Karnal, December 23, 2005.

Anonymous (2010) Dairy enterprise development, Training Manual, Smallholder Dairy Commercialization Programme, Ministry of livestock development, Kenya

Antonio Borghese; Buffalo Production and Research.

B. Shubha Lakshmi, B. Ramesh Gupta, K. Sudhakar, M. Gnana Prakash and Lt. Col. Susheel Sharma; Genetic Analysis of Production Performance of Holstein Friesian × Sahiwal Cows.

Banerjee, A (2001) "The organic dairy & Food Industry A paradigm shift", Indian Dairyman 53 (12) pp. 31-33.

Bianca Moioli and Antonio Borghese; Buffalo Breeds and Management Systems.

BLACK GOLD- Incentivizing Elite Murrah Buffalos for Germplasm and Higher Yields.

C.K. Kurar and V.D. Mudgal, Protein Requirements Of Murrah Buffaloes In The Early Stage Of Lactation.

Characteristics of Cattle and Buffalo Breeds by Indian Council of Agricultural Research.

D. Suresh Babu; Production Performance of Murrah Buffaloes under Organized Dairy Farm Production System in West Godavari District of Andhra Pradesh.

Dairy Animal Management State Institute of Vocational Education, Director of Intermediate Education, Govt. Of Andhra Pradesh.

Dairy Cattle Production Selected Readings by Baif Development Resarch Foundation.

Dairy Farmers Training Manual Produced by Ministry of Livestock Development & Kenya Dairy Sector Competitiveness Program.

Dairy India 2007, Published by Dairy India Year Book, A-25, Priyadarshini Vihar, New Delhi.

Efficient dairy buffalo production Prepared and written by: C.S.Thomas, PhD Anim.Sc. SLU, Sweden.

E-unit: Major Breeds of Dairy Cattle, AgEdLibrary.com Copyright © by CAERT, Inc.

Facts about Holstein Cattle, Holstein Association USA, Inc.

G. Kumaresan; Somatic Cell Pattern And Composition of Milk of Holstein Friesian Cross Bred Cattle.

Genetic Abnormalities in Brown Swiss Cattle.

H. M. Warriach, D. McGill, R. D. Bush and P. C. Wynn; Production and Reproduction Performance of Nili-Ravi Buffaloes Under Field Conditions Of Pakistan.

Haq Nawaz, Muhammad YAQOOB, Muhammad Abdullah; Effect of Feeding Supplemental Tallow on the Performance of Lactating Nili-Ravi Buffaloes.

http://agridr.in/expert_system/cattlebuffalo/Breed.html

http://agritech.tnau.ac.in/animal_husbandry/animhus_index.html

http://nsef-india.org

http://odishavet.com/buffalo-dairy-farm-project-report/project-report-2-buffaloes/

http://www.agriclinics.net/guidelines2010.pdf

http://www.ansi.okstate.edu/breeds

http://www.dahd.nic.in/about-us/divisions/cattle-and-dairy-development

http://www.dairyfarmguide.com/

http://www.elearnvet.net/

http://www.indiafilings.com/learn/how-to-get-nabard-subsidy-for-dairy-farming/

http://www.karnallivestocksales.com/

http://www.khuranadairyfarm.in/

http://www.modeldairyfarm.com/

http://www.nbagr.res.in/

http://www.ndri.res.in/ndri/Design/Index.html

http://www.profitbooks.net/funding-options-to-raise-startup-capital-for-your-business/

http://www.sachdevadairyfarm.com/

http://www.thehindu.com/news/national/india-leads-in-global-milk-production/article

http://www.tradeindia.com/Seller

https://www.financialexpress.com/economy/on-world-milk-day-a-look-at-how-india-became-the-largest-producer-and-why-it-continues-to-be-so/695991/

Images Source: Internet.

J. R. Wright, G. R. Wiggans, C.J. Muenzenberger, and R. R. Neitzel; Genetic evaluation of mobility for Brown Swiss dairy cattle.

J.P. Prajapati, M.J. Solanky and H.G. Patel (2005) Dairying – A Tool for Entrepreneurship. Lead paper presented in National Workshop on Entrepreneurship Development in Dairy and Food Industry held at NDRI, Karnal, December 23, 2005.

Livestock and Poultry Improvement and Management by National Bureau of Animal Genetics Resources.

Livestock Production Management by Basant Bais, G.S. Manohar and G.R. Purohit.

Livestock Production Management by N.S.R. Sastry and C.K. Thomas.

M. Afzal, M. Anwar and M. A. Mirza; Some Factors Affecting Milk Yield and Lactation Length In Nili Ravi Buffaloes.

M. P.G. Kurup; Cross Breeding of Indigenous Indian Cattle with Exotic Dairy Breeds for Improving Productivity and Increasing Milk Production: A Short Review.

M. Sarwar, M. A. Khan, M. Nisa, S. A. Bhatti and M. A. Shahzad; Nutritional Management for Buffalo Production.

M.S. Khan, G. Bilal, I. R. Bajwa, Z. Rehman1 And S. Ahmad, Estimation of Breeding Values Of Sahiwal Cattle Using Test Day Milk Yields

Madhuri Oruganti; Organic Dairy Farming – A New Trend in Dairy Sector.

Moran J (2009) The key tools of Farm Business analyses, Business Management for

R. Prendiville, L. Shalloo, K.M. Pierce and F. Buckley; Comparative performance and economic appraisal of Holstein-Friesian, Jersey and Jersey×Holstein-Friesian cows under seasonal pasture-based management.

Rao D.V., Reddy R.G. and Paul K.S.R.(2009)Practical manual Farm Management and Production Economics Department of Agricultural Economics, College of Agriculture, Bapatala, ANGARU, Hyderabad

Review of Literature on Dairy Cattle Crossbreeding in the Tropics.
Sarah Maina, Dairy Cattle Management.
Suggested Readings:
Sujeet K. Jha, Aparna, Roy, D.K.Gosain, S.Chinnadurai , Pranav K. Singh.(2005) Entrepreneurship: A Key Link for Success in Industry. Lead paper presented in National Workshop on Entrepreneurship Development in Dairy and Food Industry held at NDRI, Karnal, December 23, 2005.
T K Bhattacharya, V K Patil, J D Joshi, A S Mahapatra, S Badola; Dairy Performance of Tharparkar, Holstein Friesian And Their Crosses.
T. Usman, G. Guo, S. M. Suhail, S. Ahmed, L. Qiaoxiang, M. S. Qureshi and Y. Wang; Performance Traits Study of Holstein Friesian Cattle Under Subtropical Conditions.
Teresa Beatriz Garcia-Peniche; Comparisons of Holstein, Brown Swiss, and Jersey cows for age at first calving, first calving interval, and true herd-life up to five years in seven regions of the United States
Textbook of Preventive Veterinary Medicine by Amalendu Chakrabarti.
The Hindu(2013)Agriculture beckons Madurai's entrepreneurs MADURAI, April 2, 2013
The State of Dairy Cattle in India by Humane Society International sponsored project by the Federation of Indian Animal Protection Organizations and hosted by the Blue Cross of India.
Tropical Dairy Farmers CSIRO Publishing, Victoria, Australia.
User Guide on Dairy Husbandry by National Agricultural Advisory Services (NAADS), Ministry of Agriculture, Animal Industry and Fisheries, Uganda.
Veterinary Obstetrics and Genital Diseases by Stephen J. Roberts, Second Edition.
Vilas DONGRE, Ravindar Singh Gandhi, Avtar SINGH; Comparison of different lactation curve models in Sahiwal cows.
Working With Dairy Cattle, by Holstein Foundation, PO Box 816, Battleboro, VT 05302-0816.
www.guptadairyfarm.com
Z. Rehman, M. S. Khan and M. Aslam Mirza, Factors Affecting Performance of Sahiwal Cattle – A Review.

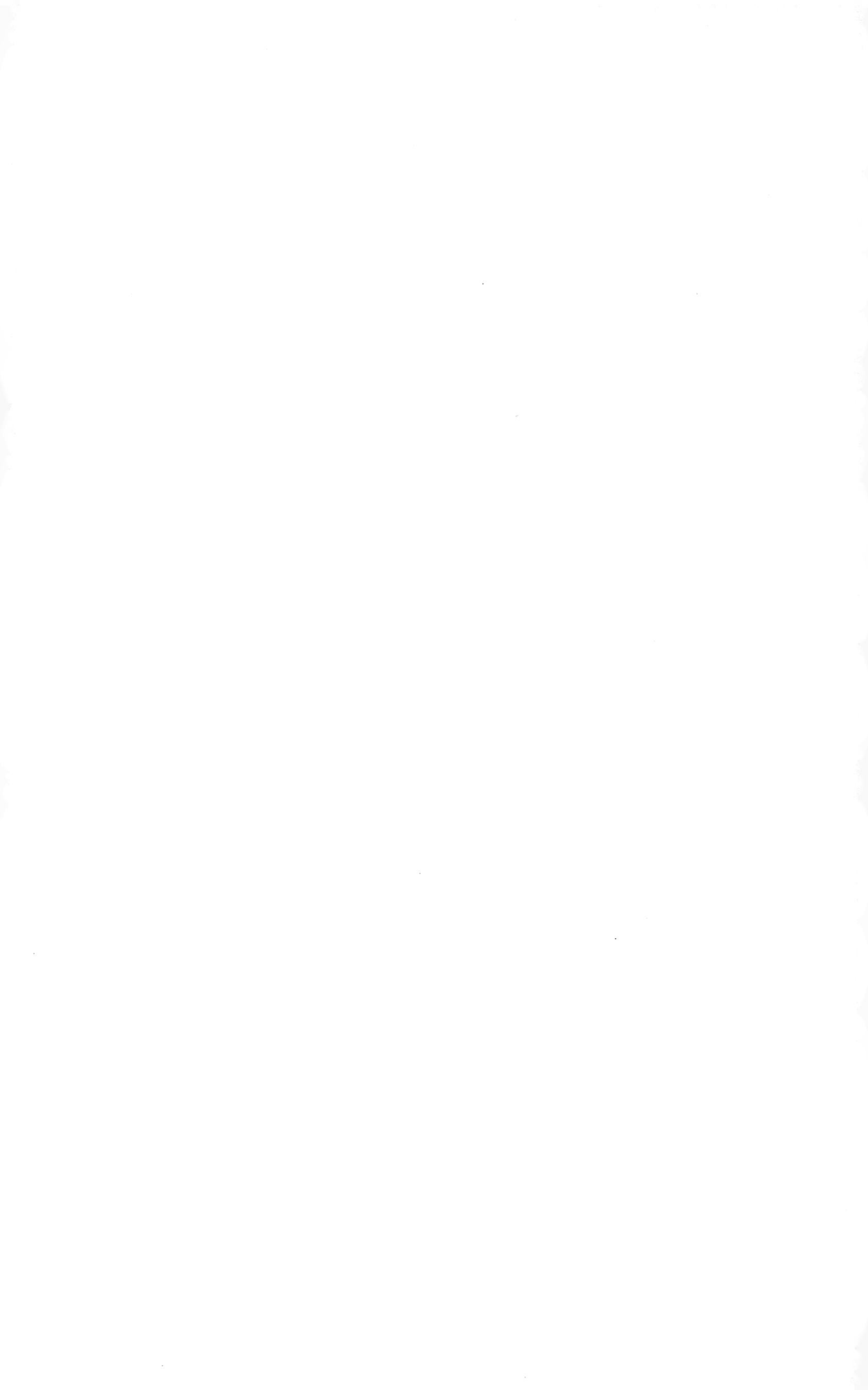